TENDON SURGERY OF THE HAND

TENDON SURGERY OF THE HAND

Edited by Claude Verdan

IN COLLABORATION WITH

J. H. Boyes
J. Cantero
A. Chamay
G. P. Crawford
D. Egloff
M. Fahrer
N. Gschwend
J. M. Hunter
H. E. Kleinert
J. M. F. Landsmeer

W. K. Lindsay
E. A. Nalebuff
A. D. Potenza
G. C. Setti
C. Simonetta
H. H. Stark
R. Tubiana
A. J. Weiland
G. Winckler
C. B. Wynn Parry

First English Edition

CHURCHILL LIVINGSTONE
EDINBURGH LONDON AND NEW YORK 1979

CHURCHILL LIVINGSTONE
Medical Division of Longman Group Limited

Distributed in the United States of America by Churchill
Livingstone Inc., 19 West 44th Street, New York, N.Y. 10036, and
by associated companies, branches and representatives throughout
the world.

First edition in French entitled *Chirurgie des Tendons de la Main*
© Expansion Scientifique Française 1976

First edition in English based on French edition
© Longman Group Limited 1979

ISBN 0 443 01881 2

British Library Cataloguing in Publication Data

Tendon surgery of the hand.—English ed.
  —(Groupe d'étude de la main. Monographs).
  1. Hand—Surgery 2. Tendons—Surgery
  I. Verdan, Claude II. Series
  617'.474 RD559 78-40943

Printed in Great Britain by
Butler & Tanner Ltd, Frome and London

Preface

Tendon repair is a *sine qua non* for the functional recovery of a wounded hand. Also, the disabilities of afflictions such as rheumatoid arthritis are directly linked to the destruction of tendons, whose repair can then produce spectacular recovery. Finally, permanent motor paralysis can be corrected by transfers of intact motor units into the paralysed musculotendinous groups that are inert.

Tendon surgery is difficult. Adequate time and care are necessary to obtain satisfactory results. Not only a general knowledge of hand surgery is necessary, but a special knowledge of the anatomy, physiology and pathology of tendons.

Well-known authors from several continents, for the most part members of GEM, were willing to be associated with this work. We have been able to include some very recent articles concerning the situation, thereby updating our work.

Since it is impossible to thank the twenty-one authors individually, I would like to express my sincere thanks to all for their precious collaboration.

My thanks also to Dr F. Cagli, scientific consultant in my service, as well as to Dr Olivier Reinberg, resident in plastic surgery, who translated several articles, particularly those written by me.

Finally, I thank my friend, Professor Raoul Tubiana, Director of Monograph Editions of GEM for entrusting me with this work, l'Expansion Scientifique Française and Churchill Livingstone for their care taken and Mr John Hueston of Melbourne for his great help with the English edition.

As a personal note, I would like to underline the great progress that has been made since the publication of my first book in 1952 'Chirurgie réparatrice et fonctionnelle des tendons de la main'. Some chapters are still valid, but many others are obsolete, and it is very rewarding to have been the author and editor of its updating twenty-seven years later.

I hope that our work will serve its purpose.

1979   C.V.

Other titles in the GEM Monograph series

Dupuytren's Disease
Edited by John T. Hueston and Raoul Tubiana
Monograph No 1, 1974, Second edition, 176 pages,
illustrated

Traumatic Nerve Lesions of the Upper Limb
Edited by J. Michon and Erik Moberg
Monograph No 2, 1974, 124 pages, illustrated

Mutilating Injuries of the Hand
Edited by D. A. Campbell Reid and J. Gosset
Monograph No 3
To be published in March 1979

General Series Editor: R. Tubiana

Contributors

J. H. BOYES, 2300 South Hope Street, Suite 400, Los Angeles, California 90007, United States of America.

J. CANTERO, Clinique Chirurgicale et Permanence de Longeraie, 9 Avenue de la Gare, CH-1003, Lausanne, Switzerland.

A. CHAMAY, Policlinique Chirurgicale Universitaire, 9 Avenue de la Gare, CH-1003, Lausanne, Switzerland.

G. P. CRAWFORD, Policlinique Chirurgicale Universitaire, 9 Avenue de la Gare, CH-1003, Lausanne, Switzerland.

D. EGLOFF, Policlinique Chirurgicale Universitaire, 9 Avenue de la Gare, Ch-1003, Lausanne, Switzerland.

M. FAHRER, Department of Anatomy, University of Queensland, St Lucia, Queensland 4067, Australia.

N. GSCHWEND, Orthopädische Klinik Wilhelm Schulthess, Neumünsterallee 3, Ch-8000, Zurich, Switzerland.

J. M. HUNTER, 275 South 19th Street, Philadelphia 19103, United States of America.

H. E. KLEINERT, 1001 Doctors' Building, 250 East Liberty Street, Louisville, Kentucky 40202, United States of America.

J. M. F. LANDSMEER, Anatomisch-Embryologisch Laboratorium, Universiteit, Leiden, Holland.

W. K. LINDSAY, The Hospital for Sick Children, Toronto, Canada.

E. A. NALEBUFF, Robert B. Brigham Hospital, Parker Hill Avenue, Boston, Massachusetts 02120, United States of America.

A. D. POTENZA, Cosmetic, Plastic, Reconstructive and Hand Surgery, 1580 East Desert Inn Road, Las Vegas, Nevada 89109, United States of America.

G-C SETTI, Instituto d'Anatomia Umana, Universita di Parma, Italy.

C. SIMONETTA, Policlinique Chirurgicale Universitaire, 9 Avenue de la Gare, CH-1003, Lausanne, Switzerland.

H. H. STARK, 2300 South Hope Street, Suite 400, Los Angeles, California 90007, United States of America.

R. TUBIANA, 47 Quai des Grands-Augustins, 75006 Paris, France.

Cl. VERDAN, Policlinique Chirurgicale Universitaire, 9 Avenue de la Gare, CH-1003, Lausanne, Switzerland.

A. J. WEILAND, 1001 Doctors' Building, 250 East Liberty Street, Louisville, Kentucky 40202, United States of America.

G. WINCKLER, Avenue de Béthusy 39, 1012 Lausanne, Switzerland.

C. B. WYNN PARRY, Department of Physical Medicine, Central Medical Establishment, Royal Air Force, Kelvin House, Cleveland Street, London, W.1., United Kingdom.

Contents

GROUPE D'ETUDE DE LA MAIN (G.E.M.)

List of Members

U.K.
D. M. Brooks (London) G. Fisk (Essex) S. H. Harrison (London) J. I. P. James (Edinburgh) F. Nicolle (London) R. G. Pulvertaft (Derby) R. H. C. Robins (Cornwall) H. J. Seddon (London) H. G. Stack (Essex) C. B. Wynn Parry (London)

U.S.A.
A. J. Barsky (New York) R. Beasley (New York) J. Bell (Chicago) J. Boswick (Colorado) J. Boyes (California) P. Brand (California) S. Brown (California) E. Clark (California) R. Curtis (Maryland) A. E. Flatt (Iowa) J. Hunter (Philadelphia) E. Kaplan (New York) C. H. Lane (California) W. J. Littler (New York) J. W. Madden (Arizona) L. Milford (Tennessee) E. Nalebuff (Massachusetts) M. Spinner (New York) A. B. Swanson (Michigan)

Australia
M. Fahrer (Queensland) J. Hueston (Victoria) W. Morrison (Melbourne)

France
P. C. Achach (Paris) Y. Allieu (Montpellier) J. Y. Alnot (Paris) J. Aubriot (Caen) P. Banzet (Paris) J. Baudet (Bordeaux) S. Baux (Paris) J. Beres (Paris) R. Bobichon (Grenoble) J. Body (Chaumont) M. Bombart (Villeneuve St Georges) M. Bonnel (Montpellier) J. Bonvallet (Paris) A. Borit (StMaur les Fosses) P. Bourrel (Marseille) J. L. Brouet (Toulon) P. de Butler (Amiens) H. Bureau (Marseille) J. Carayon (Marseille) A. Chancholle (Toulouse) P. Colson (Lyon) J. J. Comtet (Lyon) J. C. Dardour (Paris) P. Dautry (Paris) J. Dubousset (Clamart) J. L. Ducourtioux (Paris) C. Dufourmentel (Paris) J. Duparc (Paris) J. S. Elbaz (Paris) P. Esteve (Neuilly) G. Foucher (Strasbourg) Fourrier (Clermont-Ferrand) M. Gangolphe (Ste Foy les Lyon) R. Gay (Toulouse) A. Gilbert (Paris) J. Glicenstein (Paris) A. Goumain (Bordeaux) J. Gournet (Reims) J. Greco (Tours) C. Hamonet (Paris) S. Hauttier (Paris) F. Iselin (Paris) M. Iselin (Paris) M. Jandeaux (Vesoul) J. P. Jouglard (Aubagne) A. Julliard (Neuilly) A. Kapandji (Longjumeau) M. Kerboul (Paris) N. Kuhlmann (Beauvais) J. P. Lalardrie (Paris) F. Langlais (Paris) Lemerle (Paris) A. Lemoine (Paris) Le Quang (Paris) J. Lerique (Paris) J. Levans (Nanterre) J. Lignon (Nantes) R. Lisfranc (Neuilly les Toul) R. Malek (Paris) M. Mansat (Toulouse) J. P. May (Paris) C. Menkes (Paris) M. Merle (Dommartin les Toul) R. Merle d'Aubigné (Achères) J. P. Meyreuis (Toulon) J. Michon (Dommartin les Toul) C. Moitrel (Bois Guillaume) D. Morel-Fatio (Paris) R. Mouly (Paris) R. Naett (Strasbourg) C. Nicoletis (Paris) J. A. Noirclerc (Collonges au Mont D'Or) P. Oger (Garches) P. Petit (Paris) M. Pierre (Marseille) J. Pillet (Paris) J. G. Pous (Montpellier) P. Rabischong (Montpellier) J. P. Razemon (Lille) J. P. Rengeval (Paris) J. Roulet (Lyon) C. Roux (Montrouge) P. Saffer (Neuilly) T. Saucier (Grenoble) A. Sedel (Jouy en Josas) R. Souquet (Toulouse) R. Thévenin (Rouen) J. M. Thomine (Rouen) H. Tramier (Marseille) R. Tubiana (Paris) P. Valentin (Clermont-Ferrand) J. M. Vaillant (Neuilly) C. Valette (Limoges) B. Valtin (Champigny) P. Vichard (Besançon) R. Vilain (Saint Cloud)

Austria
A. Berger (Vienna) E. Trojan (Vienna) H. Millesi (Vienna)

Belgium
De Conninck (Brussels) H. Evrard (Jamioulx) H. de Frenne (Waregem) P. Van Wetter (Brussels)

Finland
K. Vainio (Heinola)

Germany
D. Buck-Gramko (Hamburg) Haimovici (Bremen) L. Mannerfelt (Villingen am Schwarzwald)

Holland
J. Bloem (Heemstede) J. F. Landsmeer (Leiden) J. Van Der Meulen (Rotterdam)

Italy
P. Bedeschi (Modena) G. Brunelli (Brescia) A. Gensini (Rome) R. Mantero (Savona) E. Morelli (Cerro Maggiore) V. Salvi (Turin)

Luxembourg
J. Y. de la Caffinière

Spain
F. Enriquez de Salamanca (Madrid) Quintana Montero (Zaragoza)

Sweden
D. Haffajee (Lund) I. Isaksson (Linkoping) E. Moberg (Göteborg)

Switzerland
A. Chamay (Geneva) A. Graedel (Schaffhausen) U. Heim (Coire) H. Ch. Meuli (Bern) V. Meyer (Zurich) H. Nigst (Basel) C. Simonetta (Lausanne) A. O. Narakas (Lausanne) I. Poulenas (Lausanne) C. Verdan (Lausanne)

Algeria
Y. Martini Benkeddache (Bainen Bologhine)

Iran
Goucheh (Teheran)

Israel
M. Rousso (Jerusalem)

Japan
M. Yashimura (Kanazawa City)

Libya
El Bacha

Argentina
E. Zancolli (Buenos Aires)

Venezuela
R. Contreras (Caras) E. Kamel (Caracas)

1. An Introduction to Tendon Surgery

C. Verdan

Just as the primary function of a muscle is to contract and then to relax, so the essential requirement of an intact tendon is to glide. Our main concern with tendon repairs will always be to get them moving, for an adherent tendon repair is a total failure. This state of affairs may be considered sometimes as a temporary stage, to be followed by a subsequent tenolysis, but, as a rule, our aim will be to obtain not merely a solid tendon, but a gliding one. The gliding apparatus, which plays so essential a part in every planning of repairing methods varies at different levels, depending on the amplitude, the direction and the situation of each tendon in relationship to bones and joints in the various anatomical arrangements of the forearm and hand. The sheaths and pulleys occur wherever tendons pass across a concave joint line—on the dorsum of the wrist or on the volar aspect of the fingers and wrist. The gliding system is then reinforced with additional fibrous pulleys, the most powerful being the palmar carpal retinaculum. At different levels, the force exerted depends on shifts of direction and the gliding amplitude; which, for the long flexor tendons is 4 cm at the base of the fingers and more than 8 cm at the wrist (Fig. 1.1).

The *nutritional system* of tendons surrounded with paratenon is supplied along the whole net of connective tissue, while the vascular organization of the free tendons within the sheaths is far more complex. This blood supply has a great importance which has just recently been fully recognized. Professor Winckler will deal with the vasculature of tendons in his contribution to this monograph.

Mr. Lindsay and Dr Potenza deal with the subject of healing in tendon injuries and their experimental works appear later in the monograph. We want to pay tribute to Marc Iselin, as he was the first, together with Lafaury, to describe the phenomenon of degeneration of cut tendons: yellow degeneration, lysis, hyaline degeneration or tendinoma, and now it is clear that these changes seem to be linked with disturbances of tendinous vascularity, as Peacock, Caplan *et al.*, Urbaniak *et al.*, and others have also confirmed.

Special attention has been given to the repair process after tendon suture and the two theories of such repair. The theory of *axial healing*, by which the tenocytes of the two tendon ends proliferate longitudinally, and the theory of *peripheral healing*, whereby new fibroblasts are derived from vessels invading the tendinous defect from the periphery, that is either from the paratenon or the synovial sheath. This problem is fundamental in endosynovial healing, since granulation tissue carrying vessels will necessarily fill all available space between the sheath and tendon and therefore create adhesions, sometimes large ones, that tend to spread far beyond the tendinous callus itself.

This peripheral healing process has been demonstrated. Axial healing has also been demonstrated but depends upon a blood supply from both cut ends. If these tendon ends are not perfectly opposed, fibres will fasten themselves onto local fixed points. Recent work of Weeks stresses the role played by hyaluronic acid in changing the order and organization of collagen fibres and of dissolving adhesions. In this respect, the synovial fluid secreted within the sheaths contains the hyaluronic acid and can thus prevent adhesions wherever the sheath is still intact, whereas adhesions are more easily formed if the synovial sheath has been opened.

Matthews and Richards, 1974, have shown experimentally on the dog's paw that flexor tendons have an active potential for repair and remodelling when partially cut and maintained in an intact sheath, without the formation of adhesions. But we know that this is not the case when the tendon has been totally cut and thereafter sewn together in a sheath which must be opened in order to repair the tendon.

The same authors have later (1976) also demonstrated on rabbits that the pathogenesis of adhesions appears to depend on other factors than the healing characteristics of the tissue itself, namely: *opening* or *excision* of the sheath, *inserting of suture material, immobilization.* The immobilization alone has no influence on adhesion formation if the sheath is intact and if the tendon is not completely severed. The trauma caused by the suturing of an incompletely cut tendon, which is subsequently reintroduced into a normal sheath does not create adhesions. The excision of an area of sheath-overlying the injured tendon does not in itself affect the reparative activity of the tendon cells, and the synovial layer of the sheath is rapidly reconstituted. The combined effect of splintage and suture in an intact sheath also allows healing mainly by tendon cell proliferation and mild to moderate adhesions were seen in one half of the specimens. These adhesions are absorbed once splintage is discarded. Combining suture of an incompletely severed tendon and sheath excision results in an adhesive response which contributes to the repair of the tendon defect. But the adhesions also tend to absorb or remodel in such a way as to allow gliding. In the same way, immobilization and removal of the sheath of the traumatized tendon leads to mild and transient adhesions.

However, when all *three variables* were introduced *simultaneously*, that is, suture, sheath excision and splintage, the result was a profuse and lasting adhesive response by the ingrowth of fibroblastic repair tissue derived from the peri-sheath layers. The intrinsic repair response of the tendon cells was suppressed.

In summary, these experiments confirm the classical clinical

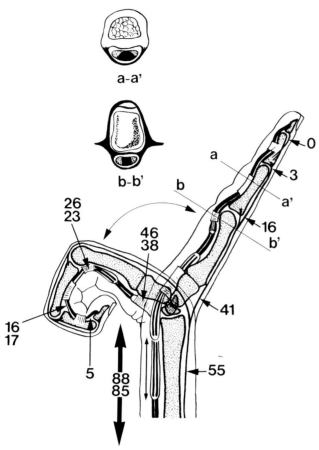

Figure 1.1
Diagrammatic sagittal-section of the hand, passing through the middle
finger and the wrist, in the extension position and complete flexion
of all articulations. The scale of movement of the flexor and extensor
tendons is expressed in millimetres, at different levels. For the
flexors, the upper figure refers to the superficial tendon, and the lower
to the deep.
a–a′: section across the pulley of the proximal phalanx. The superficial
flexor is divided into its two lateral strips and passes in depth, in contact to the phalanx. The deep flexor has thus become superficial and
continues alone until it leaves the middle third of the middle phalanx.
b–b′: section across the metacarpophalangeal volar plate and the first
annular pulley. The deep intermetacarpal ligament does not reach the
bone but merely involves the volar plate. It should be called the 'inter-
glenoidal ligament'. This point where the fibrous elements cross, on
which the hand grip is concentrated, is particularly resistant.

observation of the dominant influence of iatrogenic factors on
the healing of injured digital flexor tendons.

Studies of *tendon graft vascularity* show vessels coming from
the outside, all along the graft, in a perpendicular direction
to the tendon. However Teneff and Fonda have observed an
anastomosis appearing towards the 15th day between the perpendicular and the longitudinal networks, the latter coming
from both tendon ends. Later, the longitudinal circulation prevails and the perpendicular vessels are gradually absorbed.
That means that if the graft is to recover full mobility, a system
of mesotenons will have been shaped, as being the only physiological device capable of giving an adequate permanent blood

supply without interfering with the motion of the tendon itself.

Urbaniak, Bright, Gill and Goldner (1974), have shown in
an experimental study on dogs and chimpanzees, that vessels
bearing adhesions in flexor tendon grafts form all along the
new tendon, as well as after a two stage procedure with Hunter
rod, as after a conventional one-stage grafting, the latter giving
in general more, and denser, adhesions which restrict movements. One year after a two-stage grafting procedure, they
could observe a well developed loose reticular mesotenon
especially on the dorsal surface of the graft. This neo-meso-
tenon transmitted vessels to and from the tendon and permitted gliding, in almost the same way as with normal anatomical conditions.

A great deal of micro-anatomical studies of the vascularization of tendon and sheath have been published during
these last two years. They have brought an accurate knowledge of the vessel network inside and outside the flexor
mechanism and a better comprehension of the healing processes, but none of them have really permitted any advancement of the formerly known methods of repair. The
most baffling experiment on rabbits has recently been
carried out by Lundborg (1977) who has been able to show
that a fresh autogenous flexor tendon graft, consisting of
two segments sutured together end to end and transplanted
freely in an intact knee joint capsule, do heal. This is truly
a tissue culture *in vivo*. The two segments show a fibroblastic repair and after three weeks the resistance to rupture
seems as good as after a conventional suture, without any
adhesion to the synovial layer of the knee capsule.

Lundborg's interpretation is that these rather impressive
and technically excellent histological photos represent an intrinsic proliferation of the tenocytes, which is in contradiction to the theory which militates for extrinsic support. He
also believes that the surrounding synovial fluid was able to
nourish the graft. Taking into consideration the technical
quality of these photos, it is the author's opinion that the
fibroblastic proliferation represents a seeding of cells originating in the synovial of the knee, analogous to the free
recellularization of lyophilized heterogenous grafts described by Potenza.

The remaining tenocytes inside the tendon, along the collagen bundles, do not die. But the proliferation on the surface, especially over the cut ends and the cells invading the
suture line, seem to have their origin, either from the epitendinous layer or from free moving cells in the synovial
fluid.

It will be quite interesting to know the result of the new
series of experiments announced by Lundborg, with iso-
topic marked fibroblasts, with which it seems possible to
differentiate these different origins.

Whatever the situation may be, adhesions are until now certainly not a technically avoidable accident, but rather a con-
sequence of the physiological healing process. As long as we have
no technical solution to the problem of accurately maintaining the two cut ends in an intact synovial sheath without interfering with the blood supply (as we had searched for in 1951),
adhesions will remain a biological inevitability. The problem

consists of knowing the best means to facilitate their dissolution and disappearance, after they have occurred. A pharmacological fibrinolysis, local or by a general administration, is still largely a dream and so far the only effective treatment of adhesions is physical activity by the patient himself, supervised by a physical therapist, often with the help of some mechanical traction splintage. We will deal later in the monograph with the problem of tenolysis, or surgical adhesiotomy in this respect.

The studies of Mason and Shearon, and subsequently Mason and Allen in 1933, demonstrated that the tendinous callus undergoes many changes; a softening about the 10th day, then a hypertrophy if motion is undertaken too soon, with the implication that tendon sutures must remain at rest for three weeks. This is the standard time for the healing of a tendon. After that period, patients may be asked carefully to move their digit and increase little by little the amplitude of these movements. Quite often, this period of rest has to be prolonged rather than shortened, chiefly with the extensor tendons.

In principle, therefore, the most important thing to aim at is not the strength of suture material, but an exact opposition of the cut surfaces. To this end sutures will have to be as fine as possible, and best tolerated by the surrounding tissues.

Certain basic distinctions are necessary—such as between a *new wound* and a *scarred wound*, and between *tidy wounds* and *contused* wounds.

With old scarred wounds, one has time to consider the pros and cons before deciding upon a secondary operation.

With new primary wounds, the following three basic questions ought to be posed:

'Am I in a position to handle such a case?'
'Have I the necessary equipment?'
'Have I the time to deal with it?'

If every physician called to undertake tendon surgery would sincerely answer the foregoing questions, results would certainly become more favourable. We feel it is mandatory to raise such questions for the sake of patients with mutilated hands. A tendon repair is a difficult undertaking and it should only be entrusted to a competent team, with plenty of time and in the proper setting.

Unfortunately there is a confusion between a 'primary operation', meant as 'emergency surgery', made by anyone, anywhere, anyhow, and a 'secondary operation' as being a specialized surgery, made in a well organized centre by highly trained surgeons. If we want progress in tendon surgery, we must at all costs establish the importance of emergency surgery and organize ourselves in such a manner that it be done by competent surgeons, capable of teaching our residents the best techniques. Improvisation, still too frequent in emergency units, must henceforward be avoided.

May the following chapters safeguard the living strength of our manual workers, the masterpiece of all instruments, the hand.

REFERENCES

ISELIN, M. & ISELIN, F. (1967) *Traité de chirurgie de la main.* Paris: Flammarion.

KETCHUM, Lynn D. (1977) Primary tendon healing: A review, *The Journal of Hand Surgery,* **2**, No 6, 428–435.

LUNDBORG, Goran (1976) Experimental flexor tendon healing without adhesion formation. A new concept of tendon nutrition and intrinsic healing mechanisms, *The Hand,* **8**, No 3.

LUNDBORG, G., MYRHAGE, Ph. D. R. & RYDEVIK, B. (1977) The vascularization of human flexor tendons within the digital synovial sheath region, *The Journal of Hand Surgery,* **2**, No 6, 417–427.

MATTHEWS, P. (1976) The fate of isolated segments of flexor tendons within the digital sheath. A study in synovial nutrition, *British Journal of Plastic Surgery,* **29**, 216–224.

MATTHEWS, P. & RICHARDS, H. (1974) The repair potential of digital flexor tendons. *J.B.J.S.,* **56B**, 618.

MATTHEWS, P. & RICHARDS, H. (1975) The repair reaction of flexor tendon within the digital sheath, *The Hand* **7**, No. 1.

MATTHEWS, P. & RICHARDS, H. (1976) Factors in the adherence of flexor tendon after repair, *J.B.J.S.,* **58B**, No 2, 230.

PEACOCK, E. (1959) A study of the circulation in normal tendons and healing grafts. *Ann. Surg.,* **3**, 149.

Symposium on Tendon Surgery in the Hand. Philadelphia (Pennsylvania) (1975) March 1974. American Academy of orthopaedic Surgeons. The C. V. Mosby Company, 1975.

URBANIAK, J. R., BRIGHT, D., GILL, L. H. & GOLDNER, L. L. (1974) Vascularization and the gliding mechanism of free flexor-tendon grafts inserted by the silicone-rod method. *J.B.J.S.* **56A**, No 3, 473.

VERDAN, Cl. (1952) *Chirurgie reparatrice et fonctionnelle des tendons de la main.* Paris: Expansion scientifique française.

VERDAN, Cl. (1972) *Operationslehre.* Band X, Teil III, pp. 286–368. New York: Springer Verlag.

VERDAN, Cl. & MICHON, J. (1961) Le traitement des plaies des tendons fléchisseurs des doigts. *Rev. Chir. orthop.,* **47**, 285

ANATOMY AND PHYSIOLOGY

2. *Normal Anatomy of the Flexor and Extensor Tendons of the Hand*

G. Winckler

The palmar surface and the dorsal surface of the hand, each presents its own special characteristics.

PALMAR SURFACE

The palmar skin, well supplied with sweat glands and crease lines, is not very mobile. The subcutaneous fat, which is quite thick except in the thenar eminence, is traversed and compartmented by strands of connective tissue which connect it directly to the superficial palmar aponeurosis. There is thus very little fascia superficialis or subcutaneous areolar tissue enabling it to glide over the deeper layers.

This palmar surface can be divided into six regions with their own types of morphological and functional (and hence pathological) behaviour.

1. *The thenar eminence* is crossed by the tendon of the flexor pollicis longus muscle. The tendon follows an undulating course, first doubling back round the trapezium, then travelling the length of the first phalanx, against which it is firmly held by a fibrous flexor sheath (Fig. 2.1).

The tendon therefore passes through two zones, one of which is loose within the muscles of the thenar eminence, the other is constricted within the fibrous sheath.

2. *The hypothenar eminence*, or heel of the hand, is a support where the subcutaneous fatty layer, which encloses the palmaris brevis muscle, is quite well developed. The hypothenar muscles are skirted on the radial side by the flexor tendons of the little finger, surrounded by their common synovial sheath (Fig. 2.1).

The deep terminal branch of the ulnar nerve and the deep branch of the ulnar artery pass between the abductor digiti minimi and the flexor digiti minimi muscles.

3. *The carpal tunnel*, which extends for four centimetres beyond the distal crease of the wrist, is crossed by the solid flexor retinaculum. The tunnel encloses the flexor digitorum superficialis and profundus and the flexor pollicis longus tendons arranged on two levels as well as the median nerve. The tendon of the flexor carpi radialis muscle lies deeper, reaching the base of the second and third metacarpal after passing through an osteofibrous tunnel and synovial sheath of its own.

This osteofibrous carpal tunnel is a *constricted zone* designed for containing and allowing to glide the various tendons with synovial sheaths during wrist flexion.

4. *The palmar region*, between the thenar and hypothenar eminences, is triangular in shape. It is a *loose zone*, covered by the middle portion of the palmar aponeurosis, which is made up of longitudinal pretendinous fibres which are firmly fixed by perforating sagittal septa on each side of the meta-

carpophalangeal joint. Transverse fibres, deep to the longitudinal fibres, are more proximal than the superficial transverse (natatory) ligament.

Between the superficial transverse ligament, the pretendinous bands and the natatory ligament, situated slightly behind the metacarpo-phalangeal crease, are *three pads of fatty tissue*. These pads, with their abundant lamellated corpuscles, are traversed by the collateral nerves of the three last interdigital spaces and the beginning of the digital arteries, coming from the superficial interosseous arteries.

The distal palmar crease permits localization in depth of the metacarpophalangeal joints, which are easier to locate, however, on the dorsal surface.

The superficial palmar arch traverses the palmar region of the hand, obliquely from the lateral margin of the pisiform bone towards the second interdigital space, directly under the central portion of the palmar aponeurosis. At a deeper level are the superficial branches of the ulnar nerve and those of the median nerve; finally come the tendons of the flexor digitorum

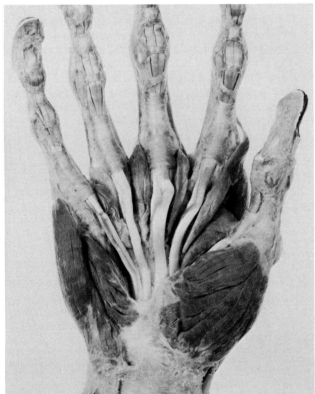

Figure 2.1
Palmar surface of the right hand.

superficialis and flexor digitorum profundus muscles arranged fanwise at their two levels.

In this loose zone the tendons are surrounded by *paratenon*. This is areolar connective tissue lying in several layers of planes and through which pass a large number of vessels. These arise from the neighbouring arches and after forming longitudinal or transverse loops, send a blood supply to the tendons. In this region only the tendons of the flexor superficialis and flexor profundus of the little finger are accompanied by a digitocarpal synovial sheath (Fig. 2.1).

Finally it is from the tendons of the flexor digitorum profundus muscle that the lumbrical muscles arise.

At a deeper level this palmar region, through which the tendons, vessels and nerves pass, is separated from the dorsal and palmar interosseous muscles, the deep palmar arch and the deep terminal branch of the ulnar nerve, by the *deep palmar aponeurosis*. This aponeurosis, which is thin, is strengthened at the level of the metacarpophalangeal joints by the *deep transverse ligament*, which separates the lumbricals and the neurovascular bundles from the interosseous muscles.

5. *The digital canals*, in which the flexor tendons of the fingers have their course, are *constricted zones* starting at the level of the metacarpophalangeal joints of the four fingers. The canals are characterized by the presence of *fibrous sheaths*, particularly well developed in the first and second phalanges but much weaker at the level of the joints with some significant strengthening elements, the cruciate and oblique ligaments. These digital fibrous sheaths, acting as pulleys, maintain the tendons against the bone surface without compressing them.

The *synovial sheaths* facilitate gliding of the tendons in the digital canals. There are three digitopalmar synovial sheaths (for the second, third and fourth digits) and two digitocarpal sheaths for the thumb and the little finger.

Each synovial sheath, essentially of connective tissue, comprises a visceral layer or *epitenon* adhering closely to the tendon and a parietal layer, lining the wall of the fibrous sheath, separated by a synovial space. The visceral layer has extensions into the inside of the tendon. These are the *endotenon*, a series of septa separating the fibre bundles from each other. Just before the end of the flexor tendons, a *mesotenon* of triangular shape joins the two layers of the synovial sheath, acting as a mesentery for the passage of vessels. Other more attenuated structures, the vinculum breve and vinculum longum, perform the same function (Fig. 2.2).

In brief, the epitenon, endotenon, mesotenon or the vincula enclose a significant number of vessels.

The tendons, covered by the visceral layer of their synovial sheath, end at the base of the distal phalanx in the case of the perforating tendon (deep flexor) and on the middle phalanx in the case of the perforated tendon (superficial flexor). On the palmar surface of the middle phalanx the two halves of the perforated tendon decussate to form a chiasma.

6. *The pulp region* corresponds to the palmar surface of the last phalanx of each digit. Here the extremely sensitive skin covers a thick, dense cellular fatty tissue. This pulp contains numerous nerve endings and vascular endings (glomi). There is no tendon or synovial sheath.

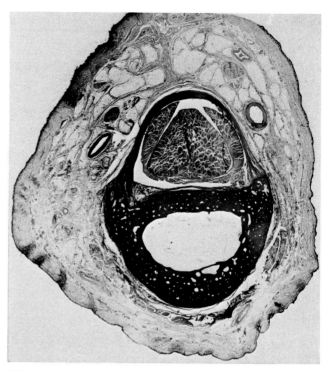

Figure 2.2
Cross-section of an adult finger. Note the phalanx on which the transverse ligament of the fibrous sheath is fixed; the synovial space; the tendon of the flexor digitorum profundus accompanied laterally by the two bands of the flexor superficialis. On the dorsal surface of the phalanx, the outspread fibrous complex of the extensor, the interossei and the lumbrical.

DORSAL SURFACE

The skin on the dorsal surface of the hand is thin, delicate and almost transparent, since the branches of the dorsal venous network of the hand are visible. Above all it is mobile. Hairs are present on the dorsal surface of the hand and of the first phalanx of the four last digits.

The fascia superficialis is very thin and in the underlying loose connective tissue lie the superficial veins and the cutaneous branches of the radial and ulnar nerves.

An aponeurosis or dorsal fascia of the hand separates these cutaneous layers from the extensor tendons.

Distal to the wrist, these tendons cross two well-defined zones.

A constricted zone, marked off by the *extensor retinaculum*, which helps to form the six osteofibrous tunnels in which the tendons are surrounded by synovial sheaths with the same general characteristics as those of the palmar surface.

A loose zone, taking up the dorsal surface of the hand, where three groups of tendons can generally be seen (Fig. 2.3).

The tendons for the thumb lie in the first and third tunnels (abductor pollicis longus, extensor pollicis brevis and extensor pollicis longus). They form the anatomical snuffbox, crossed by the median vein of the forearm accompanied by the superficial branch of the radial nerve, while deep below, against the bones, lies the radial artery.

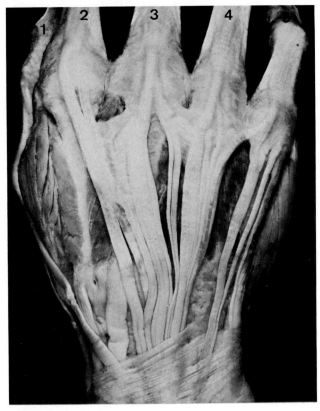

Figure 2.3
Right hand. Dorsal surface. A view of the various extensor tendons.

The two wrist extensor tendons which terminate on the base of the second and third metacarpals have passed along the second osteofibrous tunnel.

Finally, the tendons of the various digital extensors and the tendon of the extensor carpi ulnaris muscle take their course along the fourth, fifth and sixth furrows.

The dorsal surface of the digits constitutes a special region. It serves for the final passage of the extensor tendons.

The tendons intended for the thumb end on the base of the first metacarpal and the base of the first and second phalanges. As for the extensor digitorum tendons, they divide into three, then insert on the phalanges, after receiving the tendons of the interossei and the lumbricals.

The extensor carpi ulnaris tendon inserts into the base of the fifth metacarpal.

Starting from the extensor retinaculum, as soon as the synovial sheaths terminate, all these tendons are surrounded by paratenon. This loose connective tissue, which extends connective-tissue septa between the fibre bundles of the tendons (endotenon) contains the vessels which ensure nutrition of the tendons. These vessels come from the dorsal metacarpal arteries or from the digital arteries, depending on the level.

THE BLOOD SUPPLY OF THE TENDONS

After Koelliker (1850) it was accepted for some time that *adult tendons* were structures without vessels whereas *young tendons* were vascularized. Nutrition was believed to take place by imbibition through the synovia of the synovial sheaths or the interstitial fluid of the neighbouring connective tissue.

Sappey (1866) and others (Ludwig & Schweigger-Seidel (1872), Arai (1907), Rau (1914), Mayer (1916), Dychno (1936), Edwards (1946), Braithwaite (1951), Brockis (1953), Peacock (1959), Lang (1963), Guse, Erler & Loetzke (1963), Smith (1966) and Dörfl (1969)) demonstrated, in most cases by means of vascular injections, that the vessels destined for the tendons had their points of origin and entry in different places: the musculotendinous junction, the osteotendinous joining, the extrasynovial regions of areolar tissue with paratenon and the synovial regions in the constricted areas, with synovial sheaths, mesotenons or vincula.

According to Edwards & Brockis there are intrinsic intratendinous, interfascicular vessels exhibiting an internal pattern of longitudinal vessels joined by transverse anastomoses making their way through the interfascicular connective tissue (endotenon).

When the vessels have been injected through the ulnar artery with gelatine containing Indian ink, they can be observed with the naked eye, with a magnifying glass and, if necessary, under the microscope.

The tendons of the hand pass through alternate *loose areas* where they are surrounded by areolar connective tissue (paratenon) and *constricted areas* (synovial sheaths).

1. In the *dorsal and palmar loose areas* the arterial vessels coming from the neighbouring deep arteries (dorsal metacarpal arteries, collateral digital arteries or superficial palmar arch) reach the paratenon on each side of the tendons. They generally divide into a T several times. The longitudinal branches remain on the surface in the paratenon of the interfascicular furrows. The arteries on the two sides of the tendon anastomose, thus forming a superficial vascular network of very loose mesh (Fig. 2.4).

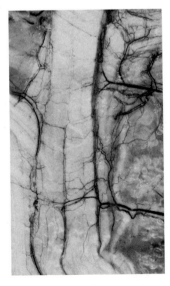

Figure 2.4
Arteries of the dorsal face of the extensor tendon of the ring finger (injected with dye).

In the palmar zone the vessels are more numerous and are contained in the various levels of the paratenon which is arranged in several layers round the tendons.

The blood supply to the tendons is mainly from these superficial vessels. Some run parallel to the tendons, while others form numerous transverse loops. Paratenon and vessels can be removed together, the latter only penetrating very shallowly into the tendon through the septa of the endotenon. These vessels remain in the perifascicular connective tissue and are never in direct contact with the fibrous bundles (Fig. 2.5).

2. In the *constricted areas* the vessels reach the tendon at the two ends of the synovial sheath (especially at the proximal 'prepucial fold' which is richly vascularized) and through the mesotenons and vincula (Fig. 2.6). The arteries which supply these vessels usually come from the arteries of the neighbouring joint.

The visceral layer of the tendon sheath or again the mesotenon near its tendon end produce extensions (villi or Haversian fringes) similar to those observed in the synovial sheaths of joints. These extensions are highly vascularized.

The microvascularization present in the visceral layer and villi of the synovial sheath is clearly visible following injection of dye into the vessels. This is very abundant on the surface of the tendons but much less so in the intermediate part between each end of the synovial sheath. It takes the form of plain or contorted skeins of vessels, sometimes under the guise of glomeruli in which the vessels consist of an arteriole, a constricted intermediate segment and a venule which passes into a vein (Fig. 2.5).

It is through the mesotenon that the vessels are able to continue their way into the endotenon. These vessels do not penetrate into the fibre bundles or come into contact with their fibres; they thus remain in the interfascicular spaces.

In some areas of the tendon, between the two ends of the synovial sheath, there seem to be few, if any, superficial or interfascicular vessels.

Further research based on serial sections of tendons would certainly provide much information.

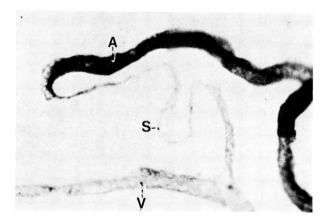

Figure 2.5
Various aspects of the microcirculation in the paratenon or the visceral layer of the synovial sheath. A: arteriole. S: intermediate segment. V: venule.

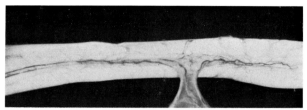

Figure 2.6
Mesotenon and vessels leading to a flexor tendon.

Nutrition of the tendons is therefore ensured mainly by a special kind of microvascular system passing through the paratenon, the visceral layer of the synovial sheath and ultimately the interfascicular connective-tissue septa or endotenon. The fibres of the tendon bundles are not in direct contact with these vessels.

To understand this pattern of nutrition of the tendons, it must be supposed that plasma dialyses through the walls of the vessels, often at some distance from the tendon fibres. Such dialysis is certainly facilitated by the special vascular apparatus of the paratenon or the synovial sheaths. The product of the dialysis forms part of the synovial fluid or the interstitial fluid of the connective tissue forming the paratenon.

The presence of these numerous vessels facilitates the *production* or, as the case may be, the *resorption* of this fluid, by means of a process analogous to that in joint cavities.

Some authors have drawn attention to the presence of hyaluronic acid in the synovial fluid. That acid is found in the connective tissue and is said also to be produced by the synovial cells. This mucopolysaccharide, which binds water, ensures normal viscosity, thus promoting the nutrition of certain tissues.

The acid is depolymerized and hydrolysed by hyaluronidase, and Maibach (1953) ascribes a role to it in the poor cicatrization of tendon sutures in synovial sheaths. As Bunnell (1956) pointed out, when a tendon is severed in a synovial sheath, its ends round over and no proliferation takes place. Bier (1949) claims that hormones peculiar to the synovia act against the healing of tendon sutures in synovial sheaths.

Certain authors assert that sutures of flexor tendons surrounded by paratenon are successful in 37 per cent of cases. In synovial sheaths, where nutrition is less well assured, the success rate is said to be only 9 per cent. Suture of the extensor tendons are usually better than those of the flexors.

It therefore seems quite obvious that the mode of vascularization or nutrition of the tendons, which varies locally in intensity and nature, is of great importance to the clinician.

THE ROLE OF LUMBRICAL MUSCLES, INCLUDING NEURO-MUSCULAR SPINDLES

These four small muscles on the radial side of fingers are important for the fine movements of the fingers. A number of variations exist, and can be summed up as follows:

1. Presence of four lumbrical muscles, two for the middle finger and none for the ring finger;

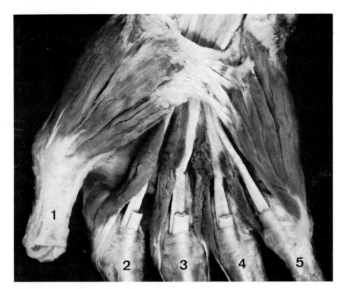

Figure 2.7
Five lumbrical muscles of the right hand, two of them for the middle finger.

2. Presence of four lumbrical muscles, two for the middle finger and none for the little finger;

3. Presence of five lumbrical muscles, two for the middle and two for the ring finger, but none for the little finger;

4. Presence of five lumbrical muscles, two for the middle finger and the remaining three for the three other fingers (Fig. 2.7).

Very frequently the middle finger is thus supplied with two lumbrical muscles and its agility and nimbleness of motion is therefore increased.

Origin: These muscles arise from a movable medium, namely the tendons of the common flexor digitorum profundus. At this level simple or feather-like origins are observed.

Insertion: Having crossed the lateral aspect of the MP joint and of the proximal phalanx, the lumbrical muscle tendon reaches the tendon of the extensor digitorum on the dorsum of the phalanges.

Innervation: They are supplied by the median and ulnar nerves, just as for the muscular body of the flexor profundus digitorum. A *muscular nerve* is found for each lumbrical muscle, and we must define it as a complex nerve, consisting of nerve fibres of different size and function.

One can successively recognize:

1. Motor fibres proceeding out of the spindles, towards the motor plates;

2. Proprioceptive fibres I^a and II, shaping the primary and possibly the secondary endings of the neuro-muscular spindles;

3. Gamma-motor fibres, bound for the muscular fibres within the spindles, for their motion;

4. Proprioceptive fibres I^b for the neuro-tendinous spindles.

Neuro-muscular spindles are numerous, i.e., up to 139 within the four lumbrical muscles (Winckler and Foroglou). Voss could reckon 156 and Cooper about 130. The first and second lumbrical muscles have the largest number of encapsulated receptors.

Neuro-muscular spindles are easily dissected and removed for further examination by silver impregnation. Some can reach the length of 12 mm. The nervous thread covering them may be divided into several branches entering the spindle at different sites or hila. A number of such spindles may also receive the same nervous twig at various levels (Fig. 2.8).

On transverse section, the neuro-muscular spindle has a characteristic shape. It is successively composed of:

1. an *external connective sheath* (consisting of several connective lamellae, concentric, providing the spindle with some consistency, allowing it to be seen and removed);

2. a *space* plasma-filled from the capillaries inside the spindle and penetrating also the layers of the external connective sheath, and the muscular fibres of the spindle as well, maintaining the spindle under some tension and thus increasing its sensibility;

3. an *internal connective sheath*, very thin;

4. *striated muscular fibres inside the spindle* itself (whose calibre is generally smaller than that of muscular fibres *outside* the spindle);

5. *capillaries* and *nervous proprioceptive fibres* (gamma-motor ones).

Silver impregnation of those neuro-muscular spindles has allowed us to demonstrate the existence of primary proprioceptive terminations forming wide loops extended on both sides as a T and also of secondary proprioceptive annular-spiral terminations and finally of gamma-motor fibres.

Function of the lumbrical muscles. The action of these muscles is shown in two ways:

1. The *voluntary contraction*, as an isolated action, producing a controlled movement, wherein the corresponding inter-

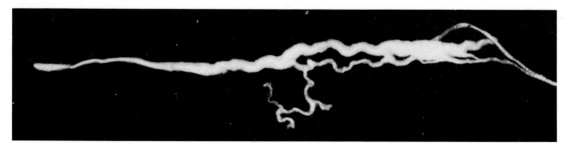

Figure 2.8
A view of a neuro-muscular spindle from a lumbrical muscle. It has a length of 12 mm and has been identified by dissection.

osseous muscle generally cooperates. The main purpose is to augment flexion of the proximal phalanx during grasp or together with the opposition of thumb pinch.

However flexion of the proximal phalanx can become more complicated and complete by flexion of the middle and distal phalanges under the force of the common flexor digitorum, or by a sudden flick extension of these same phalanges, from the thumb (fillip).

2. The *reflex contraction* of the lumbrical muscles is a result of the existence within those muscles of encapsulated receptors—neuro-muscular spindles and neuro-tendinous spindles.

The reflex commanding these movements is called myotatic, it is a reflex of extension or elongation and will act as an antagonist with the extension of the proximal phalanx of fingers. It is a reflex involving two neurons, one being centripetal, proprioceptor and the other centrifugal, motor, but nevertheless monosynaptic, unilateral and intrasegmental.

Every time the extensor muscles of the fingers contract to achieve an extension of the proximal phalanx, the lumbrical muscles undergo an elongation. Proprioceptive terminations of their receptors are stimulated and the resulting reflex is contraction of the lumbrical muscles.

Such a reflex can be considered as a control to the mechanism of extension of the proximal phalanx: its intervention is of particular import with the pianist, the violinist, the flute-player, the harpist and the typist to cite only a few examples.

REFERENCES

ARAI, H. (1907) Die Blutgefässe der Sehnen. *Anat. Hefte*, **34**, 263.

BRAITHWAITE, F. & BROCKIS, J-G. (1951) The vascularisation of the tendon graft. *Brit. J. plast. Surg.*, **4**, 130.

BROCKIS, J.-G. (1953) The blood supply of the flexor and extensor tendons of the fingers in man. *J. Bone Jt. Surg.*, **35**, 131.

BUNNELL, S. (1956) *Surgery of the Hand.* 3rd edn. Philadelphia: Lippincott.

DYCHNO, A. (1936) Zur Frage über die Blutversorgung der Sehnen. *Anat. Anz.*, **82**, 282.

EDWARDS, D. A. W. (1946) The blood supply and lymphatic drainage of the tendons. *J. Anat.*, **80**, 147.

FOROGLOU, Ch. & WINCKLER, G. (1973) Ultrastructure du fuseau neuro-musculaire chez l'homme. Comparaison avec le rat. *Zeit. Anat. Entwickl. Gesch.*, **140**, 19.

GUSE, D., ERLER, W. & LOETZK, H-H. (1963) Uber die Blutgefässanordnung an der Sehnen des Mittelfingers. *Gegenbaur's morph. Jb.*, **104**, 314.

KOELLIKER, A. (1850) *Mikroskopische Anatomie oder Geweblehre des Menschen.* Leipzig: W. Engelmann.

LANG, J. (1963) Uber die Blutgefässe der Sehnenscheiden. *Acta Anat.*, **54**, 273.

LUDWIG, C. & SCHWEIGGER-SEIDEL, F. (1872) *Die Lymphgefässe der Fascien und Sehnen.* Leipzig: Hirzel.

MAYER, L. (1916) Technique of tendon transfer. *Surg. Gynec. Obstet.*, **22**, 182.

MAYER, L. (1916) The physiological method of tendon transplantation. *Surg. Gynec. Obstet.*, **22**, 298.

MICHON, J. & VILAIN, R. (1968) *Lésions traumatiques des tendons de la main.* Paris: Masson et Cie.

PEACOCK, E.-E. (1959) A study of the circulation in normal tendons and healing grafts. *Ann. Surg.* **149**, 415.

RAV, E. (1914) Gefässversorgung der Sehne. *Anat. Heft.*, **50**, 679.

SAPPEY, Ph. (1866) *C. R. Acad. Sci. (Paris)*, **62**, 1116, or *Traité d'Anatomie descriptive.* 3rd edn. Vol. 2, p. 32.

VERDAN, Cl. (1952) *Chirurgie réparatrice et fonctionnelle des tendons de la main.* Paris: Expansion Scientifique Française.

WINCKLER, G. (1969) Les Lombricaux de la main. Remarques sur leurs variations, leurs fonctions normales et complémentaires. *Arch. Anat. (Strasbourg)*, **52**.

WINCKLER, G. (1970) Caractères des vaisseaux para—et péritendineux des fléchisseurs des doigts. *Bull. Assoc. Anat.*, **148**, (55th Congress at Nancy.)

WINCKLER, G. (1974) *Manuel d'Anatomie topographique et fonctionelle.* 2nd edn. Paris: Masson et Cie.

WINCKLER, G., FOROGLOU, Ch. (1965) Etude comparative sur les fuseaux neuro-musculaires des muscles lombricaux chez certains Mammifères et chez l'Homme. *Arch. Anat. (Strasbourg)*, **48**, 1–17.

3. Lymphatic Circulation in Tendons and Sheaths

G. C. Setti and C. Verdan

While the blood supply of tendons has been thoroughly investigated, this is not true for the lymphatic system and lymphatic circulation within tendons, particularly in the hand. Some information is available from Russian sources (Lavrentieva, 1947, 1949; Nadejdin, 1957; Guercienov, 1958) about main lymphatic vessels in some tendons. But we cannot find a precise study of the organization of the lymphatic capillary system in tendons themselves, or their connection with the reticular system of the sheaths and the synovial membrane. There are technical difficulties in demonstrating a reticular lymphatic system within tendons. Modern anatomists give the usual opinion that tendons with their well-known vascular and nervous supply, are poorly provided with lymphatic vessels.

We have undertaken a series of systematic anatomical and pathological studies on the lymph circulation within tendons and sheaths.

We report in this chapter our first results of a macro- and microscopic anatomical study of tendons in general, but mainly flexor tendons and their adventitiae.

We shall also discuss the ageing of lymphatic vessels and their alteration in pathological conditions.

MATERIAL AND TECHNIQUES

We used both animals and human tendons, ranging from the foetal to the senile, normal and pathological.

For this purpose we uniformly employed the techniques of intravascular injection, using three different materials:

1. *Gerota's mass* with some technical variations suggested by Ottaviani (Fig. 3.1);

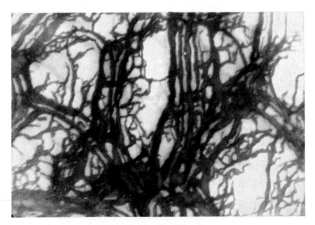

Figure 3.1
Lymphatic network of flexor pollicis longus (injected according to Ottaviani-Gerota-Setti's method: 25 × stereophotography).

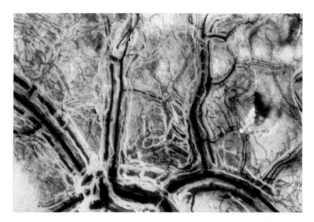

Figure 3.2
Plastic and *Neoprene* injection of vascular and lymphatic network of flexor pollicis longus (Veins and arteries in black, lymphatics in white).

2. *Neoprene* (polymerized chloropren) introduced by Ottaviani in 1974, which dyes arteries red, veins blue and lymphatic white (Fig. 3.2);

3. and the *special Du Pont* diluted dye, introduced by Setti in 1971. All the specimens were dehydrated with alcohol and then treated with xylol or methylsalicylate for microscopic examination.

The tendons injected with Neoprene and fixed, were treated in HCl solution in different concentrations.

These preparations were studied and photographs were taken with a Zeiss stereomicroscope.

Some microtomical slices were made, longitudinal and transverse and treated with Van Gieson stain after the vascular system had been injected.

RESULTS

LYMPH VESSELS OF TENDONS

We demonstrated a very rich lymphatic system in tendons. We investigated mainly flexor tendons, both their superficial network and the deeper lymphatic capillaries (Fig. 3.3)

1. *Superficial lymphatic network:* In the former, vessels were intersecting to produce various geometrical shapes—triangular, rectangular, even circular—over the whole surface of the tendon. Larger lymphatic collectors followed the blood vessels which enter the tendon substance through the mesotenon. There is a close relation between the lymphatic circulation of the tendon itself and of both surfaces of its sheath.

2. *Deep lymphatic network:* The deeper lymphatic vessels

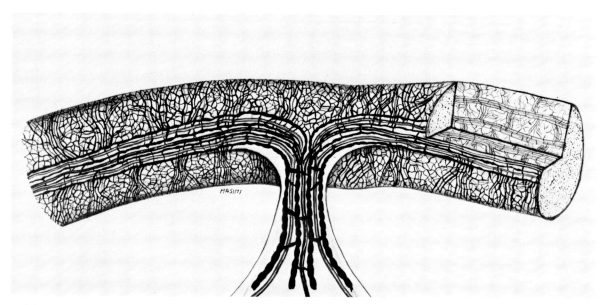

Figure 3.3
Model of the whole blood supply and lymphatic system of a flexor tendon from microscopic preparations.

surround the blood capillaries like cuffs or run together with them to ramify within the tendon substance (Fig. 3.3).

LYMPH VESSELS OF TENDON SHEATHS

Both the visceral and the parietal layers of the sheath have their own lymphatic circulation. The lymphatic vessels are to be seen at all levels, with numerous anastomoses forming a closed reticulum with polygonal and rounded interspaces. Their calibre varies with the depth. Comparatively wide vessels serve as efferent lymphatics. These efferent vessels are to be seen throughout the fibrosynovial sheath and are continuous with the efferent lymphatics proper in the mesotenon which accompany the arterioles and venules.

EFFERENT LYMPHATICS OF TENDONS

They originate from the mesotenon. All the lymph from the tendon substance and from the synovial sheath is collected by vessels of medium size and carried out to the main efferent lymphatics, which run longitudinally in the fibrous sheath with the blood vessels.

These efferent lymphatics merge to some extent with other efferent vessels coming from the intrinsic muscles. They are mainly directed towards the dorsum of the hand.

AGEING OF LYMPHATIC VESSELS

Lymphatic vessels undergo modifications with age. Obvious evidence of senility was noticed in tendon lymphatics at all levels, similar to the findings in the lymphatics of other organs made by other workers (Ottaviani *et al.*; Setti *et al.*; Zdanov *et al.*).

Senility is obvious not only in a vascular network but also in lymphatics within *tendons* themselves. Whereas the pattern regularly found in young adults is geometrical, in elderly patients this pattern is characteristically disorderly and irregular as age advances. The vessels become sinuous and dilatations appear along their course, as shown by comparative studies. If inflammation is present, polymorphism and hyperplasia are the rule as may be seen in cases of rheumatoid arthritis.

CONCLUSIONS

Our investigations revealed an unsuspected extent of lymphatic vessels and capillaries within tendons. This plays an important role, both under normal conditions and in pathological states, as these vessels are intimately related to adjacent tissues such as bone, articular cartilage, synovial membrane, muscles, subcutaneous tissue and skin.

Under normal circumstances the lymphatic plexus of the tendon sheaths facilitates the reabsorption of the synovial fluid in conjunction with the venous system.

In morbid states, particularly in acute rheumatic disease, deep modifications occur in both the smaller and the larger lymphatic vessels, in the tendon sheaths and throughout the tendon substance. The inflammation leads to microscopic lymphangiectasia and other irregularities, with lymphangitis leading to vascular hyperplasia.

In connection with tendon repair and grafting, alterations of this important plexus of lymphatics within and around tendons, may be of great importance in the maintenance of their optimal local metabolism.

We wonder also whether pathological changes could be found in the so-called Sudeck dystrophy. The opportunities to study this are obviously difficult to encounter.

REFERENCES

GUERCIENOV, A.-P. (1958) *Arkh. Anat. topogr. Anat.* (Tomsk).
LAVRENTIEVA, A.-P. (1947) *Diss. Samarcanda, Tomsk.*
LAVRENTIEVA, A.-P. (1949) *Probl. Anat. (Leningrad)*, **3**, 141.
NADEJDIN, V.-N. (1957) *Arch. Istol. Embriol.*, **34**, 90.
OTTAVIANI, G. (1954) *Ateneo parmense*, **25**, 109.
ZDANOV, D.-A. (1964) *Arkh. Anat. Gistol. Embriol.*, **10**, 13.

4. The Anatomy of the Deep Flexor and Lumbrical Muscles

M. Fahrer

The deep plane of flexors in the forearm is represented by three groups of muscles, all of them spindle shaped, prolonged by long tendons, and inserting into the distal phalanges of the five digits of the hand. They are classically described as two separate muscles:

1. Flexor digitorum profundus, which includes:
   (a) The medial group, with tendons ending in the medial three fingers, and
   (b) The middle group, whose tendon inserts into the index finger.
2. Flexor pollicis longus.

M. FLEXOR DIGITORUM PROFUNDUS

M. Flexor digitorum profundus arises from:

1. the upper 2/3 of the anterior surface, the anterior border, the medial surface and the posterior border of the ulna;

2. the intermuscular septum, which attaches to the posterior border of the ulna, and from the continuing aponeurosis, which also gives origins to the flexor carpi ulnaris and extensor carpi ulnaris muscles;

3. the interosseous membrane.

Proximally, the origins of the muscle will reach as far as the base of the coronoid process, the medial aspect of the olecranon and the arch formed by the brachialis and the supinator (Fig. 4.1a). The distal limit of the origins reaches the upper border of the M. pronator quadratus.

The muscular mass is divided in the middle third of the forearm into two distinct segments: one lateral (Fig. 4.1b), taking its origins from the interosseous membrane, one medial, arising from the ulna.

In the lower third of the forearm, corresponding to Zone VII of Verdan (1964), the muscular fibres run forward and downward into two groups of tendons: the lateral segment into a separate tendon, the digital tendon of the index; the medial segment into a variable number of tendons, seven to twelve or more, joined into a common mass by paratenon. The paratenon is loose enough to allow ample longitudinal movements of the individual elements of the tendinous mass. The digital tendons exist as distinct entities only distal to the flexor retinaculum. Interdigital tendinous slips from the middle and little finger converge distally into the digital tendon of the ring finger, forming an 'M' shaped pattern (Fig. 4.1c). This slip can only be seen by removing the synovial sheath, dividing the relevant lumbricals and pulling the tendons apart (Fahrer, 1971).

At the level of the carpal canal, the tendons of the flexor digitorum profundus (FDP) and of the flexor digitorum superficialis (FDS) are surrounded by a common synovial sheath attached to the posterior wall of the canal by its parietal layer, and to the flexor tendons by mesotenons.

The lumbrical muscles take their origins at the same level—Zone VI of Verdan. The digital tendons of the FDP are situated in a coronal plane between the middle and posterior folds of the synovial carpal sheath. The tenuous interdigital tendons, contained within the common tendon complex of the medial segment of the FDP end at the level of the carpal canal:

1. by direct continuation with the lumbrical muscular fibres (Fig. 4.2A) forming digastric elements (Bossy and Gondy, 1961; Fahrer; 1971, 1975; Testut, 1884).

2. by bifurcating into a tendinous slip joining the digital tendon and a slip of origin for lumbrical muscular fibres (Fig. 4.2B);

3. by dispersing into the synovial membrane (Fig. 4.2C).

The origin of the first two lumbricals is by means of concentric tendinous lamellae, less than 1 mm long. It is impossible to trace accurately by micro-dissection these lamellae within the digital tendons. Lumbricals III and IV take origin from a fibromembranous reticulum formed by:

1. the digital tendons of the medius, anularis and minimus;

2. their interdigital tendinous connections;

3. membranous elements belonging to the carpal synovial sheath.

Up to a quarter of the muscular mass can arise directly from the synovial membrane (Fahrer, 1971, 1975) (Fig. 4.3). Direct synovial origins of lumbrical muscular fibres were noted in rheumatoid hands during synovectomies (Backhouse, 1972).

In the palm—Zone V—the digital tendons are surrounded by a stratified paratenon. Together with the tendons of the superficialis, to which they are posterior, the tendons of the profundus run into digital osteofibrous tunnels in Zones II and I. At this level, the tendons are surrounded by digital synovial sheaths. Each of the tendons of the superficialis divides sagittally into two separate slips, at the level of the shaft of the proximal phalanx (Zone II). The resulting tendinous slips run posteriorly and distally and pass round the sides of the profundus tendons, which are converted thus into perforating tendons (Fig. 4.1d). Further distally, the paired slips of the superficialis join and then decussate at the level of the proximal IP joint, and insert into the palmar aspect of the base of the middle phalanges. The tendons of the profundus continue their course distally, present an incomplete sagittal division at the level of the middle phalanges and end in a fan-shaped insertion into the base of the distal phalanges (Fig. 4.1e). Careful dissection of a FDP digital tendon demonstrates the existence of four discrete longitudinal fibre bundles. These

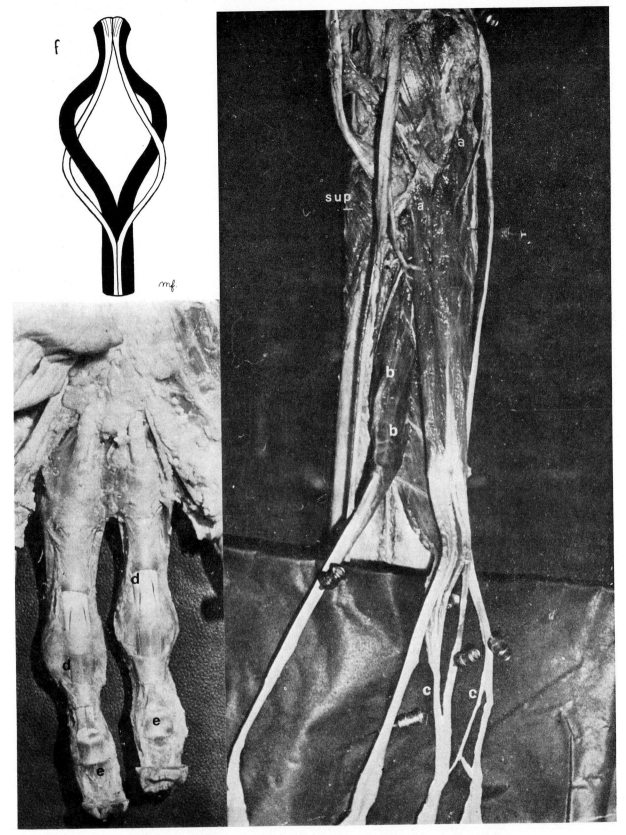

Figure 4.1
Dissection of the common deep flexor muscle of the fingers with its proximal insertions, its division into two muscular masses, which both end in two different tendon systems.

It must be noted that on the ulnar side the connections between the three digital tendons converge distally towards the annular tendon.

In the large diagram the digital canal with the two flexor tendons and the system of pulleys.

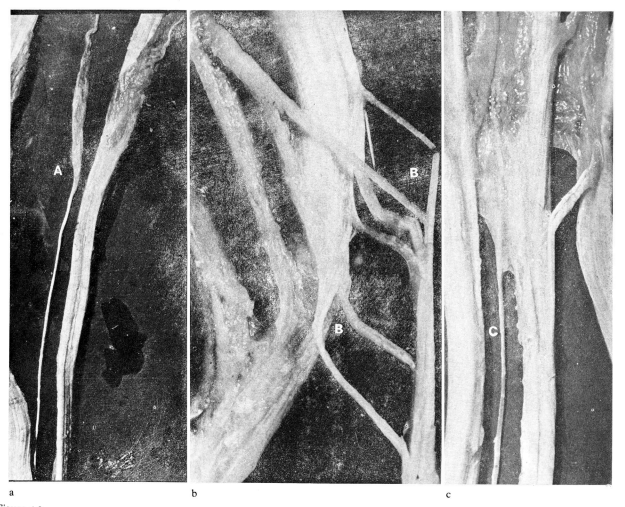

a   b   c

Figure 4.2
Dissections of the attachments of the lumbrical muscles to the deep flexor tendons.

(A) On the ulnar side, the deep flexor tendon may have small interdigital tendons which are in direct continuity with the muscular fibres of the lumbricals, thus forming digastric elements.

(B) The deep flexor tendon partially branches off into multiple tendinous elements leading to a lumbrical muscle.
(C) Certain interdigital tendon fibres will be scattered in the synovial membrane.

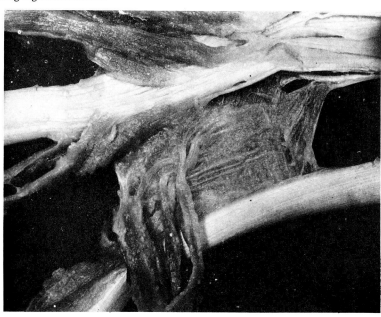

Figure 4.3
The lumbricals III and IV may be inserted into a tendino-membraneous plexus losing themselves in places with the synovial sheath.

bundles, symmetrical to the middle sagittal plane of each finger, present a spiral course. From proximal to distal, the volar bundles run lateral, then dorsal to the other bundles and end up, after penetrating medially and forward, by inserting volar and medial into the distal phalanx (Fig. 4.1f). The spiral arrangement, described in detail by Hueston and Wilson (1972), Martin (1958), Rouviere (1938), Wilkinson (1953) and Wilson and Hueston (1973), explains the changes in shape of the tendinous cross sections at various digital levels: it increases the elasticity of the tendons (Rouviere, 1938) but exposes the profundus tendon to trigger finger nodules (Hueston and Wilson, 1972).

BLOOD AND NERVE SUPPLY

FDP derives its blood supply from muscular branches of the ulnar and anterior interosseous arteries. The tendons are supplied by longitudinal arteries running inside the endotenon, without direct contact with the tendinous fibres. The proximal part of the tendons receive descending branches from the muscular arteries. In the Zones V and VI, the arteries of the tendons, paratenons and synovial sheaths are given off from the superficial palmar arch. In the Zones I and II, the blood vessels running through the vincula arise from the articular branches of the palmar digital arteries.

Winckler (1970) has recently noted the extraordinary richness of arteriovenous anastomoses in the para and peritendinous vascular plexuses of the flexors as well as the complexity of the apparatus controlling the blood circulation.

The nerve supply of the FDP comes from the ulnar nerve and from the anterior interosseous branch of the median nerve.

In 30/36 cases of Brash (1955), the branch of the ulnar nerve, sometimes duplicated, enters the muscle by its medial side, at the proximal end, 6–7 cm below the medial epicondyle: the branch of the anterior interosseous nerve enters the muscle on the anterior surface, 2–4 cm below the hilus of the ulnar nerve.

An anastomosis between the median and ulnar nerves is recorded in 15–20 per cent of the cases, crossing the anterior surface of the FDP.

The index and medius segments are supplied by the median nerve, the anularis and minimus by the ulnar nerve.

The lumbricals are, as a rule, supplied by the same nerves as supply the muscular bellies of their deep flexor tendons: first and second lumbricals by the median, third and fourth by the ulnar. Variations are as frequent as the standard innervation, for the FDP as well as for the lumbricals. Sunderland (1968) finds a standard nerve supply in about 50 per cent of his cases. In the other half, the median nerve encroaches on the territory supplied by the ulnar nerve twice as often as the latter extends laterally. While complete substitution is exceptional, overlapping nerve supply is common.

FUNCTIONAL ANATOMY

FDP is the only flexor of the distal phalanx. This movement is usually associated with the flexion of the middle phalanx by the flexor superficialis. In rare cases of articular laxity, hyperextension of the middle phalanx can allow independent flexion of about 30–45 degrees of the distal IP joint (Kaplan, 1965), thus imitating the 'swan neck' type of deformity. The range of flexion of the distal phalanx is 80 degrees. Flexion of the distal phalanx produces passive flexion of the middle phalanx by the distal gliding of the extensor expansion and by the subsequent pull of the oblique band of the retinacular ligament of Landsmeer (1949). It is quite possible that the co-ordinated flexion of the two IP joints starts as a result of the passive actions of the retinacular ligament. Nevertheless, the FDP can flex completely (120 degrees) the middle phalanx. With the wrist stabilized in extension, the FDP can flex the MP joints to 90 degrees, after having fully flexed the IP joints. This sequence of actions is impossible with a fully flexed wrist joint. Finally, with the fingers stabilized in extension, the FDP flexes the wrist with a force of 4.5 mkg (Von Lanz and Wachsmuth 1959) being, together with FDS, the strongest flexor of the wrist. This last action is contested by a number of authors (Basmajian, 1967; Duchenne, 1867; Kaplan, 1965). In a coronal plane, the FDP adducts the fingers towards the medius and adducts the hand towards the medio-sagittal plane (Braus, 1954).

A Colles' fracture or a subluxation of the lower radio-ulnar joint after destruction of the articular disc by rheumatoid arthritis can straighten the normal ulnar deviation of the hand or even invert it into radial deviation. The changed direction of traction results in a loss of useful muscular power of the flexors (Forgue, 1948); it also sends the fingers at the MP joints into ulnar drift (Flatt, 1971; Millroy, 1966; Schapiro et al., 1971; Stack and Vaughan-Jackson, 1971) to compensate, by a Landsmeer (1968) type of zig-zag mechanism, for the loss of the ulnar deviation. The amplitude of gliding of the tendons of the FDP varies with the finger and the topographical zone. The average figures, according to Verdan (1964) are summarized in the following table:

Zone:	I	II	V	VI	VII
Medius:	5 mm	45 mm	45 mm	45–85 mm	85 mm
Minimus:	3.5 mm	29.5 mm	29.5 mm	29.5–70 mm	70 mm

The division of the FDP into two elements, one for the index and one for the three ulnar fingers is functional as well as anatomical in 90 per cent of the cases. The separation of flexor indicis, as well as the separation of flexor pollicis longus, represents a distinctly human characteristic. The author has never yet found tendinous connections between index and medius. In 5/50 dissections, the muscular bellies of index and medius presented wide areas of fusion in the upper 2/3 of the forearm. In 1/15 microdissections, a bipennate second lumbrical represented the only connection between the index and medius tendons (Fig. 4.4A). Occasional oblique tendinous slips may connect the tendons of the pollex and index: the direction of these tendinous connections will mechanically determine the loss of independent action of the index (Fig. 4.4B) or of the thumb (Fig. 4.4C) (Fahrer, 1971; Rank and Wakefield, 1960; Rank, Wakefield & Hueston, 1973).

The three ulnar fingers are connected by a double intertendinous system:

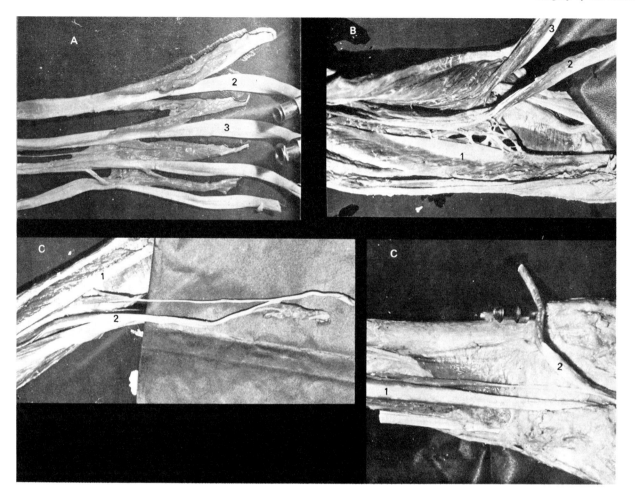

Figure 4.4 (1 – thumb; 2 – index; 3 – middle finger)
(A) Microdissection of the lumbrical system. Note the 2nd bipenniform lumbrical muscle, inserted into the tendons of the index and middle fingers, which represents the only connection existing between these two tendons.

(B) and (C) Oblique tendinous strips sometimes link the tendons of the thumb and the index finger: their direction will determine mechanically the loss of independence of action of one or other of the two fingers.

1. At the level of Zone VII, the tendinous slips converging distally towards the anularis tendon will prevent active flexion of the medius and minimus if anularis is passively extended. This manœuvre, described by Verdan (1960, 1961, 1972) eliminates the action of FDP in order to allow the examination of the FDS. The corollary of Verdan's sign is impaired extension of the anularis at the MP joint while the fingers III and V are fully flexed (Fahrer, 1969, 1971).

2. At the level of Zone VI, digital tendons, interdigital slips and areas of synovial membrane fused to the tendons form a distal fibrous reticulum, which provides a relatively rigid frame for the lumbricals III and IV.

This complex intertendinous apparatus causes the three ulnar fingers to move together. The role of this system seems to be to check independent gliding in opposite directions of the digital tendons and by so doing, to protect the origins of lumbricals III and IV from traction. The fine proprioceptive organs are not under undue strain and the balance between flexor and extensor tendons is not interfered with. While agree-

ing with Bruner (1970) on the importance of the double origins of lumbricals III and IV in the interdependent action of the last three fingers, the author considers that this passive action of the lumbricals comes into play only in the absence of both the proximal and the distal reticular systems. The author has seen one such case in a series of 31 microdissected specimens of lumbricals with multiple origins.

The elimination of the action of the FDP at the level of the distal IP joint by Verdan's manœuvre leaves a flail distal phalanx in extension (Fig. 4.5A). If, however, one tries to elicit Verdan's sign, starting from the position of full flexion of the fingers, the result is a flexed distal IP joint (Fig. 4.5B). Landsmeer (1976) ascribes this paradoxical phenomenon to the pull of the perforated tendon of the FDS. Contraction of the muscle tightens the noose around the perforating tendon and blocks it in passive flexion. The distal IP joint can be passively extended, yields with a slight click and will not go back to the flexed posture. This physiological 'trigger' finger view is confirmed by pathological cases of trigger fingers in which the

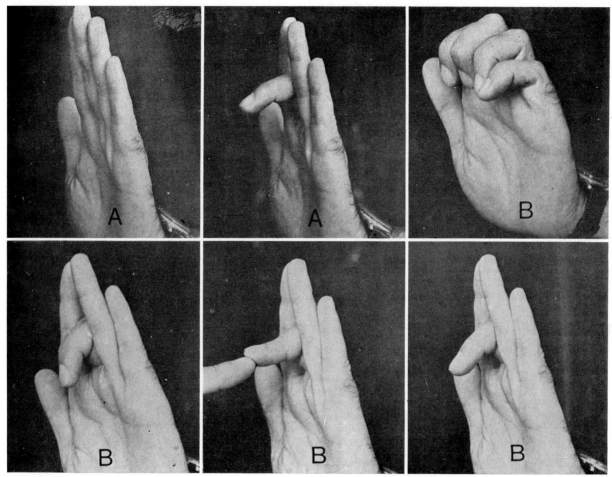

Figure 4.5

(A) Verdan's manœuvre. At the level of the three last fingers, one can neutralize the deep flexor the better to examine the superficial flexor. It is enough to extend the three fingers to block the deep flexor and to individualize the action of the superficial flexor on IPP.

(B) If one uses Verdan's manœuvre, starting from a position of active flexion of the IP articulations and if one stretches the index finger and the annular, one establishes that the IPD of the middle finger remains fixed in flexion; if one now passively straightens this distal phalanx, one feels a slight resistance which can give way with a click of elasticity. Landsmeer attributes this paradoxical phenomenon to the decussation of the superficial flexor tendon, which put the deep flexor tendon into acute tension as if across a real running knot, preventing it from sliding.

nodules on the profundus are trapped between the slips of the perforated tendon (Flatt, 1971; Helal, 1970; Hueston and Wilson, 1972).

FLEXOR POLLICIS LONGUS

Flexor pollicis longus arises:

1. From the medial epicondyle of the humerus and the base of the coronoid process, by a superficial head running laterally and distally, surrounded by the fibres of the FDS. Described as a variation and noted by Ganzer as early as 1813 this head is present in more than 50 per cent of the cases (Fig. 4.6A).

2. From the anterior surface of the radius and from the interosseous membrane by a deep head, which represents the principal mass of the muscle. On the interosseous membrane, it is separated from the index segment of the FDP by the anterior interosseous vessels and nerve.

The muscular fibres, about 50 mm long, run distally and medially into a more or less cylindrical tendon which lies, surrounded by paratenon, on the anterior surface of the M. Pronator Quadratus (Fig. 4.6B) in the Zone VII. Behind the flexor retinaculum—Zone VI—the tendon is surrounded by a synovial sheath, and occupies the lateral side of the carpal canal. At this level, the FPL tendon uses as a pulley, besides the flexor retinaculum, also the tendon of flexor carpi radialis, around which it spirals from posterior to anterior and from medial to lateral (Verdan and Poulenas, 1975; Wilson and Hueston, 1973). In the palm of the hand, the FPL tendon runs deep between the thenar muscles—Zone IV—then enters the digital osteo-fibrous tunnel and inserts into the base of the distal phalanx. The structure of the fibre bundles of the tendon and their spiral arrangement, similar to the tendons of FDS and FDP, was studied by Hueston and Wilson (1972), Wilkinson (1953) and Wilson and Hueston (1972). The carpal

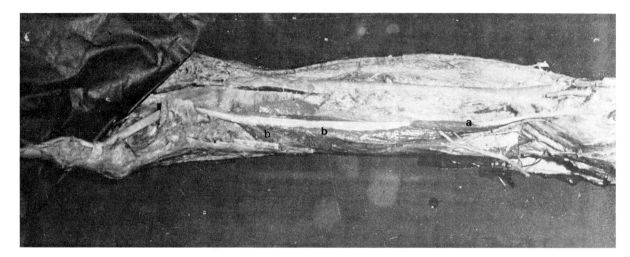

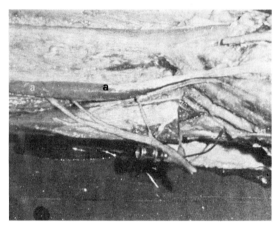

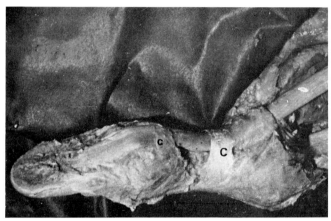

Figure 4.6
Anatomical plate of the individual long flexor of the thumb.
(A) This muscle inserts itself from the proximal side by a superficial head on the epitrochlea and the base of the coronoid process, and by a deep head on the anterior surface of the radius and of the interosseous membrane.

(B) The muscular mass terminates on a single tendon which slides surrounded by paratenon, on the anterior surface of the quadrate and the distal extremity of the radius.
(C) Dissection of the osteofibrous tunnel of the thumb, which shows only two pulleys of transverse fibres.

synovial sheath of FPL extends through the whole length of the digital tunnel, in Zones III and I. As the thumb has only two phalanges, the tunnel has only two pulleys (Fig. 4.6C). The proximal pulley (sometimes congenitally constricted) and the spiral structure of the tendinous fibre bundles make the trigger thumb more common than any trigger finger.

The tendinous connections of the FPL have already been discussed. Occasionally, the tendon of the FPL can send tendinous slips to the first lumbrical and very seldom may give origin to a lumbrical muscle.

BLOOD AND NERVE SUPPLY

The FPL is supplied by the radial artery on its proximal and lateral aspects, and by the anterior interosseous artery on the medial side. The tendon is supplied by the muscular arteries in Zone VII, by the radial artery and the superficial palmar arch in Zone VI, by A. princeps pollicis and its digital branches in the Zones I, III and IV.

The nerve supply is given off by the anterior interosseous nerve, which sends a separate branch to the superficial head and 1–3 branches to the deep head. The nerves run for a few mm on the anterior surface of the muscle, before penetrating it in 16/30 cases (Brash 1955) in the upper third, near the medial border.

FUNCTIONAL ANATOMY

The FPL flexes the distal phalanx of the thumb at 90 degrees and the MP joint at 80 degrees. It is also a flexor of the trapezometacarpal joint and flexes the wrist with a force of 1.2 mkg (1959). According to Braus (1954), the FPL is also a weak abductor of the wrist.

The amplitude of gliding is, according to Verdan (1964): Zone I: 12 mm; Zone III: 32 mm; Zone IV: 40 mm; Zone VI: 40–52 mm; Zone VII: 52 mm. As the amount of contraction is relatively small, the amplitude of gliding can be used completely only in association with opposed movements of the wrist. Similar to the FDP, the thumb cannot flex the IP joint if the MP and wrist joints are fully flexed.

THE LUMBRICAL MUSCLES

The lumbrical muscles, situated between the profundus tendons and the extensor expansions of the fingers, are a peculiar element of the locomotor system. Based on the situation of the lumbricals as well as on the huge concentration of proprioceptive receptors contained by this muscle, Rabischong (1961) who had given an exhaustive description of the nerve endings in the lumbricals, considers as their main function the recording and regulation of tensions between the extrinsic muscles of the fingers. This function seems to prevail over the potential muscular actions determined by electrical excitation (Duchenne, 1867) or computed by traditional methods.

The origins of the lumbrical muscles have already been described with the tendons of the FDP. The insertions are into the radial aspect of the extensor expansions of the fingers, distal to the interossei and to the MP joints. Kopsch (1933), on a series of 110 dissections, finds 39 per cent of cases corresponding to the standard description. The variations in nerve supply and eventually in numbers (absence of one or more of the muscles, but more frequently duplication, especially of the third lumbrical) have been revised by Winckler (1969). The lumbricals run usually along the lateral side of the corresponding profundus tendon, cross the MP joints usually on the radial side, sometimes on the ulnar side and occasionally on both sides, and are separated from the interossei by the deep transverse metacarpal ligament.

BLOOD AND NERVE SUPPLY

Muscular arteries derive directly from the superficial palmar arch or from the digital branches and enter the palmar aspect of the lumbrical muscles. The posterior branches arise from the deep palmar arch, enter the posterior aspect of the muscles, and represent the principal supply.

In standard cases, lumbrical muscles I and II are supplied by digital branches of the median nerve through their palmar surfaces. Lumbricals III and IV by the deep branch of the ulnar nerve by their deep surfaces. The variations, more frequent than the norm, incline, according to Sunderland, towards predominance of the ulnar nerve and do not necessarily coincide with the supply of the corresponding segments of the FDP (Sunderland, 1968).

FUNCTIONAL ANATOMY

The proprioceptive role of the lumbricals has already been discussed. The conventional action of the lumbricals is classically equated to that of the interossei on the radial sides of the fingers: flexion, radial inclination and some medial rotation at the MP joint and extension of the IP joints. By direct excitation during operations, Kaplan (1965) noted that, on fingers maintained passively in extension, the contraction of the lumbricals produces a distal gliding of the tendons of the FDP. Electromyographic studies show a dissociation between the actions of the lumbricals and FDP. Lumbricals contract in association with extensors (Backhouse, 1968; Long and Brown, 1964). The 'up stroke' movement in writing, which illustrates so perfectly the potential action of the lumbricals, does not contract these muscles (Backhouse, 1968). We can consider the lumbricals as extensors of the IP joints and the interossei as flexors of the MP joints.

The lumbrical muscles have very long muscular fibres—90 mm—and have an amplitude of contraction of 50 mm. A considerable tension is needed to produce an extra passive elongation of 10–15 mm (Stack, 1970). This extra passive elongation can occur only in complete divisions of the FDP tendon in the Zones I or II, and, according to Parkes (1970) will be responsible for the paradoxical extension of the IP joint when contracting the divided flexor. The 'lumbrical plus' finger is usually the medius. The treatment, division of the insertion of the 2nd lumbrical, produces instant improvement. It is interesting to note that the lumbrical is really inhibited and acts passively as an insertion of the flexor into the extensor expansion: contraction of the proximal belly of a digastric system in the hand (Fahrer, 1975) doesn't trigger a reflex myotatic contraction in the distal belly.

The lumbricals of the thumb arising from the tendon of FPL were considered by the classics as exceedingly rare (Testut, 1884). Goldberg (1941) finds in 1/50 cases a double origin for the first lumbrical, the second origin being from the FPL. The absence of a lumbrical muscle acting as tensiometer and tension regulator between the extrinsic tendons in the thumb is remarkable in a digit capable of such precise movements. However, in a more superficial plane, the abductor pollicis brevis takes origin from the palmaris longus, from the abductor pollicis longus or from both, and inserts into the extensor expansion. In a series of 30 dissections, the author has constantly found the APB to take origin from at least one of the long tendons. Considering:

1. the large number of neuro-muscular spindles in the abductor pollicis brevis, higher than in the lumbricals (Cooper, 1960);

2. the joint action of APB, APL, and PL in the sagittal flexion of the thumb, and

3. the situation of the APB or, at least of its collateral borders, as muscular bridges between extrinsic tendons, the similarity with the lumbricals is striking (Fahrer, 1975; Fahrer and Tubiana, 1976).

REFERENCES

BACKHOUSE, K. M. (1968) The mechanics of normal digital control in the hand and an analysis of the ulnar drift of rheumatoid arthritis. *Ann. Roy. Coll. Surg, Engl.* **43**, 154.

BACKHOUSE, K. M. (1972) Personal communication.

BASMAJIAN, J. V. (1967) *Muscles Alive.* 2nd edn. Baltimore: Williams and Wilkins Co.

BOSSY, J. & GONDY, B. (1961) La vertitable origine des muscles lombricaux palmaires. *Bull. Assoc. Anat.*, **167**.

BRASH, J. C. (1955) *Neuro-Vascular Hila of Limb Muscles*. Edinburgh: Livingstone.

BRAUS, H. (1954) *Anatomie des Menschen*. Vol. 1. Dritte Auflage (Elze). Berlin: Springer.

BRUNER, J. M. (1970) The dynamics of Dupuytren's disease. *The Hand*, **2**, 172.

COOPER, S. (1960) Muscle spindles and other muscle receptors. In *The Structure and Function of Muscle*, ed. Bourne, G. H. Vol. 1. New York: Academic Press.

DUCHENNE, G. B. (1967) *Physiologie des Mouvements*. (Translated by E. B. Kaplan, 1959.) Philadelphia: W. B. Saunders Company.

FAHRER, M. (1969) The range of movement of the 4th metacarpo-phalangeal joint: a problem for pianists and anatomists. *J. Anat. (Lond.)*, **104**, 410.

FAHRER, M. (1971) Considérations sur l'anatomie fonctionnelle du muscle fléchisseur commun profond des doigts. *Ann. Chir.*, **25**, 945.

FAHRER, M. (1971) Observations on the origin of the lumbrical muscles in the human hand. *J. Anat. (Lond.)*, **110**, 50.

FAHRER, M. (1975) Considérations sur les insertions d'origine des muscles lombricaux: les systèmes digastriques de la main. *Ann. Chir.*, **29**, 979–982.

FAHRER, M. & Tubiana, R. (1976) Palmaris longus anteductor of the thumb. An experimental study. *The Hand*, **8**, 287–289.

FLATT, A. (1971) Personal communication.

FORGUE, E. (1948) *Précis de Pathologie Externe*. Vol. 1. 11th ed. Paris: G. Doin & Co.

GOLDBERG, S. (1941) The origin of the lumbrical muscles in the hand of the South African native. *The Leech (Johannesburg)*, **12**, 35. Reprinted in *The Hand*, **2**, 168, 1970.

HELAL, B. (1970) Distal profundus entrapment in rheumatoid disease. *The Hand*, **2**, 48.

HUESTON, J. T. & WILSON, W. F. (1972) The aetiology of trigger fingers. Explained on the basis of intratendinous architecture. *The Hand*, **3**, 257–260.

KAPLAN, E. B. (1965) *Functional and Surgical Anatomy of the Hand*. 2nd edn. Philadelphia: J. B. Lippincot Company.

KOPSCH, F. (1933) *Rauber-Kopsch Lehrbuch und Atlas der Anatomie des Menschen*. Vol. 3, 14th edn. Leipzig: Georg Thieme.

LANDSMEER, J. M. F. (1949) The anatomy of the dorsal aponeurosis of the human finger, and its functional significance. *Anat. Rec.*, **104**, 35.

LANDSMEER, J. M. F. (1968) Les cohérences spatiales et l'équilibre spatial dans la région carpienne. *Acta Anat.*, 1–84. Supl. 54/1 ad vol. LXX.

LANDSMEER, J. M. F. (1976) *Atlas of Anatomy of the Hand*. Edinburgh: Churchill Livingstone.

LONG, C. & BROWN, E. (1964) Electromyographic kinesiology of the hand: Muscles moving the long finger. *J. Bone and Joint Surg.*, **46A**, 1683.

MARTIN, B. F. (1958) The tendons of flexor digitorum profundus. *J. Anat. (Lond.)*, **92**, 602–608.

MILLROY, P. (1966) Surgery of the rheumatoid hand. *J. Bone and Joint Surgery*, **48B**, 593.

PARKES, A. R. (1970) The 'Lumbrical Plus' finger. *The Hand*, **2**, 164.

RANK, B. K. & WAKEFIELD, A. R. (1960) *Surgery of Repair as Applied to Hand Injuries*. 2nd edn. Edinburgh: Livingstone.

RABISCHONG, P. (1961) Recherches sur la morphologie et la répartition des organes neurotendineux et des récepteurs épitendineux et intramusculaires encapsulés dans les muscles lombricaux de l'Homme. *Arch. Anat. Embryol.*, **44**, 329.

ROUVIERE, H. (1939) *Anatomie Generale*. Paris: Masson.

SCHAPIRO, J., HEIJNA, W., NASATIR, S. & RAY, R. (1971) The relation of wrist motion to ulnar phalangeal drift in the rheumatoid patient. *The Hand*, **3**, 68.

SMITH, J. W. & CONWAY, H. (1966) La dynamique du glissement des tendons normaux et greffes. *Rev. Chir. Orthop.*, **52**, 13.

STACK, H. G. (1970) Tension in the lumbrical muscle. *The Hand*, **2**, 166.

STACK, H. G. & VAUGHAN-JACKSON, O. J. (1971) The zig-zag deformity in the rheumatiod hand. *The Hand*, **3**, 62.

SUNDERLAND, SIR S. (1968) *Nerves and Nerve Injuries*. Edinburgh: Livingstone.

TESTUT, L. (1884) *Les Anomalies Musculaires Chez l'Homme*. Paris: Masson.

VERDAN, C. (1960) Syndrome of the Quadriga. *Surg. Clin. North Amer.*, **40**, 425.

VERDAN, C. (1964) Practical considerations for primary and secondary repair in flexor tendon injuries. *Surg. Clin. North Amer.*, **44**, 951.

VERDAN, C. (1972) Half a century of flexor tendon surgery. *J. Bone and Joint Surg.*, **54A**, 472 491.

VERDAN, C. & POULENAS, I. (1975) Etude anatomique et fonctionnelle des tendons du grand palmaire et du long fléchisseur propre du pouce. *G.E.M. Communications Programme Montpellier*, **11**.

VON LANZ, T. & WACHSMUTH, W. (1959) *Praktische Anatomie*. Vol. 1/3, 2nd edn. Berlin: Springer.

WILKINSON, J. L. (1953) The insertion of the flexores pollicis longus et digitorum profundus. *J. Anat. (Lond.)*, **87**, 75–87.

WILSON, W. F. & HUESTON, J. T. (1973) The intratendinous architecture of the tendons of flexor digitorum profundus and flexor pollicis longus. *The Hand*, **5**, 33–38.

WINCKLER, G. (1969) Les lombricaux de la main. *Arch. Anat. Embriol.*, **52**, 381.

WINCKLER, G. (1970) Caractéres des vaisseaux para et péritendineux des fléchisseurs des doigts. *Bull. Assoc.* **148**, 581.

The great diversity of movement of fingers and of the hand can be reduced to a number of key phenomena.

In this paper, we will deal with the important role these key-motions play in the analysis of the extensor apparatus and of flexion and extension patterns. We shall thus cite, among others:

1. The coordination of interphalangeal movements (Landsmeer, 1955, 1958) easily observed both with extension and flexion of the digits.

2. The independence of the interphalangeal joints from the metacarpophalangeal (MP) ones and vice-versa.

3. The flexion of the proximal interphalangeal joint alone, leading to a loose distal phalanx.

4. The phenomenon whereby the flexor profundus can be trapped together with the sublimis.

ANATOMY OF THE EXTENSOR APPARATUS

PALMAR INTEROSSEI

They resemble each other quite closely as to the formation of their tendons. The palmar interosseus at the radial side of the ring finger is the simplest in structure: one tendon emerges from this muscle and fans out as the radial wing of the extensor assembly. There is only a small attachment of this muscle through the transverse lamina into the palmar pad of the joint. The two other palmar interossei, on both sides, are similar to each other and have a major tendinous insertion upon the wing of the assembly, while smaller tendinous fascicles reach on to the palmar pad and even into the base of the proximal phalanx.

DORSAL INTEROSSEI

These display a much more complicated internal disposition, due mainly to the formation of their tendons (Landsmeer, 1965, 1966). The first dorsal, though the most massive of them all, is comparatively simple in structure. One strong tendon emerges from this two-bellied muscle and inserts, in most cases, on to the base of the proximal phalanx. The deep portion of the muscle from the first metacarpal spirals around the main tendon, shaping the transverse proximal portion of the assembly. The radial wing of the extensor assembly of the index finger is thus somewhat underdeveloped, this being partially compensated for by a well-developed first lumbrical.

With the second and fourth dorsal interossei, the muscular

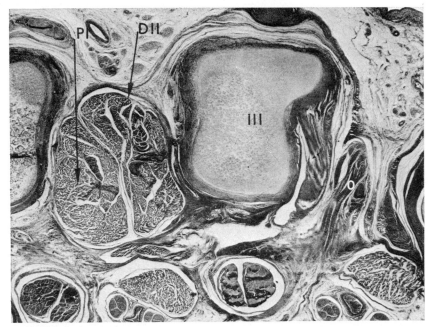

Figure 5.1
Transverse section across the head of the third metacarpal (III). On the right side, the tendinous complex of dorsal interosseus III is anchored into the interosseous metacarpal ligament. On the left, ten-dinous structures in dorsal interosseus II (DII) and in the palmar interosseus I (PI).

arrangement of the most dorsal two-bellied part leads to a pha-langeal tendon, while a more anterior portion originating from the homonymous metacarpal accounts for a strong, dorsally reinforced, wing-tendon.

The third dorsal interosseous differs from the others in that the tendon fascicles emerging from this muscle do not part into a phalangeal and a wing-tendon, but are unified, finally radiat-ing on to the wing of the assembly, and anchoring themselves into the transverse intermetacarpal ligament (Fig. 5.1).

Taking into account the position of the lumbrical muscles, it is obvious from the foregoing that both the lumbrical and the dorsal and palmar interossei aid in shaping the wings in a specific pattern according to each digit. The same can be said for their phalangeal insertions.

THE EXTENSOR ASSEMBLY (FIG. 5.2)

This basically consists of the interweaving of an extensor tendon with two wings. Over the dorsum of the proximal pha-lanx, the extensor assembly forms a hood ('dossière des inter-osseux', Montant and Baumann, 1937). The lateral borders of the hood converge slightly towards the dorso-lateral aspects of the PIP area, while its proximal portion, being transversely arranged, is continuous with the transverse lamina. The extensor tendon sends its lateral fibres on to the lateral borders of the assembly. The middle band of the assembly is thus rein-forced by the wing fibres from the interossei. The middle band runs over the trochlea of the first phalanx so as to insert on to the base of the middle phalanx.

The lateral bands bridge the PIP joint running on the dorso-lateral aspects of the trochlea of the proximal phalanx (Fig. 5.3) and gliding in two shallow grooves on both sides of the dorsal tubercle, at the base of the middle phalanx (Fig. 5.4).

Over the dorsum of the second phalanx the two bands inter-weave into a flat tendon, which is finally inserted into the dorsal

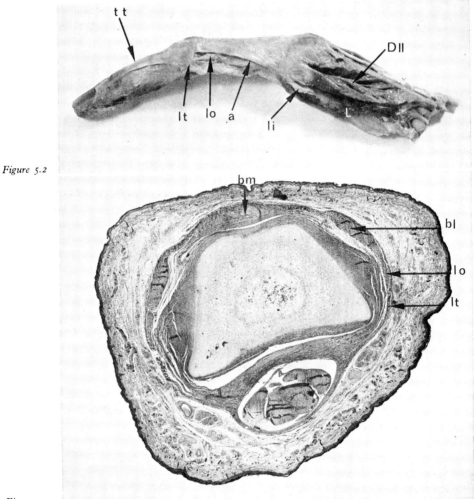

Figure 5.2

Figure 5.3

Figure 5.2 (*Top*)
Dissection of the extensor assembly. Radial aspect of the middle finger. L = lumbrical; l.i. = interosseous metacarpal ligament; DII = Dorsal Interosseus II; l.t. and l.o. = transverse ligament and oblique ligament of the retinacular ligament; a = lateral band; t.t. = terminal tendon.

Figure 5.3 (*Bottom*)
Transverse section across the trochlea of the first phalanx. Notice the position of the middle band (b.M.) and of two lateral bands (b.l.) and the retinacular ligament, wherein a transverse ligament (l.t.) and an oblique (l.o.) one are distinctly seen.

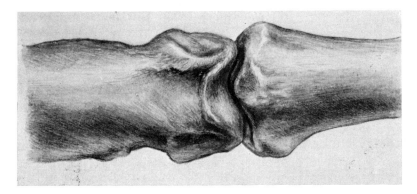

Figure 5.4
The bones of the PIP joint. Notice the shallow grooves on both sides of the base of the middle phalanx and their position with respect to the lateral aspect of the trochlea.

tubercle at the base of the terminal phalanx, whereas the middle band has its insertion on the dorsal tubercle of the middle phalanx.

THE RETINACULAR LIGAMENTS

The terminal portion of the extensor tendon is reinforced by the so called retinacular ligament: this can be looked upon as its volar reins. A careful dissection will demonstrate an oblique part, and a longitudinal bundle originating from the volar crest of the proximal phalanx that joins the terminal part of the tendon running just to the palmar side of the axis of flexion of the PIP joint (Fig. 5.2). This tiny cord is covered by a transverse, fascia-like layer that radiates from the terminal tendon and merges volarly into the flexor sheath.

A FUNCTIONAL ANALYSIS OF THE EXTENSOR MECHANISM

The anatomical disposition of the extensor assembly, and the flexor system as well, can be reduced even further (Fig. 5.5).

THE COORDINATION OF THE INTERPHALANGEAL MOTIONS

To assess the mechanism of the extensor assembly, we may start irrespectively from an extended or a flexed position of the finger, extended position being quite adequate to demonstrate the significance of the extensor apparatus for normal flexion of the interphalangeal joints. Flex the PIP joint, either by the superficialis or by external force. The middle phalanx by virtue of the middle band will pull the extensor assembly distally over the dorsum of the proximal phalanx, over a distance roughly equal to the product of angular rotation in radians and the distance held by the middle band to the centre of curvature of the PIP joint. The lateral bands will obtain a tolerance of the same magnitude, owing to the intercrossing of fibres, but since those bands run closer to the centre of curvature of the trochlea (Figs. 5.3 and 5.5), the lateral tendons use only a portion of the imparted tolerance to permit flexion of the PIP joint, so that the surplus can be used in no other way than to flex the DIP joint. The crucial point is that the lateral bands, in the given situation, cannot be put under tension by a proximal pull, either by the extensor or the interosseus. They will only be put under tension by a distal pull, and this can be accomplished only by flexing the terminal phalanx. If this phalanx is not taken into flexion, some slack remains in the lateral bands, a condition that accounts for the remarkable phenomenon of the *loose third phalanx*.

TRAPPING OF THE DEEP FLEXOR TENDON IN THE FORK OF THE SUPERFICIALIS

From a totally extended position of all fingers, if one finger is allowed to flex in the PIP joint only, the others being kept firmly extended in all their joints, the *loose third phalanx* of the flexed digit will easily be observed (Fig. 5.7A). This pha-

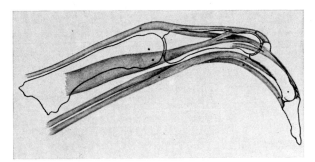

Figure 5.5.
Scheme of the extensor apparatus and flexor tendons of a digit. Draft taken from a radiography, where the different tendons have been surrounded with a copper wire.

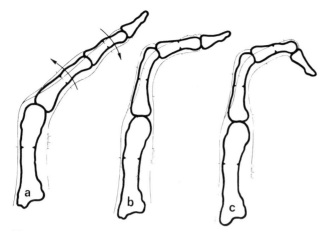

Figure 5.6
A scheme explaining the functioning of the extensor assembly. From (a) to (b) is shown flexion of the PIP joint, whose range is determined by the amount of extension of the MP joint. Note the distal gliding of the extensor assembly on the dorsum of the PIP, with consequent relaxation of both lateral bands. The DIP joint can then be flexed and the flexor tendon is pulled proximally. The arrows show the tendency to anteversion and retroversion of the phalanges.

lanx will be beyond control of both the flexor and the extensor whenever the flexor profundus is out of action (Fig. 5.6C). By flexing all fingers and then slowly extending all of them but one, one can see that in this latter finger the third phalanx will remain flexed (Fig. 5.7B). This remaining flexion of the DIP joint can be easily overcome by an outside force; its mechanism is explained only by the profundus tendon being trapped in the fork of the superficialis. These phenomena are inherent to the anatomy of the extensor assembly and to the well-known decussation of the flexor superficialis tendon.

PATTERN OF THE DIGITAL ARTICULATED CHAIN

THE INTERPHALANGEAL CHAIN

We have so far taken for granted that the middle and distal phalanges are constantly under control of the extensor assembly, provided the flexor profundus keeps its function. Although that may sound somewhat trivial, the question becomes immediately meaningful by considering some well-known malfunctions. To be more specific let us examine the '*swan-neck*' *deformity*.

In this situation the middle phalanx is fully out of control from the middle band of the extensor assembly. The lateral bands bowstring the hyperextended PIP joint and with increasing DIP joint flexion, the more slack will occur in the middle band. This deformity is further complicated by the locking of the PIP joint through the oblique retinacular ligaments, acting with flexion of the distal joint as dorsal reins to the PIP joint. This deformity demonstrates the effects of the relative distances held by tendons with respect to the centres of curvature of the concerned joints. As we have previously pointed out (Landsmeer, 1955, 1961a & b) the so-called articulated chain is an appropriated model to digital function. Briefly stated, *this chain consists of two joints* bridged by two bi-articular tendons. More details on this mechanism are provided by Thomas (1965), Crochetiere (1964) and Fisher (1969).

Such a system can be characterized by the distances the respective tendons run from the axes of the curvature, provided we omit the middle band of the extensor assembly. An articulated chain (Fig. 5.8) possesses some specific qualities: If *a, b, c, d* are the respective distances between tendons and the centres of curvature: if

$$\frac{a}{b} \gtreqless \frac{c}{d},$$

the system cannot be kept in equilibrium. It is quite logical that a proximal shift of the tendon imposed by its muscle can be arrested only by the other tendon of the system, the muscle of the other tendon opposing itself to lengthening. In this condition, the two muscles will increase their tensions in a mutual sense and therefore we term this condition '*reciprocal loading*'. A static equilibrium is thus achieved.

It is an exclusive quality of an articulated chain that a proximal pull of one of the tendons can be made while the other keeps its length. This accounts for the so-called *collapse* or

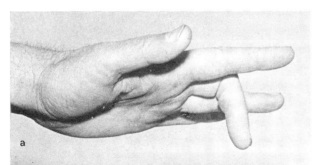

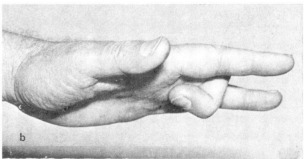

Figure 5.7
The phenomenon of the 'loose third phalanx'. (a) The medius is flexed, while the other fingers keep in extension. The extensor assembly has no more control upon the distal phalanx, which is under the sole action by the flexor profundus. (b) All fingers are flexed, then extended but the middle one. The flexor profundus is then kept trapped in the fork of the superficialis and the DIP joint remains in flexion. The situation (a) can be restored passively.

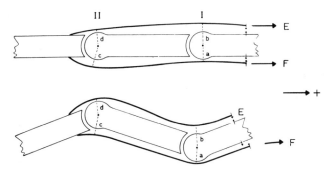

Figure 5.8
Collapse of the digital articulated chain. The muscle pulling the tendon E is in a condition of isometric contraction. When a pull is exerted on the tendon F, a zig-zag will be brought about according to the scheme shown, since

$$\frac{b}{a} > \frac{d}{c}$$ (inequality, unbalance).

zig-zag of the system. The direction of the zig-zag is determined by the inequality:

$$\frac{a}{b} \gtrless \frac{c}{d}.$$

If

$$\frac{a}{b} < \frac{c}{d}$$

(Fig. 5.8), flexion of the DIP joint and extension of the PIP one, will lead, according to the ratio

$$\frac{a}{b} : \frac{c}{d}$$

to a proximal displacement of one of the tendons, while the other keeps its length.

This motion in the system will be arrested at the very moment that, in one of the joints, the *functional end-position* is attained, because a mono-axial joint has always two *anatomical end-positions*, generally termed extension and flexion. As part of an articulated chain, under the conditions described above, for each of the two joints involved only *one* functional end-position exists. The two end-positions flexion and extension of the two joints are always opposite (Fig. 5.8).

As soon as one of the joints has reached its end-position, the other joint can be moved at will, and when this second joint happens to be in its end-position (functional), the first one is free to move again. This is termed the *alternating* or *marginal* pattern.

As a result of the fact that the relative flexion arc in the PIP joint is relatively (in relation to the extension arc) larger than the flexion arc in the DIP joint, the middle phalanx is subjected to a rotation within the chain (Fig. 5.6A). This can be termed *anteversion*, and is just a different formula for the 'zig-zag of the system'. The intercalated bone, namely the middle phalanx, is regularly arrested in this anteversion by the middle slip. The middle slip is responsible for any resistance to collapse

and is regularly loaded with tension. Both middle and distal phalanges, are suspended by offshoots from the extensor assembly. The respective positions of the middle slip and of the lateral bands on the trochlea of the proximal phalanx ensure a coordinated pattern of movement whereby useful flexion and extension of these phalanges can take place.

Rupture or division of the middle slip will disturb the co-ordinated pattern and enhance the anteversion tendency of the middle phalanx. In fact, the button-hole deformity without volar displacement of the lateral bands is evidence for the anteversion tendency of the middle phalanx.

THE MP AND PIP BIARTICULAR CHAIN

This system represents a bimuscular and biarticular chain. As soon as we remove the influence of the intrinsic muscles from this system its motion pattern is strictly of the *alternating* or the *marginal* type. The inequality

$$\frac{a}{b} < \frac{c}{d}$$

(Fig. 5.6A) prescribes a retroversion of the proximal phalanx, with hyperextension of the MP joint and flexion of the PIP joint as functional end-positions.

Whereas the tendency to the zig-zag or collapse of the distal or IP part of the chain can occur only as a result of a traumatic disturbance, in the proximal part of the chain (MP) the collapse and marginal movements can be produced voluntarily.

ELECTROMYOGRAPHICAL STUDY

Long and Brown (1964) have given ample electromyographical evidence that both the collapse of the system (extension of the MP joint and flexion of the PIP joint) and the alternating motions such as curling and decurling of the fingers are characterized by typical extrinsic EMG patterns and a silence of the intrinsics. On the contrary, a bimuscular system is required to maintain MP extension with interphalangeal joint extension. Interossei and lumbricals may be considered as antagonists of the extrinsics. All motions in the chain are feasible by regulation of the length of the three components involved, the two joints being able to move independently from each other.

THE IMPORTANCE OF THE LUMBRICALS

Backhouse and Catton (1954) were able to demonstrate through intramuscular electrodes that interphalangeal extension, no matter what the position of the MP joint, invariably yielded activity of the lumbricals. This was later confirmed by Long and Brown (1964). Landsmeer and Long (1965) distinguished four classes of free unresisted motions, namely opening, closing, clawing, and reciprocal motions. Each class consists of various components, but is strictly characterized by its own EMG pattern of activities.

1. Closing of the hand, in a natural and unconstrained manner requires primarily the activity of the flexor profundus. But in six out of 10 people tested the extensor showed an activity level of three (scale 0–4).

2. The curling of a finger, which is a much more constrained flexion (flexion of the IP joints, while the MP joint is held extended), required a much higher activity of the extensor. Three out of nine people tested demonstrated a score of three (scale 0–4) and six out of nine tested level four (scale 0–4) extensor activity (Long and Brown, 1967).

All these exercises were executed with the palm down, so that gravity had to be resisted by the extensors.

Recognition of the fact that motions of the marginal or alternating type are much more constraining than non-marginal flexion motions is all important, because it seems to be in contradiction to the behaviour of the model system, where the marginal motions required just two muscles, while the three independent motions required intervention of three muscles, two extrinsic and one oblique. We must conclude that counter-clawing factors are built into the normal finger, which are naturally conditioned towards unconstrained motion. The lumbricals play such a role, both actively and passively and their function derives from their exclusive position, coupling the extensor to the flexor (Crochetiere, 1964; Thomas, 1965; Thomas *et al.*, 1968). It is apparent that interphalangeal flexion requires considerable lengthening of the lumbrical. This passive break of lumbrical activity will favour MP flexion in flexor profundus contraction. In the same way, contraction of the lumbrical will release the distal portion of the profundus feeding its traction on to the extensor. So, lumbrical activity results in instantaneous interphalangeal extension and the action of the extensor and the lumbrical combined, represents an extremely efficient mechanism towards opening of the hand.

THE NORMAL CLAWING (MULDER AND LANDSMEER, 1968)

With maximal metacarpophalangeal hyperextension full IP extension may be inhibited. This phenomenon can be attributed to the transverse laminae which limit the proximal shift of the extensors. Full use of this hyperextension can be made only by interphalangeal flexion. In turn, interphalangeal extension can only be achieved by limiting full metacarpophalangeal extension. MP hyperextension, through lumbrical activity, is limited by the amount of the proximal shift of the extensor.

The ability to demonstrate the clawing posture in a normal hand is a prerequisite for pathological clawing position, to result from intrinsic paralysis. In the latter case, in addition, clawing requires the absence or insufficiency of other counter-clawing mechanisms in the finger, among which the rich development of soft tissues must be cited. Therefore clawing as a pathological phenomenon might rather be expected in lean fingers.

HANDLING, GRIPPING AND GRASPING

The MP joints play a primary role in the positioning of the digits in handling and gripping. The obliquely running lateral ligaments permit abduction of these joints, imposing a rotation component upon this abduction (Landsmeer, 1955; Landsmeer and Ansingh, 1957). More specific positioning of fingers with respect to the palm are often required; in these mechanisms, both abduction and rotation are necessary and it is essential to assess the activity of each particular interosseus for the performance of the important postures or motions.

Precise investigations on interosseus and in general intrinsic behaviour took place recently in Highland View Hospital, Cleveland, Ohio. If we want to use pronation and supination in the handling of a tool, it is quite advantageous to use a tool with a cylindrical handle, representing, as it were, the lengthened part of the fore-arm. This cylindrical grip, with the fourth and fifth fingers flexed and rotated toward the thenar mass is the pattern of choice and screwdriving is the classical

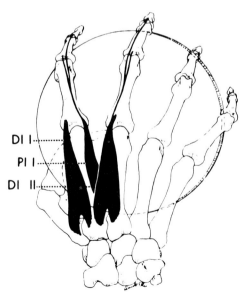 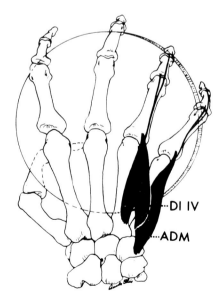

Figure 5.9
Activity of the intrinsic muscles in the 'power grip'. On the left, with the rotation counter-clockwise. On the right, with the rotation 'clock-wise'. (See E. A. Hall, 1968—reproduced with permission from the author.)

example. Elizabeth Hall (1968) recorded electromyographically the interosseus activity during screwdriving and turning a disc against a larger or smaller load (Fig. 5.9). In clockwise motion (for the right hand), dorsal interosseus IV and the abductor digiti V were extremely active, while in counterclockwise turning, both dorsal I and II dominated the EMG picture.

Susan Meibuhr (1969) investigated the role played by the intrinsics of index and thumb in eight types of precision handling, in which the medius was also involved. On each of these exercises two phases were recorded, the handling phase, and the return phase in which the fingers are released from the object, so as to regain the starting position. The following types of pinch were tested, both as two-jaws and as three-jaw-grip or pinch:

1. Tip-to-tip and pad-to-pad rotation
2. Pad-to-side rotation
3. Translation away from or toward the palm
4. Tip-to-tip and pad-to-pad pinch
5. Pad-to-side pinch.

All rotations were carried out in a clockwise and counter-clockwise motion with EMG recordings of both the handling and return-phase. Only some of the most salient points will be mentioned here. As for rotations, there seems to be great resemblance in the EMG pattern, no matter whether the rotation is being performed with the hand loaded or unloaded. There is however a marked difference between the handling and the return-phase in each motion. In the right hand, clockwise rotation (handling-phase) requires only intrinsic activity of palmar I. This muscle quits in the return-phase and keeps silent in a handling-phase with counter-clockwise rotation, however, in the handling-phase with counter-clockwise rotation all other intrinsics, dorsal I, lumbrical I, opponens pollicis, abductor pollicis and flexor pollicis brevis show activity.

Continuing a clockwise pad-to-pad rotation into a pad-to-side rotation during the handling-phase, next to palmar I, dorsal I, lumbrical I and adductor pollicis are also brought into the picture. This pattern seems somewhat inhibited when the same motion is performed as return-phase of counter-clockwise pad-to-side handling rotation.

The handling-phase of counter-clockwise pad-to-side motion requires activity of the opponens, the abductor pollicis brevis and of the flexor pollicis brevis ('thenar triad') while the index intrinsics completely drop out.

It may be useful to combine into one continuous motion both the clockwise and counter-clockwise movements, pad-to-pad and pad-to-side, executed as handling-phases without dropping the tool. We can thus observe:

Clockwise
Tip-to-tip } palmar I (dorsal I)
Pad-to-pad }

Pad-to-side   dorsal I, palmar I, lumbrical I, (flexor pollicis brevis) and adductor pollicis

Counter-clockwise (handling)
Pad-to-side   (opponens), abductor pollicis brevis and flexor pollicis brevis

Pad-to-pad } dorsal I, lumbrical I, opponens, abductor
tip-to-tip } pollicis brevis and flexor pollicis brevis.

When we consider the motion of index and thumb toward the palm, there is a marked difference in the activity of the intrinsics, whether the motion is a free return-phase or a handling-phase, executed against a resisting spring. For example, the handling-phase requires cooperation by dorsal I, palmar I and the 'thenar triad' (the opponens, flexor brevis and abductor brevis); whereas, in the return phase, not one single intrinsic, neither of the index nor of the thumb is active.

It seems justified to interpret this remarkable result as the counterclawing effect of the intrinsics, in order to ensure secure contact with the object. The same was observed by maintaining the arch of the finger in tip-to-tip and pad-to-pad positions.

The intrinsic triad of the index (dorsal I, palmar I and lumbrical I) and the thenar triad as well, contribute both to maintaining the proper position of digits and to obtaining a good pinch effect. The arches are sustained by a specific counterclawing effect as soon as the fingers and thumb are handling a tool, and this explains the extremely disabling condition following an intrinsic paralysis (Mannerfelt, 1966). Clawing in the thumb and other clinical signs of ulnar nerve paralysis involving the thumb require further analysis.

Ebskov (1970) has recently dealt with the analysis of thumb movements by electromyography. A spatial goniometer of great technical refinement, called a hexatron, was used in order to precisely locate the thumb in its various positions with respect to hand (Ebskov and Boe, 1966). The data collected by EMG give a picture of the maximal activity of each muscle, according to location and function of this digit in its diverse motions.

To summarize, we have tried to comment upon some points of practical and theoretical importance to the function of fingers and the hand. We have stressed in particular the importance of the lumbricals for normal function, and of clawing and counterclawing tendencies in the fingers both in free motion and in acts of gripping and pinch.

REFERENCES

BACKHOUSE, K. M. & CATTON, W. T. (1954) An experimental study of the functions of the lumbrical muscles in the human hand. *J. Anat.*, **88**, 133–141.

CROCHETIERE, W. J. (1964) *A preliminary analysis of the dynamics of the human finger*. Thesis. Case Institute of Technology, Cleveland.

EBSKOV, B. (1970): *De motibus motoribusque pollicis humani*. Thesis. Copenhagen.

EBSKOV, B. & BOE, C. (1966) The hexatron, a new thumb goniometer. *Acta Orthop. Scand.*, **37**, 58.

HALL, E. A. (1968) *Electromyography of the intrinsic hand muscles in power grip*. Thesis. Case Western Reserve University, Cleveland.

LANDSMEER, J. M. F. (1955) Anatomical and functional investigations on the articulation of the human finger. *Acta Anat.*, 1–69. Suppl. 24 = 2 ad vol. XXV.

LANDSMEER, J. M. F. (1958) A report on the co-ordination of the interphalangeal joints of the human finger and its disturbances. *Acta Morphol. Neerl.-Scand.*, **2**, 59–84.

LANDSMEER, J. M. F. (1961a) Studies in the anatomy of articulation. I. The equilibrium of the 'intercalated' bone. *Acta Morphol. Neerl.-Scand.*, **3**, 287–303.

LANDSMEER, J. M. F. (1961b) Studies in the anatomy of articulation. II. Patterns of movement of bi-muscular, bi-articular systems. *Acta Morphol. Neerl.-Scand.*, **3**, 304–321.

LANDSMEER, J. M. F. (1965) Structural analysis of the fourth dorsal interosseus of the human hand. *Acta Anat.*, **62**, 176–214.

LANDSMEER, J. M. F. (1966) Analyse de la structure des interosseux dorsaux II et III. *Compt. Rend. Ass. Anat.*, **132**, 590–595.

LANDSMEER, J. M. F. & ANSINGH, H. R. (1957) X-ray observations on rotation of the fingers in the metacarpo-phalangeal joints. *Acta Anat.*, **30**, 404–410.

LONG, C. & BROWN, M. E. (1964) Electromyographic kinesiology of the hand: muscles moving the long finger. *J. Bone and Joint Surgery*, **46**, 1683–1706.

LANDSMEER, J. M. F. & LONG, C. (1965) The mechanism of finger control, based on electromyograms and location analysis. *Acta Anat.*, **61**, 330–347.

MANNERFELT, L. (1966) Studies on the hand in ulnar nerve paralysis. A clinical-experimental investigation in normal and anomalous innervation. *Acta Orthop. Scand. Suppl.* **87.**

MEIBUHR, S. L. (1969) *Electromyography of intrinsic muscles of the hand during precision handling*. Thesis. Case Western Reserve University, Cleveland.

MONTANT, R., & BAUMANN, A.: (1937) Recherches anatomiques sur le système tendineux extenseur des doigts et de la main. *Ann. Anat. & Path.* **14.**

MULDER, J. D. & LANDSMEER, J. M. F. (1968) The mechanism of claw finger. *J. Bone and Joint Surgery*, **30B**, 3, 664–668.

THOMAS, D. H. (1965) *The physical properties of the human finger*. Thesis. Case Institute of Technology, Cleveland.

THOMAS, D. H., LONG, C. & LANDSMEER, J. M. F. (1968) Biomechanical considerations of lumbricalis behaviour in the human finger. *J. Biomechanics*, **1**, 107–115.

EXPERIMENTAL SURGERY AND TENDON HEALING

6. Tendon Healing: A Continuing Experimental Approach

W. K. Lindsay

With injuries to different tendons we have come to expect different results. Extensor tendon injuries, with proper care, give good to excellent results in 90 per cent of cases. Injuries to the long straight flexor tendons give similar results. However, injuries to the flexor tendons in the digital fibrous sheath region, or 'No man's land', where the tendons work over pulleys and have to glide free for long distances give good results in only 60 per cent of cases and rarely give a normal result. This does not matter whether direct suture techniques are used, or, free tendon grafts are used. To improve these results is one of the great challenges left for modern reconstructive surgery.

There has been little opportunity to study the pathophysiology of human tendon healing because of the waiting period before secondary procedures are undertaken. Consequently, it has been necessary to turn to animal experimentation. To a large extent, we have used the chicken (Fig. 6.1) as the standard laboratory preparation to investigate the various parameters of tendon healing. As well as being anatomically similar, it also offers an opportunity for in vivo appraisal of the functional result which is most important in this type of work. Hopefully, through detailed and controlled experimental study, factors can be elaborated that will lead to a better understanding of the problems and ultimately to a more adequate human clinical functional return.

Our initial work dealt with the role of the individual components of the tendon mechanism (Lindsay and Thompson, 1960). With elevation of the skin flap alone (Fig. 6.2), or combined with the excision of the synovial sheath and the fibrous tunnel, chicken profundus tendon action is unaffected. When the sheath is excised, it regenerates with amazing rapidity and completeness. It was not possible to demonstrate a difference in tendon healing, adhesion formation, or clinical function when the sheath was excised. Therefore, it is unlikely that sheath excision is a worthwhile addition to the flexor tendon repair.

Excising the sublimis tendon from otherwise normal chicken feet, produces a clinical picture much as in humans. In some cases, you cannot detect its absence. In others, the proximal

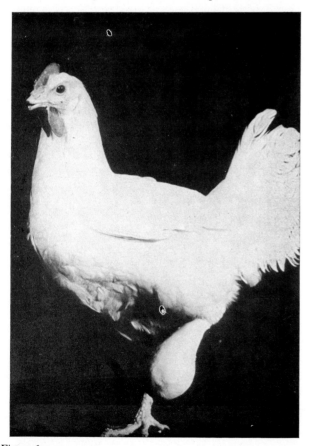

Figure 6.1
The chicken experimental model.

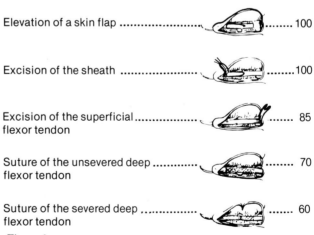

Experimental technique	% of function
Elevation of a skin flap	100
Excision of the sheath	100
Excision of the superficial flexor tendon	85
Suture of the unsevered deep flexor tendon	70
Suture of the severed deep flexor tendon	60

Figure 6.2
Controlled experimental surgical interference of increasing severity. Five types of experimental technique of growing importance have been undertaken. The percentage of functional recovery is in inverse proportion to the importance of the surgical lesion.

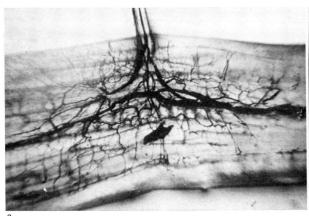
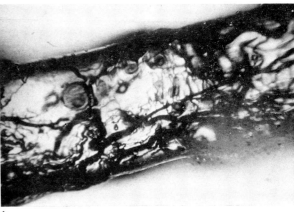

a   b

Figure 6.3
(a) Normal flexor tendon blood supply

interphalangeal joint is held in some extension with the digit at rest. Excision of the sublimis tendon reduces the overall functional return to 85 per cent (Fig. 6.2).

Various grades of trauma to the profundus tendon itself produce a closely related amount of reaction with subsequent adhesion formation with loss of function. If a Bunnell-type suture is put through the intact profundus tendon and all other parameters are held constant, the functional result is reduced to 70 per cent. If the profundus tendon is first divided and then sutured, the functional return is reduced to 60 per cent. Thus, the functional result would seem to be inversely proportional to increasing increments of trauma above a baseline level. Mild trauma, consistent with standard plastic surgical technique, does not affect the clinical result. More severe trauma, above this baseline level, proportionately impairs function (Lindsay and McDougall, unpublished data). There is a place for atraumatic surgery, but atraumatic surgery alone is not the whole answer.

The blood supply of the flexor tendons has been the subject of considerable interest. Our study using liquid silicone rubber injection techniques confirms the four generally accepted major sources as being at the osseotendinous junction, the vincula brevi, the vinculum longum (Fig. 6.3A) and, at a proximal level *outside* the sheath from the surrounding paratenon. Generally, the more central vessels are straight and parallel to each other while at the periphery, superficial vessels show an arcuate and intracommunicating formation. Between these major sources of blood supply are zones of apparent avascularity.

Chicken experimentation has shown that occlusion of each of these sources is followed by a loss of the normal vascular pattern and replacement by abundant but haphazard arrangement of small vessels which seem to supply a similar area to that supplied by the normal vasculature (Fig. 6.3B). In trauma experiments, revascularization is mediated by adhesions from the surrounding tissues. The new vessels were generally arranged in a haphazard manner with frequent cross-communications. Fat interposition predisposed to a more abundant revascularization, with a large calibre of vessels. Revascularization in traumatized areas remains a major problem in flexor

(b) Flexor tendon blood supply after injury or tendon suture.

tendon surgery (Lindsay and Freiberg, unpublished data).

Considerable time has been spent in our laboratory delineating the source and role of the fibroblast in tendon healing. Histological appraisal (Fig. 6.4) shows the tendon to be composed of the peritendinous tissue—a slippery layer of transparent areolar-like tissue closely applied to the epitenon. This represents a 1–3 cell fibroblast layer on the surface of most tendons. The endotenon is the structure dividing tendons into bundles or fasciculae and carrying blood vessels. It is composed of loose relatively acellular collagen. The tendon bundles are collections of longitudinally aligned cells and collagenic material.

In our original histological studies, fibroblastic proliferations and contribution to the healing response seemed to follow a set pattern. Immediately after trauma, an inflammatory cell exudate accumulates in the perisheath tissue and the gap zone, accompanied by a specific fibroblastic proliferation. In 48 hours, the epitenal cells proliferate vigorously and contributed to the healing process. Subsequently, in an additional two days, the endotenal cells and then finally the tendon cells themselves,

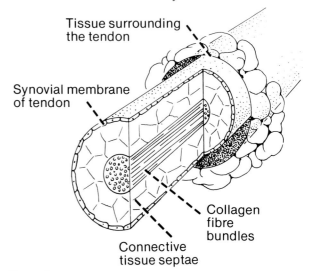

Figure 6.4
Intrinsic tendon anatomy.

took part in this proliferative reaction (Lindsay and Thomson, 1960). As in any histological study, the observations are valid only for a given instant of time and extrapolative interpretation must be used to determine whether or not cells in a proliferating tissue are increasingly *in situ*, or whether the observed increase is due to the migration of extraneous cells.

To resolve this controversy, we used thymidine, a DNA 1 c precursor labelled with a radioactive isotope (Lindsay and Birch, 1964). For approximately one hour post-injection those cells engaged in DNA synthesis became labelled and by an autoradiographic technique, their location can be detected. This study showed that with injection and sacrifice on day 1 postoperatively, the fibroblasts in the peritendonous tissue became labelled showing that at this time these were the most rapidly dividing cells. Injection and sacrifice on day 12, showed the label present in fibroblasts of the gap, adhesive and tendonous tissues with a marked decrease of label of the peritendonous tissue. To trace any migration of cells, we injected on day 1 knowing that this would label the fibroblasts of the peritendonous tissue and sacrifice the specimen on day 12 to locate these original fibroblasts or their descendants (Fig. 6.5). Again, the labelled cells were located almost completely in the gap zone, tendon proper and adhesions with little or no activity in the peritendonous tissue. It is apparent that this work supports the theory that tendon healing is mitigated

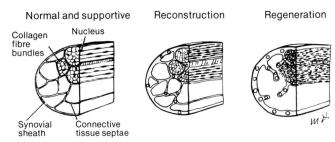

Figure 6.6
Three types of tendon healing reaction seen with light microscopy.

through fibroblasts originating in the peritendonous tissue. Also, any impervious interposition substance would block this migration and consequently interfere with primary tendon healing.

Again, radioactive isotopes subtantiated this histological picture. The problem was approached from two opposing points of view. Using radioactive proline, an amino acid found almost exclusively in collagen, the rate and extent of incorporation into traumatized tendon was measured. The uptake (Fig. 6.7) was directly proportioned to the amount of trauma, being maximal in the zone of severe trauma and the junction-gap

As the healing response is studied the investigation undoubtedly approaches the question of the autografts, as to its function in terms of being a living transplant and supplementing the healing response, or being merely a strut through which living tissue can migrate. Histological studies allowed us to clarify the overall response by separating it into three merging processes (Lindsay and McDougall, 1960). Firstly, in areas of severe trauma such as occur at the zone of suture or the zone of approximation of the cut ends, there is complete replacement of old lysed tendon elements by new fibres. We term this 'regeneration'. Secondly, in areas of moderate trauma somewhat removed from the zone of suture or the cut ends of the tendon, repair is mediated through new fibroblasts producing new collagen, but the whole process is not nearly as voluminous. We term this, 'reconstitution'. Lastly, in areas removed from the zone of injury, fibroblasts already in the area contribute largely to the healing response. We term this 'maintenance' (Fig. 6.6).

UPTAKE OF THYMIDINE

inject on day 1   sacrifice on day 1

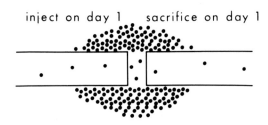

inject on day 12   sacrifice on day 12

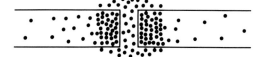

inject on day 1   sacrifice on day 12

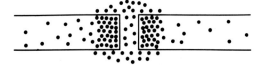

Figure 6.5
Tracing the migrating fibroblast during tendon healing. Dividing fibroblasts are labelled with thymidine.

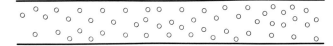

NORMAL

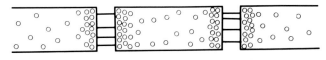

GRAFT

Figure 6.7
The uptake of tritiated proline in normal tendon and in a tendon graft preparation.

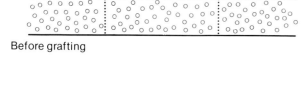

Before grafting

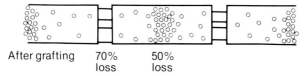

After grafting   70%   50%
                  loss   loss

Figure 6.8
The loss of tritiated proline from a normal labelled tendon subsequently used as a free tendon autograft.

zone with minimal uptake in the central area of the graft. Also, we labelled the collagen prior to autogenous graft replacement and recorded the disappearance of isotope in the graft segment (Fig. 6.8). This showed that 70 per cent of the labelled collagen was lost at the graft ends and 50 per cent in the central portion. Therefore, 30 to 50 per cent of the original collagen remained or was re-utilized in the healed tendon.

A repetitive complication in tendon surgery is the occurrence of a gap at the suture line (Lindsay, Thomson and Walker, 1960). Our work implies that this is the cause of poor clinical results, which is probably impossible to recognize at any secondary procedure after three months. Gap formation is associated with increased callus size, increased adhesion formation, and disoriented fibroblastic proliferation (Fig. 6.9). A major causative factor is proximal muscle pull. To alleviate this, division of the tendon at a more proximal level, with secondary suture after the flexor mechanism has healed was proposed. This was carried out, and in addition, radioactive proline was used to detect any change in collagen synthesis. The corporation of new collagen decreased and adhesion formation was lessened (Douglas, Jackson and Lindsay, 1967). However, later suture at the site of relaxing incisions compounds the

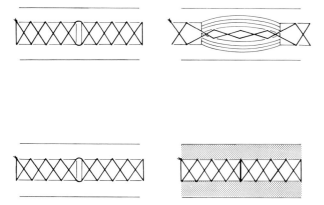

Figure 6.9
To illustrate the gap (top right) which commonly occurs when a tendon is sutured (top left). To illustrate the adhesion problem (bottom right) occurring about a sutured tendon (bottom left).

problem. Adequate external immobilization appears to be the best answer.

Adhesions are the nemesis of flexor tendon surgery (Fig. 6.9). Their devious behaviour assists in the healing response, and revascularization, but immobilizes the tendon preventing a satisfactory functional return. Various biochemical agents including antihistamines (Walker, Bensley and Lindsay, 1967), anabolic agents and steroids, have been investigated in an attempt to modify the adhesive response in order to retain this beneficial aspect, while decreasing its adverse reaction. Presently, much attention has been focused on the lathrogenic drug, beta-aminopropryonitril (BAPN) (Herzog, Lindsay and McCain, 1970). Other investigators have shown a reduction of 50 per cent of work necessary to flex a digit after a tendon repair with a secondary tenolysis and administration of BAPN. In our series, the ultimate functional return was not significantly different from the controls, although several untoward effects were noted, including a marked increase in spontaneous rupture and bony changes.

Another attempt at control of adhesions has been the use of interposition substances. Any attempt to use homologous or autogenous tissue resulted in dense adhesion formation. The synthetic interposition substances were generally disappointing with an increased incidence of gap formation and spontaneous rupture. Of note, are the facts that polyethylene gave rise to a new sheath formation while silastic evoked little tissue foreign body reaction. In this case, the function was impaired because of growth of adhesions around the end of the silastic. Since vascular and cellular infiltration are integral parts of primary tendon healing, it is unlikely that impervious interposition substances will be of much value. (Table 6.1.)

It is unfortunately apparent, that the ultimate solution has not yet been achieved. With this in mind, an investigation of the more basic biochemical components of tendons has been undertaken, in order to delineate the various roles in the healing response. Tendon is composed of a few cells, the fibroblasts, and the extracellular material—collagen, elastin and reticulum, embedded in an amorphous material ground substance which contains mucopolysaccharides. The strength of collagen is dependent not only on its own crosslinkage, but also upon the surrounding environment, the most important part of which is mucopolysaccharides.

Our studies using both isotope incorporation and quantitative biochemical analysis show that in a healing tendon, collagen deposition commences about the fourth day while mucopolysaccharide concentration peaks at about four to eight days, then declines. Thereafter, both substances gradually accumulate in the healing area and reach a peak at about 21 days. Subsequently, they both gradually decline. The amount of new collagen deposition is directly related to the amount of trauma being greatest in the most traumatized area. However, in a completely healed tendon, the total amount of collagen present is not equal to the total amount in a normal tendon at the same area. Also, the collagen and mucopolysaccharide deposition in adhesive tissue closely parallels that of healing tendon. Unfortunately no selective difference could be determined to dif-

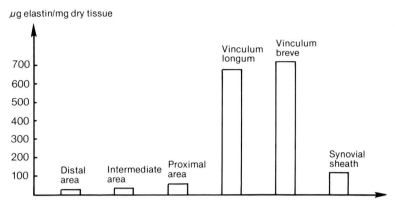

Figure 6.10
The content of elastin material in various regions of the tendon mechanism.

ferentiate the adhesive tissue from the tendon (Douglas *et al.*, 1967; Lindsay *et al.*, 1964; Tustanoff *et al.*, 1965; Munro *et al.*, 1970).

A constituent that to the present time has attracted little attention in tendon healing studies, is elastin (Fig. 6.10). Desmosine and isodesmosine, which are specific for elastin, were estimated by fluorescent techniques and these levels used as the relative values in our tendon study. Normal tendon itself contains a minimal amount of elastin material (4 to 6 per cent) whereas the vinculii contain up to 70 per cent and the pulley-sheath region contains up to 20 per cent. Operated or traumatized tendon showed increased elastin material content most marked and sustained in the zone of the greatest trauma. Ad-

hesions contained 45 per cent elastin (Lindsay, McCain, Hurst *et al.*, unpublished data). Hopefully, a selective difference will be found to explain the restrictive action of some adhesions while other equally voluminous ones allow adequate glide.

One of the most aggravating aspects of flexor tendon reconstruction is the wide individual variation of functional return when as many variables as possible are held constant. This as yet unexplained individual variation leads to a superb result in one case, and a completely unsatisfactory result in what seems to be a comparable case. Perhaps with more accurate knowledge of the basic biochemical alterations in a healing wound, we will be able to modify this response in order to gain a more beneficial clinical result.

TABLE 6.1   Interposition substances tested to decrease adhesion formation

	Function	Adhesions	Gap	Spontaneous rupture
1. Homologous vein	0	Dense	+2	Increased
2. Homologous artery	0	Dense	+2	Increased
3. Autologous vein	Poor	Dense	+2	Increased
4. Polyethylene	Poor	Formation of a new sheath	+3	Increased
5. Teflon	Poor	Dense	+3	Increased
6. Silastic	Poor	At the margin	+2	Increased

REFERENCES

DOUGLAS, L. G., JACKSON, E. R. & LINDSAY, W. K. (1967) The effects of Dexamethasone, Norethandrolone, Promethazine and tension relieving procedure on Collagen synthesis in healing flexor tendons as estimated by tritiated proline uptake studies. *Can. J. of Surg.* **10**, 36–46.

HERZOG, M., LINDSAY, W. K. & McCAIN, W. G. (1970) Effects of Beta-aminoproprionitrile on adhesions following digital flexor repair in chickens. *Surgical Forum*, **21**, 509–511.

LINDSAY, W. K. & BIRCH, J. R. (1964) The fibroblast in flexor tendon healing. *Plast. & Reconst. Surg.*, **34**, 223–232.

LINDSAY, W. K. & FREIBERG, A. Unpublished data.

LINDSAY, W. K. & McDOUGALL, E. P. Unpublished data.

LINDSAY, W. K. & McDOUGALL, E. P. (1960) Direct digital flexor tendon repair. *Plast. & Reconst. Surg.*, **26**, 613–621.

LINDSAY, W. K. & THOMSON, H. G. (1960) Digital flexor tendons: An experimental study. Part I. The significance of each component of the flexor mechanism in tendon healing. *Brit. J. Plast. Surg.*, **12**, 289–316.

LINDSAY, W. K., McCAIN, G., HURST, L. N., *et al.* Unpublished data.

LINDSAY, W. K., THOMSON, H. G. & WALKER, F. G. (1960) Digital flexor tendons: An experimental study. Part II. The significance of a gap occurring at the line of suture. *Brit. J. Plast. Surg.*, **13**, 1–9.

LINDSAY, W. K., TUSTANOFF, E. R. & BIRDSELL, D. C. (1964) The uptake of Tritiated Proline in tendon healing. Surgical Forum Proceedings. *Am. Coll. of Surg.*, 459.

MUNRO I. R., LINDSAY, W. K. & JACKSON, S. H. (1970) A synchronous study of Collagen & Mucopolysaccharide in healing flexor tendons of chickens. *Plast. & Reconst. Surg.*, **45**, 493–501.

TUSTANOFF, E. R., BIRDSELL, D. C. & LINDSAY, W. K. (1965) In vivo incorporation of Proline—H_3 and its subsequent hydroxylation during Collagen synthesis in regenerating tendon. *Proc. Can. Fed. Biol. Soc.*, **8**, 54.

WALKER, F. G., BENSLEY, S. H. & LINDSAY, W. K. (1961) The effects of an Antihistamine (Promethazine) on the reaction of tendons to trauma—a histological study. *Can. J. Biochem. Physio.*, **39**, 89–101.

7. The Healing Process in Wounds of the Digital Flexor Tendons and Tendon Grafts. An Experimental Study.

A. D. Potenza

The repair of flexor tendons in the fingers remains one of the most complex problems in hand surgery, for here the tendons are surrounded by synovial sheaths and are opposed to the metacarpals and phalanges by circular ligaments called pulleys. Following trauma and surgical repair, the two sliding surfaces of this complex system can adhere, and consequently impede the free play of the system.

In order to better understand the vagaries of flexor tendon surgery, since 1959 the author has undertaken a detailed study of the healing of flexor tendons.

At present, disagreement still persists on the exact nature of the healing process. Some authors think that the tendon heals by cellular regeneration arising from the two ends of the cut tendon, whilst others (Adams, 1860; Skoog & Persson, 1954; Hank, 1924; Narvi, 1924) state that the tendon heals only due to the cellular activity of the peritendon tissues. Others (Mason & Shearon, 1932; Mason & Allen, 1941; Flynn & Graham, 1962) believe that the two processes play an equally important role.

As for the behaviour of tendon grafts, the polemic is equally lively. Some researchers (Skoog & Persson, 1954; Flynn & Graham, 1962) state that auto-grafts are subject to degeneration and gradual replacement. Others (Mason & Shearon, 1932; Bunnell, 1955; Lindsay & McDougall, 1961) believe that these transplanted tendons can survive in entirety within their new bed.

In order to make progress in the surgery of the flexor tendons in the hand, it is essential to study the healing of tendons and of tendon grafts in a biological context comparable to that of the human finger.

The dog has been chosen in which to study this healing process because of the anatomical similarity between the two digital flexor systems. In fact, in the dog forefoot one finds a flexor mechanism comparable to that of the human hand (Fig. 7.1). Each digit possesses a superficial flexor tendon and a deep flexor tendon both encased within the synovial sheath extending from the metacarpal phalangeal joint to the insertion of the deep flexor tendon at the base of the distal phalanx. These two tendons run into a rigid osteofibrous tunnel at the MP articulation. Within the digital sheath the superficial flexor tendon divides—as in the hand—into two divisions which completely encircle the deep flexor, before becoming inserted into the base of the middle phalanx. These two divisions are lined with a synovial membrane joined to the synovium of the fibrous sheath by vincula comparable to those of the human finger. A short, triangular vinculum joins the dorsal aspect of the deep flexor to the synovial membrane which covers the distal phalanx at the insertion of the tendon. At the proximal end of the digital sheath the synovium is reflected off the superficial and deep flexors in a single membranous fold. The skin, the subcutaneous cell tissue and the neurovascular pedicles of the dog's paw are comparable to those of the human finger.

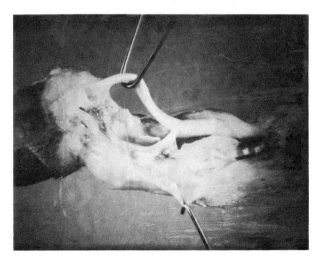

Figure 7.1

HEALING OF THE DEEP FLEXOR TENDON IN THE DIGITAL SHEATH

In this series of experiments we have tried to define in a precise manner the healing process of the deep flexor tendons within the sheaths. The greatest possible number of variables were eliminated by using the least traumatic techniques and rigorously controlling the surgical conditions. In all the experiments the author himself carried out the tendon division and repairs. The methods and techniques described were used in all the experiments. Those experiments which required special techniques will be described separately.

Material and method. Adult dogs of both sexes, whose weight varied between 10 and 14.5 kg were anaesthetized using an intravenous injection of 32 mg of sodium penthobarbital per kg of body weight. After shaving, the paw and forefoot were cleansed for three minutes with Hexaclorophene. After the application of an Esmarch bandage the operation was carried out using a tourniquet. All the usual precautions of asepsis were applied at the time of each operation.

Operating technique. 70 deep flexor tendons were studied

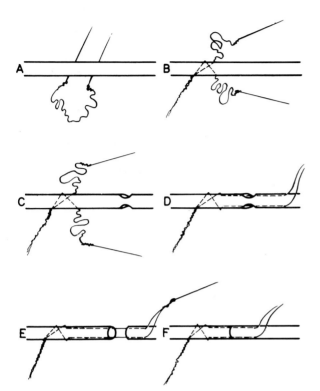

Figure 7.2

in 35 dogs, taking care not to damage the superficial tendons. Mid lateral incisions were used identical to those on the hand. The tendons of the second and fifth digits of each forefoot were preferentially selected. These tendons were dissected only with a scalpel and handled in the least traumatic way possible. They were never held by forceps or any other traumatising instrument.

After the tendons were cleanly cut they were brought into exact apposition, suturing the two ends with a stainless steel suture using a 'pull-out' technique (Fig. 7.2). During the operation the vincula were preserved. Finally both the sheath and the skin were sutured with No. 36 monofilament stainless steel suture. The paw was dressed with a sterile dressing and was then encased in a padded plaster, reinforced with a wire mesh. The plaster was used to immobilize the sutured tendon and to maintain the paw in a functional position. The sutures and the plaster were retained until the animal was sacrificed. In this series of experiments 35 dogs (each having two tendon sutures) were sacrificed at intervals between one and 128 days.

Preparation of tissues. Immediately before the animal was sacrificed, the tissue to be studied was excised under general anaesthetic and placed in a solution of 10 per cent formalin. From each of the specimens obtained within 12 days of the operation, the phalanges were amputated and fixed *en bloc*. The histological preparations were stained with hematoxylin and eosin with Wilders silver stain for the collagen fibres and Rheinehart's modification of Hale's colloidal iron stain.

MICROSCOPICAL OBSERVATIONS

Normal anatomy. Under normal conditions the functioning adult deep tendon within its sheath has no continuous synovial lining in contrast to the parietal synovial layer of the sheath. After cutting and repairing a deep flexor tendon within its sheath in the dog, granulation tissue can be seen arising directly from the parietal layer. This granulation tissue invades the interior of the tendon suture line. On or about the fourth or fifth day after operation the synovium encasing the sheath completely disappears in the vicinity of the tendon section. The progressive regeneration of this synovial membrane begins about the fourteenth day after operation and ends about the twenty-first day, except for some adhesions which persist at the suture line.

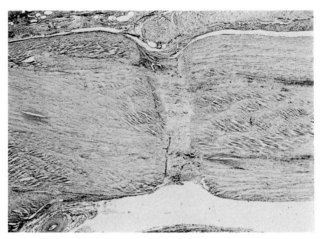

Figure 7.3

On the seventh day following operation fine collagen fibres appear in the granulation tissue around the tendon wound. Towards the tenth day, the fibroblasts and collagen tissues proliferating within the suture zone are lying in a plane perpendicular to the longitudinal axis of the tendon, whilst at the same time on the surface of the suture zone the cells as well as the collagen fibres lie in a direction parallel to the long axis of the tendon. Towards the twenty-first day after tendon section the collagen fibres and the cellular elements of the scar begin to align in a direction parallel to the longitudinal axis of the tendon. Towards the twenty-eighth day after operation this process is completed. All the fibroblasts and the young collagen fibres are oriented in the longitudinal axis of the tendon. It is not until after the ninetieth day that the collagen fibres group together in bundles. These groups increase in density to take on the appearance of a normal tendon towards the 112th day after operation. The adhesions at the tendon's suture line remain loose, thin and filmy (Fig. 7.3). The cells belonging to the tendon (tenocytes) remain inactive during the process of healing.

STUDY OF THE HEALING OF FLEXOR TENDONS INSIDE ARTIFICIAL SHEATHS

With the aim of preventing formation of adhesions of flexor tendons during healing, numerous surgeons have searched for an ideal, inert material, which could be placed between a ruptured or wounded tendon and its anatomical environment. Experimental as well as clinical techniques, have employed numerous metal, plastic or natural materials which have been introduced between the two sliding surfaces to prevent the formation of adhesions on the flexor tendons during healing. Nylon, cellophane, teflon, polythene, millipore, invalon, silastic, stainless steel, vitallium have been used, as well as a number of natural anatomical structures. Initial experiments with these materials were promising but alas experimental hypotheses have not been confirmed by clinical experience.

SURGERY OF TENDONS OF THE HAND

In order to place different materials between the synovial sheath and the tendon repair it was necessary to cut the superficial flexor tendon. Before introducing any material we studied the healing of the tendon after simple excision of the superficial flexor. Fifteen tendons were thus treated and studied over periods of between one and 56 days.

In this series of experiments, the deep flexor tendon healed at the same rate and in the same way, after excision of the superficial flexor tendon as when the superficial flexor tendon had been preserved. However the adhesions that formed about the suture zone were slightly denser than in the preceding experiments.

HEALING OF THE DEEP FLEXOR TENDON INSIDE POLYTHENE TUBES

After total excision of the superficial tendon and cutting the deep one, a polythene tube 2 cm long was drawn over the two ends of the tendon before carrying out the Bunnell suture technique using monofilament stainless steel. The tube was then slid along the tendon and centred over the stitch line. The digital sheath and the skin were sutured and the postoperative management were identical to that used in the experiment de-

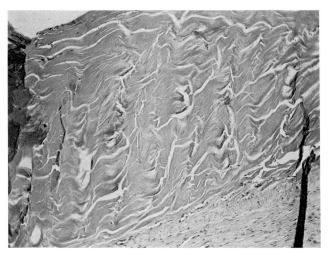

Figure 7.5

scribed above. Fifteen tendons were excised and studied at intervals varying between six and 56 days.

The polythene tube was found intact in all the animals but with adhesions at each end. There was an aseptic necrosis of the tendon within the tube in one animal sacrificed on the thirty-second day. The tube was filled with an amorphous gelatinous substance in which the 'pull-out' type of suture was found to be intact. This substance seemed to be the product of tendon degeneration.

The microscopic features of the tendons within the polythene tube were interesting. The longitudinal sections of all the specimens studied showed that granulation tissue arising from the healing synovial sheath proliferated and grew beneath the end of the polythene tubes (Fig. 7.4). This granulation tissue, composed of fibroblasts and capillaries, spread gradually along the tendon's surface from the two ends of the tube to the level of the tendon anastomosis. Correctly speaking it is at the moment this tissue reaches the suture zone that the tendon healing process begins. Intrinsic healing arising from the two ends of the cut and repaired tendon was never

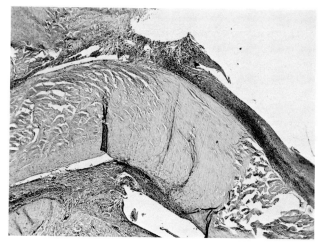

Figure 7.4

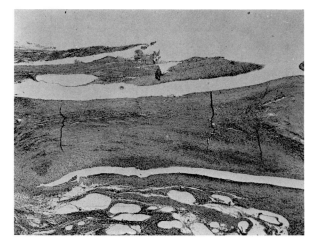

Figure 7.6

observed. The healing of these tendons was exclusively by granulation tissue from the synovial sheath and actual tendon healing was therefore delayed by precisely the time necessary for the granulation tissue growing beneath the tube, along the surface of the tendon to reach the suture zone. The two tendon segments in the polythene tube showed signs of degeneration in the form of cellular depopulation evident by the presence of karyorrhexis and karyolysis of the tenocytes (Fig. 7.5). The tendon, thus rendered acellular is later invaded and recellularized by fibroblasts introduced by the granulation tissue proliferating on the surface and filtering between the collagen groups and the suture line. In those instances when tendon degeneration is complete, healing is achieved through a long scar of vascularized fibrous tissue filling the space between the remaining viable tendon ends (Fig. 7.6).

HEALING OF DEEP FLEXORS INSIDE MILLIPORE TUBES

In this experiment the technique described above was applied but using 2 cm long tubes of Millipore reinforced with nylon. The Millipore filter is a cellular membrane which has pores of constant dimensions (0.54, 0.02 microns). These tubes are made by the firm of Millipore Filters, Bedford, Massachusetts.

In this series fifteen tendons were examined at intervals between four and 111 days. Microscopic examination revealed that the Millipore was an effective barrier between the tendon and the surrounding tissues since no tissue invasion was observed through the walls of the tube. However thick adhesions similar to those observed with the polythene tube developed at each tube end. In these cases healing was clearly delayed compared with the control group because the healing granulation tissue from the synovial sheath was delayed in reaching the tendon wound by the Millipore tube.

Histological examination revealed that the tendon surrounded by a Millipore tube became acellular from the fourteenth day. It is then gradually revascularized and invaded by cells from the granulation tissue proliferating on its surface. Likewise the collagen groups degenerate and are replaced by granulation tissue which thickens and becomes scar tissue. This tissue assures the continuity between the two living ends of the tendon. Macroscopically the tendon still looks granular and moderately hyperemic after 56 days. After 111 days the regenerated tendon still does not have its normal lustre. Microscopically the collagen bundles reappear but the neotendon remains abnormally cellular and vascularized.

These experiments clearly show that if a sectioned tendon is isolated by a tubular membrane from its sheath and surrounding tissues, thick vascular adhesions between the tendon and its sheath are formed at the ends of the tube. These adhesions provide nutrition for the granulation tissue which is necessary for the healing of the tendon. However, these adhesions remain thick and restrict gliding of the tendon. This is in sharp contrast to the loose filmy adhesions which are formed at the suture zone when no tubes are used; these do not restrict tendon gliding. Thus the use of a pseudo-sheath to avoid adhesions is illusory since on the one hand the sheaths delay the healing of the tendon and on the other they produce adhesions that are

even thicker, more rigid and more widespread than if the tendon were left to heal in its own natural tissue surroundings.

EFFECT OF ASSOCIATED TRAUMA ON THE HEALING OF A DIVIDED TENDON

In this series of experiments we tried to evaluate the specific effects of trauma on the healing of the tendon. A detailed macroscopic and microscopic study of the material obtained from the experiments described above showed that the granulation tissue which arises from the digital sheath and which proliferates in the tendon wounds, also penetrates the tendon where sutures perforate its surface. This process, never previously described, therefore suggested that even minor trauma to the tendon could be a very important factor in the formation of adhesions. The following experiments were therefore undertaken to evaluate the effect of physical trauma on the healing of tendon.

The surgical technique used was identical to that described in the first section. After non-traumatic section and suturing of the deep flexor tendon, various forms of artificial trauma were inflicted on the tendon. Thirty deep flexor tendons in the digits of dogs were subjected to specific and controlled episodes of trauma. Following repair using a 'pull-out' technique, 10 tendons were pierced 12 times on each side of the suture line with a Bunnell tendon needle. 20 other tendons were crushed on one occasion at a point 0.5 cm on each side of the suture line. They were crushed using the same haemostatic forceps and in the same manner. The animals were sacrificed at periods varying between 14 and 70 days after the operation.

Microscopic examination showed adhesions between the tendons and the surrounding tissues, at each point where the physical integrity of the tendon surface had been previously disturbed by trauma, whether this was by holes created by the needle (Fig. 7.7) or by crushing produced by the haemostatic forceps (Fig. 7.8). After crush injury there was a much more intense inflammatory response than in non-traumatized wounds, and the resultant adhesions were denser and thicker in direct proportion to the area of tendon surface injured. Ad-

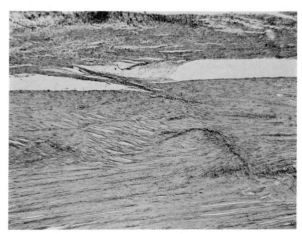

Figure 7.7

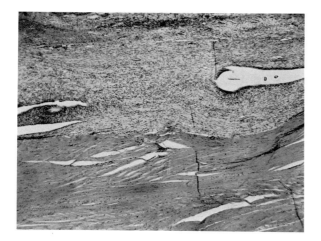

Figure 7.8

hesions to needle puncture wounds were discreet and occurred only in relation to the individual puncture wounds.

Observations made after this series of experiments contribute further proof that physical trauma inflicted on tendon surfaces is responsible for the majority of adhesions observed after the repair of digital flexor tendons. These adhesions can be prevented or limited by meticulous and atraumatic surgical technique.

RELATION BETWEEN THE SURGERY OF ADJACENT TISSUES AND THE FORMATION OF ADHESIONS ON THE HEALING FLEXOR TENDONS

The practice current at the time of these experiments was to excise the tendon sheath and the superficial tendon at the time of the primary repair or free grafting of the deep flexor tendon. The results of the experiment described in the second section showed clearly that the adhesions on the sutured deep flexor were much greater when the superficial tendon was excised than when it was preserved. It was therefore essential to study in an objective and critical manner the effects which excision of the superficial flexor and of the digital sheath can have on the healing of the deep flexor tendon.

As in all previous experiments we used digital flexor tendons of the forefoot of the dog as our experimental model. The selection of animals, preoperative preparation, surgical techniques, and postoperative management, were similar to those previously described.

EXCISION OF THE SHEATH

In this series of experiments 30 deep flexor tendons, divided into two groups of 15, were studied following non-traumatic section and suture. In the first group the digital sheaths of the flexor tendons were completely excised. In the second control group the sheath was left in place. The superficial flexors were left intact in both groups. The animals were sacrificed at intervals between three and 56 days. The results in the control

group following non-traumatic section and repair of the tendon were identical in every respect to those obtained in the first group of experiments reported here dealing with our original standard wound technique.

Results in both groups were identical in every respect. The tendon wound heals by local cellular proliferation from the sheath. No proliferation of tenoblasts was noted as in experiments described in the first section. The adhesions formed in the immediate vicinity of the wound. The lesions created by sutures appeared as the synovial layer of the sheath regenerated. These adhesions did not restrict the movements of the tendon within the digits compared to unoperated tendons in the same paw.

In the experimental group in which the digital sheaths were excised the following was observed:

Initially there is an outpouring of blood from the subcutaneous tissues surrounding the freshly cut and sutured deep flexors. Haematoma is invaded by granulation tissue which forms a new fibrin pseudo-sheath about the tendon. Fibroblasts and capillaries from the granulation tissue surrounding the tendon deposit new collagen in the suture zone effecting tendon union. The process is identical to that which we described initially. Simultaneously fibroblasts also arrange themselves parallel to the tendon surface, forming a fibroblastic layer over the precipitated fibrin to form a new gliding tendon sheath. Ultimately this fibroblastic layer takes on the appearance of synovium, so that a new synovial-like sheath develops about the repaired tendon. Adhesions at the suture line remain loose and filmy. Whether the new synovial sheath represents a metaplasia of the maturing tissue about each repaired tendon or a regeneration from microscopic remnants of the synovial sheath is not resolved. The new sheath provided a new gliding mechanism about each tendon.

EXCISION OF THE SUPERFICIAL FLEXOR TENDON

In this group, we studied problems created by excision of the superficial flexor tendon, a common clinical practice.

The two insertions of the superficial flexor are connected to the periosteum of the phalanx by two vascular vincula. It is therefore quite evident that total excision of both insertions of the tendon has the effect of destroying the integrity of the periosteal floor of the digital canal, not only at the insertions on the base of the middle phalanx but also on the proximal phalanx as well as the volar plate of the proximal interphalangeal joint.

This important alteration of the vascular and cellular floor of the digital canal could therefore logically be responsible for the considerable formation of adhesions occurring after the excision of the superficial flexor experimentally and clinically.

In order to verify this hypothesis, we carried out the following experiment.

Forty dogs' digits were divided into two groups of 20, after non-traumatic section and suture of their deep flexors by our standard technique as previously described. The following techniques were adopted for cutting the superficial flexors. In the first group the superficial flexor tendons were completely excised, including the insertions into the base of the middle

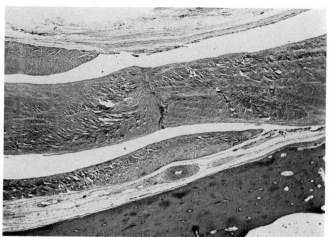

Figure 7.9

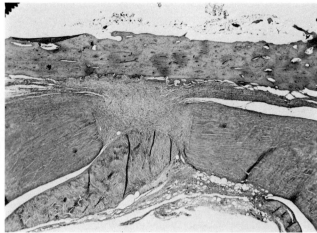

Figure 7.10

phalanx and the vincula from the middle phalanx. In the second group, the two insertions of the superficial flexor were left in place to allow the preservation of the vincula as well as the integrity of the periosteal floor of the digital canal by dividing the superficial flexor transversely immediately proximal to the proximal reflection of the vinculum breve. The animals were sacrificed at regular intervals between the third and sixty-second day. The results are now presented.

In the two groups the healing process of the tendon was identical to that already described for our standard wound technique. However, there is a very important difference between the two experimental groups. In the second group where the superficial flexors were cut proximal to the vincula (preserving vincula, periosteal floor and sublimis slips of insertion), granulation tissue did not form from the floor of the periosteal digital tunnel as the latter was preserved in its entirety. In this group no adhesions were therefore seen between the tendon and the osseous floor of the digital tunnel (Fig. 7.9). No adhesions were seen between the cut ends of the superficial flexor tendon slips and the repaired deep flexor tendon.

In the group in which we completely resected the superficial flexor tendon we observed the formation of granulation tissue, not only from the digital sheath as expected, but also arising from the periosteal floor of the tunnel. This prolific cellular reaction arising from the periosteum contributes equally to the healing of the deep flexor, as does the cell reaction arising from the digital sheath. (Fig. 7.10.)

In conclusion, total excision of the superficial flexor and its vincula provokes a disturbance of the vascular bed of the digital canal on the distal half of the proximal phalanx and at the base of the middle phalanx. The granulation tissue arising from this bed produces wide adhesions to the deep flexor tendon. Since these adhesions arise from the periosteum of the underlying phalanx they firmly anchor the healed profundus tendon to the bone, preventing tendon gliding. Subtotal excision of the superficialis immediately proximal to the reflexion of its vincula breve does not disturb the periosteum and thus allows the profundus tendon to heal without adhesions to the under-

lying phalanx; profundus tendon gliding is therefore not impaired under this circumstance.

In summary, the formation of adhesions to the deep flexor tendons after division and repair within the digital sheath is not an inexplicable occurrence after tendon surgery. The experiments described above demonstrate that adhesions form on the tendon surface wherever it has been traumatized. It is therefore necessary to handle the tendon as little as possible even by so-called atraumatic surgical technique. As far as the true healing of the tendon is concerned our experiments tend to prove that the vascular and cellular support necessary for the healing arises from the neighbouring tissues, either from the synovial sheath, or from the subcutaneous cellular tissue after the sheath has been excised. The adhesions are therefore both necessary and physiological. They are largely resolved at the end of the healing process and become loose and filmy.

We have seen that excision of the digital sheath does not produce undesirable effects on the healing of the tendon or on subsequent adhesion formation if the superficial flexor tendon is not excised. However, if the two tendinous insertions of the superficial flexor are removed with the vincula which run between them and the periosteal floor of the canal then a marked inflammatory reaction results provoking the formation of thick adhesions and causing adherence of the deep flexor tendon to the proximal phalanx. In cases where excision of the superficial flexor tendon is necessary it seems preferable to leave the two tendon insertions *in situ* together with their vinculum.

HEALING OF AUTOLOGOUS TENDON GRAFTS WITHIN THE DIGITAL SHEATH OF THE FLEXORS

These series of experiments were designed to determine the fate of autogenous tendon grafts in the fingers. Experimental protocol has been responsible for eliminating certain previous variables which were uncontrolled and badly defined (Peer, 1955).

It is essential to study tendon grafts within the digital

sheaths rather than in those places where the tendons are surrounded by loose cellular tissue or by paratenon. It is in fact
in the digital sheath that the adhesions so feared by the surgeon
are actually formed. It is important to study the fate of tendon
grafts whilst preserving their natural bed. If the pulleys and
the superficial flexors are all excised one cannot hope to discern
normal healing processes. The normal anatomy of the canine
digit was preserved in our experiment.

It is equally important that a biologically inert suture
material be used. The reaction of tissues to silk (the material
formerly used by many surgeons) is very marked. To avoid
this reaction we only used stainless steel sutures. The slides
were not only stained with hematoxyline-eosine but also with
specific collagen stains. Hematoxyline and eosine does not
show up collagen fibres very well and thus alone does not allow
an accurate assessment of the healing process.

As with the preceding experiments we utilized the digital
flexors of dogs as experimental models.

Fifty-four autologous tendon grafts of the deep flexors were
studied on 27 dogs' paws. The second and fifth digit of one
forefoot of each dog was opened by mid-lateral incisions
extending into the hollow of the paw to demonstrate the deep
flexor above the level of the tendon sheath. The sheaths were
only opened at their distal end in the distal phalanx so as to
expose only the most distal part of the deep flexors. The deep
flexor tendons were then cut at the distal insertion and in the
pad of the paw. The tendons were stripped of the tissue connections and completely withdrawn from their bed. They were
then re-introduced into their original bed and sutured at the
proximal and distal ends with No. 36 monofilament stainless
steel using the same technique as shown in Fig. 7.11. All traumatic manipulation of the tendons was avoided. Only fine,
sharp surgical needles were used. The surface of the tendon
grafts were injured only by suture needle pricks and the injuries left by cutting the vincula. Care was taken to spare the
tendon sheath, the superficial flexor and the pulley so as to preserve the greatest possible integrity within 'No man's land'.
The animals were sacrificed at regular intervals between seven
and 160 days, after the tissues had been excised under general
anaesthetic. Four types of histological sections were made on
the flexor mechanism—longitudinal cuts of the proximal tendon anastomosis, longitudinal sections of the distal anastomosis, transverse sections within 'No man's land' and longitudinal sections in 'No man's land'. These sections were
stained with hematoxyline-eosine or with Wild's silver stain
for collagen and Rheinehart's modification of Hale's colloidal
iron stain.

RESULTS

*The proximal and distal anastomoses in the palm and the digital
tendon sheath.* The healing of the anastomoses in the suture
zones was due exclusively to the activity of cells from the neighbouring tissues; that is to say from paratenon in the palm and
from the synovial layer of the sheath in the digits. The healing
of the tendon graft anastomoses progressed according to a well-
ordered process identical to that described for simple wounds
of the deep flexors. The suture sites of the proximal and distal

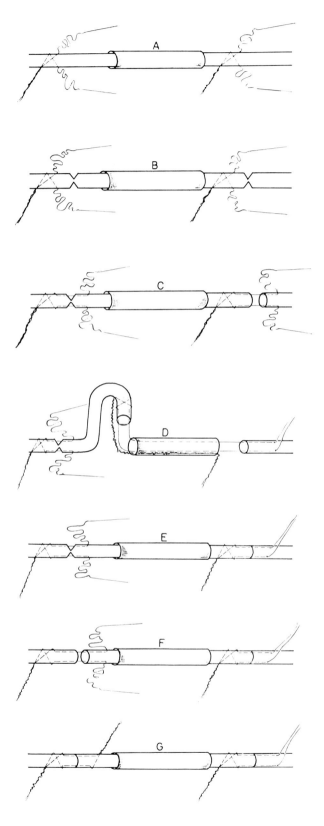

Figure 7.11

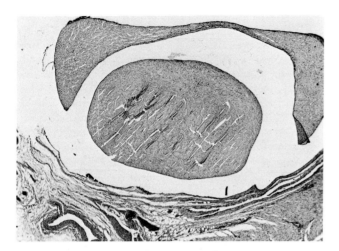

Figure 7.12

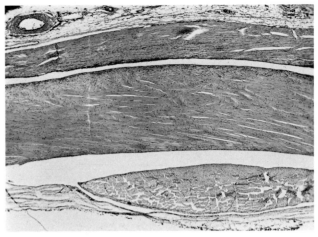

Figure 7.13

ends of the grafted tendon remain viable; on histological examination there was no trace of karyolysis or of karyorrhexis. The tendon cells (tenocytes) do not take part in the real healing of the tendon. The collagen remains quantitatively unchanged at the two ends of the graft. The adhesions which form between the suture zones and the neighbouring tissues gradually become less fibrotic by the process already described. After 106 days the healing of the tendon wounds was complete and the tendon regained a perfectly normal macroscopic and microscopic appearance, identifiable only by the very slight increase in the number of its cells and vessels. At every control stage in our experiments, the cells of the tendon grafts had retained their viability according to all the histological criteria. We were not able to show the slightest trace of degeneration or the replacement of the collagen of the grafts.

THE FATE OF FREE GRAFTS OF THE DEEP FLEXOR IN 'NO MAN'S LAND'

The experimental protocol already described permitted us to assess what happened to tendon grafts within the tendon sheaths in a very precise manner. In these cases we took care to save the superficial flexor, the pulleys and the sheath itself. It was thus possible to compare the structure of the whole superficial flexor with the free graft in the same histological section. In these experiments there were no observed adhesions between the graft on the one hand and the superficial flexor tendon, the pulleys and the digital sheath on the other. No quantitative or qualitative changes were observed in the cellularity or the nature of the collagen of the grafts. The cells maintained their viability and the collagen its integrity without evidence of oedema, degeneration or replacement (Figs. 7.12, 7.13).

Formation of adhesions. Since no adhesion had formed within the tendon sheath in 'No man's land' (Fig. 7.14) no further comment regarding this is indicated. The adhesions which formed at the distal tendon anastomoses site are necessary for they contribute the vascular and cellular basis of tendon healing. With the establishment of union, vascularization diminishes, the adhesions become thin and loose and the

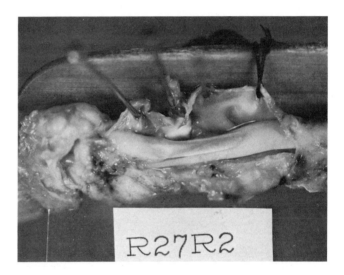

Figure 7.14

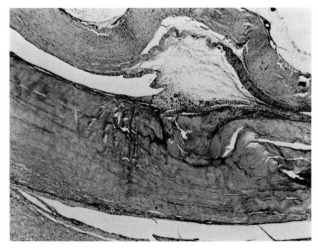

Figure 7.15

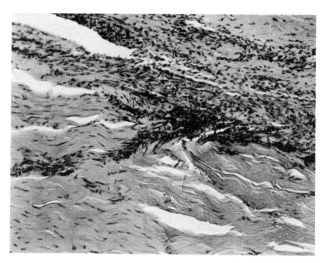

Figure 7.16

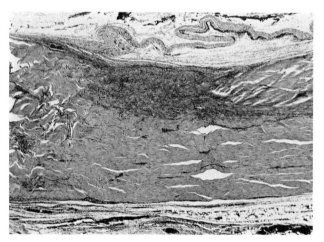

Figure 7.17

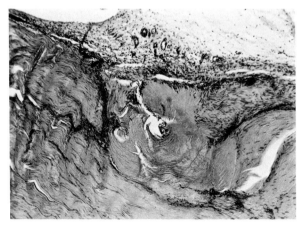

Figure 7.18

sheath re-establishes its continuity. The study of adhesion formation in the palm and at the proximal level of the digital sheath was informative. When one removes the deep flexors here one must necessarily injure the proximal digital sheath and tear the proximal vinculum of the tendon. This injury involves a proliferation of the sheath's synovial layer extending from its proximal limit to the basal pulley surrounding the superficial flexor and the profundus graft. Synovial proliferation thus closes the sheath and reconstitutes its integrity (Fig. 7.15). The synovium is later partly re-absorbed becoming reduced to a single layer of very loose cells which cover the proximal end of the graft. We have also noticed that the tendon graft injury is caused by sutures. (Fig. 7.16). In fact there is a localized tendon degeneration in those areas where the tendon surfaces are subjected to considerable pressure from the knots and pull-out stitches. These areas are then invaded by fibroblasts arising from the paratenon or the sheath (Fig. 7.17) as the case might be. These fibroblasts secrete new collagen fibres and thus contribute to the re-establishment of the anatomical integrity of the tendons. As in all other cases, adhesions which develop within the sheath eventually resolve and become thin and loose with no noticeable restraint on the function.

In certain cases we noted zones of cellular degeneration at the ends of the central portion of the grafts (Fig. 7.18) in 'No man's land'. Since these zones of degeneration always occur about suture tracts we think that they can be attributed to an excessive tension of stitches on the tendon grafts which has repercussions in the graft. No zone of tendon degeneration was observed at a distance from the sutures. These degenerative zones were invaded by granulation tissue and repopulated with new cells. When the tension on the suture is sufficient to produce degeneration of the collagen, the metallic suture may actually cut through longitudinal axis of the graft. This diminishes the tension within the system. The injuries left by the metallic suture are repaired by granulation tissue which grows into the suture tract (Fig. 7.19). This tissue produces new collagen and repopulates the damaged zone with cells.

If one pays very particular attention to the anatomical and microscopic details, one notices that the zones of tendon degeneration do not occur spontaneously but that they are generally due to too violent traction or to pressure or to surgical trauma. However, in most of our cases following the process of repair and healing, the adhesions become partially or completely reabsorbed.

It is essential to state that the tendon grafts remain viable: in fact comparing them with the superficial flexors left intact inside their common sheath, one notices that tenocytes keep their histological characteristics. There is no collagen oedema, degenerative zones or remodelling of the graft noted. However, after a tendon injury, secondary to abnormal compression, a specific, very localised tendon degeneration can occur. These specific zones always heal in the same way, by fibroblasts and vascular tissue arising within granulation tissue originating from the synovial sheath. We have never observed intrinsic healing of the tendons. This process is therefore extrinsic, it involves adhesions which become attached to those places where the integrity of the tendon surfaces is destroyed by sutures

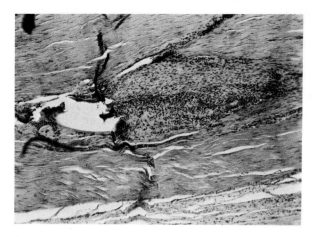

Figure 7.19

or by excessive handling. These adhesions tend to disappear or become very thin when the healing process is completed.

These experiments are contradictory to those of Flynn and Graham which seem to indicate that tendon autografts are subject to complete necrosis followed by replacement by fibroblasts arising from the anastomotic zones of the graft. These differences may be explained by the use of reactive silk thread instead of inert material and the fact that they used extensor tendon grafts instead of the digital flexor tendons and they exclusively used hematoxyline and eosine as a stain. On the other hand, our results agree with the results of Lindsay and McDougall (1961) who maintain that tendon grafts as such can survive. However, these authors describe an excessive adhesive state which limits the movement of the graft whereas our are practically devoid of adhesions. It is possible that the differences are due to the fact that Lindsay and McDougall selected the chicken for their experiments rather than using mammals. It must also be noted that these authors cut out the digital sheaths and the superficial flexors contrary to the technique used in our experiments. It is possible that this technical difference explains the excessive adhesive state noted by these authors.

COMPARATIVE STUDY OF THE HEALING OF PARATENON-COVERED AND NON-PARATENON-COVERED TENDON GRAFTS

Our results using flexor autographs are very satisfactory. However, it is extremely rare in current practice to have a deep flexor tendon at one's disposal with which to carry out a free graft. Usually autologous paratenon-covered tendons are used (palmaris longus, long extensor of the toes etc.). This series of experiments is done to compare the healing and fate of autogenous profundus flexor grafts with that of autogenous paratenon-covered tendon grafts.

As with the other experiments described in this work, the flexor mechanism of the dog's digit was used as our experimental model. The techniques are identical to those previously described. Sixty autogenous tendons were studied, 30 deep

digital flexors and 30 flexor carpi ulnaris tendons; the latter tendons are covered with paratenon. The index and the fifth digit of one of the forepaws of each dog was exposed using a mid-lateral incision, extending into the proximal aspect of the palm. The digital sheaths were only opened at their two ends. One of the two deep flexors thus exposed was entirely extracted from its bed, freed of all tissue attachment and then replaced within its original anatomical position within the sheath and sutured at both ends with stainless steel pull-out type stitches.

In the other digit of the same paw the deep flexor tendon was freed and extracted from its sheath in exactly the same way; but in this case it was replaced by an autograft covered with paratenon, in this case the flexor carpi ulnaris tendon. The latter graft was taken from the foreleg using longitudinal incisions. It was done without being traumatised and freed from neighbouring tissues by careful sharp dissection taking care to preserve the paratenon. The graft was then introduced into the digital sheath, proximal and distal anastomoses were carried out using Bunnell's pull-out technique with No. 6 stainless steel wire suture. Thus in each operated paw there was a controlled experiment with grafted deep flexor tendon without paratenon in one digit and fresh autologous graft covered with its paratenon in another digit.

The 30 animals each having had two tendon autografts were sacrificed at successive intervals of three to 77 days after the operation.

RESULTS

Scarring and healing were similar in the two groups. These processes were identical to those described in the earlier part of this article dealing with autologous profundus tendon grafts. Tendon graft anastomosis whether proximal or distal heal due to cellular activity from the neighbouring tissues arising from the digital sheath for the distal anastomosis or from the subcutaneous tissue in the case of the proximal palmar anastomosis.

The grafts covered with paratenon show extensive adhesions to the neighbouring tissues after the inflammatory stage of healing. The paratenon is not an essential element for the healing of grafts because the grafted deep flexor tendons heal in the same time and in the same manner without paratenon. They are not involved in extensive adhesions to the surrounding tissue, however. In this series of experiments the tendon grafts all remained viable and normal according to all the histological criteria used.

No necrosis of a graft was noted whether the tendon was a paratenon covered or a non-paratenon covered graft. Those autografts covered with paratenon showed diffuse adhesions along their length both in the palm as well as in the flexor digital sheaths. These irregular widely spread adhesions seem to arise in part from the paratenon itself. They are particularly marked in the region of the pulleys and the vincula of the superficial flexors. Granulation tissue arising from the subcutaneous tissue within the palm also proliferates along the paratenon of the graft well beyond the palm into the digital sheaths themselves. It seems that the paratenon is therefore a biologically active tissue favouring the formation of granulation tissue and subsequent adhesions. In our experiments the adhesions observed on the grafts with paratenon remained filmy and low in collagen. They do not appear to restrict tendon gliding. However, in cases where the graft might be traumatised adhesions can be expected to be more dense and restrictive.

From our experiment, the paratenon does not appear to be essential to the survival of free tendon grafts. On the contrary, its conservation in such grafts leads to the formation of more widespread adhesions which can jeopardize the final functional result. Our conclusions agree with the clinical results of experienced hand surgeons (Littler) who have found that the preservation of paratenon on a free graft gives poorer results with greater adhesion to the graft than if the paratenon is carefully removed.

THE HEALING OF HOMOLOGOUS LYOPHILIZED TENDON GRAFTS IN FLEXOR SHEATHS

From the experiments described above it appears that the best grafts seem to be grafts of the flexor profundus tendons themselves. Unfortunately, in normal practice, such tendons are often not available. That is why we have been interested in the possible use of homologous flexor tendon grafts in the hope of being able to use them in clinical practice.

EXPERIMENTAL METHOD

Flexor tendons were excised surgically from the donor dogs using strictly atraumatic techniques. They were then sutured at either end to hooked pyrex rods so as to allow atraumatic handling throughout the lyophilization process and their subsequent introduction into the digits of new dogs.

Immediately after being removed they were fixed between the two hooks of the glass rods and were immersed into a nutrient medium for a maximum of 45 minutes. During this time they were taken to the Tissue Bank of the Naval Medical School, Bethesda, Maryland and then lyophilized in the standard manner used at this Institute. Before being transplanted into new animals, the lyophilized autografts were soaked in a

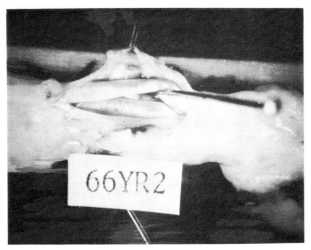

Figure 7.20

sterile saline solution containing no antibiotic or antiseptic for a period of half an hour. These tendons were then transplanted atraumatically into the digital flexor sheaths of the recipient dogs. The sheaths, pulleys and superficial flexors of the hosts were preserved in each case. The grafts provisionally sutured to the ends of the flexor tendons were then drawn into the sheaths when the latter were extracted. The proximal and distal anastomoses were carried out with a classic Bunnell pullout technique using No. 36 stainless steel suture material. Seventeen dogs were studied, each with two lyophilized deep flexor tendons in one paw. The dogs were sacrificed variously between seven and 180 days later. The microscopic sectioning and staining techniques were identical to those used in our earlier experiments on fresh autogenous flexor profundus grafts.

RESULTS

Macroscopically no adhesions were noted between the lyophilized grafts and the digital sheaths nor annular ligaments nor superficialis tendons of the recipients in any of the 17 operated specimens (Fig. 7.20). There was no macroscopic evidence of graft degeneration or replacement. The lyophilized grafts could not be distinguished *in situ* from normal profundus tendons.

HISTOLOGICAL ASPECTS

The microscopic findings were divided into two categories— the observations made at the two points of anastomosis and those made of the events within the flexor digital sheath. As no significant difference was observed between the healing reactions at the proximal and distal anastomosis sites, they are described together.

HEALING OF THE ANASTOMOSES

In the first week the connective tissue around the points of anastomosis showed a pronounced inflammatory reaction. The wounds were rapidly surrounded by granulation tissue rich in capillaries, erythrocytes, histiocytes and fibroblasts. This granulation tissue spread over the tendon graft surface and entered between the tendon ends at the suture line.

The presence of collagen fibres within the tendon wound together with the progressive invasion of granulation tissue along suture tracts ends was noted on the 14th day. Cells arising from the granulation tissue are responsible for cellularising the homograft. Those areas adjacent to the suture tracts are more quickly repopulated with cells than the more distant parts because of the fibroblast-rich tissue which grows into the suture tracts.

On the 21st day after the operation the collagen fibres in the tendon graft anastomosis lies in the longitudinal axis of the tendon. The suture zones at the anastomoses become attached to the neighbouring tissues by adhesions which contain little collagen whilst the inflammatory reaction of healing diminishes progressively. There is a progressive maturation of the healing wounds so that at 35 days union of the two ends is moderately advanced and comparable to that seen in the case of profundus tendon autografts.

By the sixth week all microscopic signs of acute inflammation have resolved. A few sparse adhesions persist between the grafts and surrounding tissues at the suture sites. Cellularization of the grafts is complete for 1 cm on either side of the anastomosis.

After 93 days, the anastomosis is barely identifiable histologically. The postoperative adhesions necessary for healing become very loose and filmy.

The specimens taken at 160 and 180 days after operation show complete collagenization of the anastomotic zone. This collagen matches perfectly with that of the host tendon. There is no difference detectable between the lyophilized graft and the host tendon to which it has been sutured. There were no signs of collagen degeneration of the lyophilized grafts. The collagen staining reactions remained identical on the two sides of the anastomosis with all three staining techniques used in this study.

No evidence of degeneration of the grafts was noted. There was no sign of degeneration of the lyophilized collagen and its substitution by elements from the host. The collagen of the lyophilized tendon graft is fully accepted and incorporated by the host and recellularized by host cells.

THE FATE OF LYOPHILIZED GRAFTS WITHIN THE FLEXOR SHEATH

In the region classically known as 'No man's land' far from the anastomotic points, the lyophilized acellular grafts were examined by serial longitudinal histological sections of the digital flexor mechanism. In that way it was possible to compare the tendon graft with a normal tendon *in situ* since the superficial flexor tendon lay in its normal position within the digital sheath and was, therefore, present in the same histological section.

In successive samples taken between the seventh and the 108th day, there was no evidence of necrosis, fragmentation or degeneration of the collagen of the grafts, when compared to that of the superficial flexor tendon and the collagen of the pulleys in the same *en bloc* sections. The histological characteristics of the lyophilized collagen bundles using the three stains previously mentioned, remained identical to those of the superficial flexor tendons of the recipient except for an initial absence of cells.

The following histologic changes were observed:
Areas of proliferation of the synovial cells of the flexor sheath are seen in apposition to the lyophilized grafts.

In these immediate areas, matching collections of cells were observed on, and invading the surfaces of the lyophilized grafts. These histologic sections revealed that the grafts were recellularized by the seeding of cells from the proliferative areas of the synovial sheath. Early recellularization of the lyophilized grafts always occurred in direct relation to the areas of synovial cellular proliferation. In some of these areas bridges of proliferating synovial cells can be seen extending from the synovium to the graft surface.

Special stains (Rheinehart and Wilder) show that there is no deposition of collagen within these cellular cords passing from the synovial sheath to the grafts throughout the synovial space. At the end of our experiment, 180 days after implantation, with the graft remaining immobilized throughout this whole period, the graft was incompletely cellularized and areas of acellularity persisted.

Significantly, however, there were two cases which were sampled on the 56th day which showed normal cellularity in the centre as well as on the periphery of the graft. This represents an example of biological variability.

It is important to note that although there is a heavy cellular and vascular proliferation within the synovial sheath, no blood vessels entered the tendon in 'No man's land'. Throughout the 180 days that the experiments lasted, vascular injections did not reveal blood vessels in this part of the graft.

Thus it would seem that the synovium of the sheath constitutes the only source of cellular repopulation of the frozen grafts within 'No man's land'.

All through the experiment there was no evidence of rejection of the homografts. The inflammatory cells of wound healing present in the tendon wound disappeared as normal healing progressed. They did not appear at areas removed from the tendon wounds or about the grafts within the digital sheaths. The entire process observed was one of complete host acceptance and recellularization of the lyophilized grafts with structural and anatomic incorporation of the graft collagen.

DISCUSSION

This is certainly not the first experimental study devoted to the possible use of preserved tendons for implantation as tendon grafts. Cordrey and his associates (1963) have reviewed these attempts. However, few authors have studied the possible use of lyophilized tendon grafts and none have done this within the digital sheath.

We have been able to show that lyophilized flexor tendon homografts, implanted within the flexor sheath, are fully accepted by the recipients without degeneration or rejection of the collagen. Moreover, the cells of the recipient synovial sheath repopulate the grafts by a process of cell seeding that originates within the synovial cells of the digital flexor sheath. This is done without the formation of collagenous adhesions. The recipient accepts these lyophilized tendon grafts and incorporates them into his flexor mechanism. They are recellularized by the host and remain free of adhesion in 'No man's land'.

Cordrey and his associates (1963) in a study of the homologous tendon grafts preserved by different methods and carried out on the Achilles tendon of the rabbit report that the homografts of lyophilized tendon are gradually surrounded by scar tissue and reabsorbed. He reports that the tendon graft junctions are in a good state after seven weeks, but there are zones of fragmentation of the collagen fibres and centres of necrosis within the grafts. However, these authors were unable to answer the question of whether the collagen of the grafts is preserved or reabsorbed.

Flynn and Graham (1963) in a study of lyophilized heterologous tendon grafts described total necrosis and degeneration of the grafts with ultimate replacement by host inflammatory cells. Their microphotographs support this view. Significantly they found no anatomical evidence of immunological rejection of the grafts.

Since the results obtained by Flynn and Graham are diametrically opposed to those of the present report, it is essential to emphasize that these authors used lyophilized heterografts and not homografts. Moreover, they used carpal extensors and not deep digital flexors as in our experiments. The grafts used by these authors were washed in saline solution for five days, and then chemically sterilized in betaproproiolactone before dry freezing them, whereas the tendons in this report were never subjected to such chemical denaturation. All these differences are perhaps at the basis of the variations in results.

While the cells of lyophilized tendon grafts have been destroyed, the collagen which is an extracellular protein fibre with no clinically significant immunologic competence, should be perfectly integrated within a new host. There is no compelling reason for its being rejected or subjected to a progess of reabsorption or remodelling. In fact, our study shows that the collagen can be completely accepted by the recipient and become an integral and normal complement of that individual once it has been recellularized. The dry freezing process apparently does not denature the collagen protein.

The process of lyophilizing profundus tendons permits the preservation of flexor tendons for use in other hosts. Lyophilized flexor tendon profundus homografts are better tolerated than fresh autografts of tendons which are covered with paratenon. It is essential that the tendons are removed in a strictly atraumatic fashion and are not subject to chemical denaturation. If these tendons are treated carefully and reimplanted with full atraumatic precautions, such grafts are fully accepted by the recipient and produce a gliding flexor profundus mechanism with no adhesions within 'No man's land'.

CONCLUSIONS

This work, based upon experiments on dogs, can help achieve a better understanding of the problems of flexor tendon injuries in the human hand and help to effect better treatment of such injuries.

In the first instance it was shown that a deep flexor tendon when cut and sutured within its sheath, heals as a result of the cellular activity of the synovial sheath and the surrounding tissues and not because of an intrinsic healing reaction of the tendon itself. The second series of experiments confirms this observation, for if the zone of tendon repair is isolated from its neighbouring tissues by an impermeable membrane, healing is delayed or prevented entirely. This delay represents the time lapse necessary for the granulation tissue from the sheath to proliferate under the tube to the level of the suture zone. Flexor tendons thus possess no intrinsic reparative function. This fact is also confirmed in the fourth section of our work. In fact, these experiments show that the stumps of the cut flexor tendons do not produce any fibroblastic proliferation at their ends. This observation is confirmed by what can be observed clinically when a cut tendon retracts proximally into a non traumatized zone of the digital canal. There is no adhesion to the sheath, nor is there an intrinsic tenoblastic reaction.

It is frequently said that flexor tendons when repaired within their sheaths become swollen and that they tend to necrose if the synovial sheath and the superficial tendon are removed. We have never seen oedema of repaired flexor tendons in these experiments nor have we seen any tendon necrosis secondary to oedema or swelling.

It is generally acknowledged that when a flexor tendon is divided and repaired within the flexor digital sheath, poor functional result often occurs because of the adhesions forming between it and neighbouring tissues. However, it is not appreciated that the adhesions form only at the immediate wound sites and at those points where the surface of the tendon is damaged and that adhesions occur quantitatively in direct proportion to the extent of injury to the tendon surface. In relation to tendon adhesions the trauma inflicted on the neighbouring anatomical structures is likewise extremely important. When the superficial tendon is completely excised, the periosteal floor of the traumatized digital canal takes part in the healing reaction and gives rise to granulation tissue which helps to heal the tendon. The adhesions thus formed between bone and tendon completely immobilize the tendon and destroy all hope of achieving useful function. A flexor tendon requires an extrinsic source of granulation tissue to heal and that is why it tends to adhere to all injured neighbouring tissues which are capable of giving rise to granulation tissue. Consequently an intact superficial tendon should not be sacrificed to repair a damaged profundus tendon within the same digit, for this gives rise to adhesions between the bony floor of the digital tunnel and the deep tendon. If the superficial tendon is seriously damaged, then it is preferable to remove it by subtotal excision immediately proximal to its vincula without damaging the vincula and the periosteal floor of the digital tunnel for these structures if they are damaged become the source of disastrous adhesions.

In brief, the surgeon must be meticulous throughout surgery in order to preserve the integrity of the neighbouring structures which could become a source of adhesions.

The experiments on tendon grafts described in this report have clearly shown that tendons covered with paratenon, are not very satisfactory when used as free grafts. The paratenon constitutes both a source of adhesions and a fertile site for the ingrowth of granulation tissue arising from neighbouring tissues.

It is preferable to excise the paratenon without damaging the tendon surface before grafting it within the flexor sheath.

There is no better substitute for a flexor tendon than a free graft of another flexor tendon. If a tendon of this type is available (rarely) then it may be given preference.

Our tendon autografts, whether of the deep flexor or of flexor carpi ulnaris tendon, all remained viable; they remained cellularized and without the least trace of degeneration of collagen. With regard to lyophilized flexor profundus homografts, the process of cellular repopulation by proliferation of the synovium of the digital sheath constitutes a unique phenomena not previously described.

It is interesting to note that lyophilized flexor tendon homografts give better results than autografts of paratenon-covered tendons. The lyophilized tendon grafts remained intact equal in appearance and function to those of the normal deep flexor tendons found in the same limb in non-operated digits. The grafts remained free of adhesions and the anastomotic zones within the palm were identifiable only by the presence of a few sparse translucent adhesions with no signs of degeneration or alteration of the collagen. On the contrary, the collagen of lyophilized homografts was completely accepted by the host tissues and was repopulated with new host cells. The grafts are completely integrated within the distal flexor mechanism of the recipient on an anatomical as well as functional basis. It is impossible to distinguish them *in vivo* from normal tendons.

REFERENCES

ADAMS, WILLIAM (1860) On the reparative process in human tendons after subcutaneous division for the cure of deformities. With an account of the appearances presented in fifteen post-mortem examinations in the human subject; also a series of experiments in rabbits, and a resume of the English and foreign literature on the subject. London: J. Churchill.

ANGEL, S. H., LIBSCOMB, P. R. & GRINDLAY, J. H. (1961) Construction of artificial tendon sheaths in dogs. *Am. J. Surg.*, **101**, 355–356.

ASHLEY, F. L., POLAK, TEODOR, STONE, R. S. & MARMOR, LEONARD (1962) An evaluation of the healing process in avian and mammalian digital-flexor tendons following the application of an artificial tendon sheath (silastic). In Proceedings of the American Society for Surgery of the Hand. *J. Bone and Joint Surg.*, **44A**, 1038.

ASHLEY, F. L., STONE, R. S., EDWARDS, J. W. & SLOAN, R. F. (1960) Further studies on the application of monomolecular cellulose filter tubes to create artificial tendon sheaths in the hand and wrist. *Western J. Surg.*, **68**, 156–161.

ASHLEY, F. L., STONE, R. S., ALONSO-ARTIEDA, MIGUEL, SYVERUD, J. M., EDWARDS, J. W., SLOAN, R. F. & MOONEY, S. A. (1959) Experimental and clinical studies on the application of monomolecular cellulose filter tubes to create artificial tendon sheaths in digits. *Plast. and Reconstruct. Surg.*, **23**, 526–534.

BENJAMIN, H. B., WAGNER, M., ZEIT, W. & AUSMAN, R. K. (1955) The use of an endothelial cuff in tendon repair. *Med. Times*, **83**, 697–699.

BOYES, J. H. (1950) Flexor-tendon grafts in the fingers and thumb. An evaluation of end results. *J. Bone and Joint Surg.*, **32A**, 489–499.

BUNNELL, STERLING (1955) Hand surgery in World War II. Washington, D.C.: Dept. of the Army.

BURMAN, M. S. (1944) The use of a nylon sheath in the secondary repairs of torn finger flexor tendons. *Bull. Hosp. Joint Dis.*, **5**, 122–133.

CARSTAM, N. (1953) The effect of cortisone on the formation of tendon adhesions and on tendon healing. An experimental investigation in the rabbit. *Acta Chir. Scandinavica*, Supplementum **182.**

CORDREY, L. J., McCORKLE, H. & HILTON, E. (1963) A Comparative Study of Fresh Autogenous and Preserved Homogenous Tendon Grafts in Rabbits. *J. Bone and Joint Surg.*, **45B**, 182–195.

DAVIS, LOYAL & ARIES, L. J. (1937) An experimental study upon the prevention of adhesions about repaired nerves and tendons. *Surgery*, **2**, 877–888.

FLYNN, J. E. & GRAHAM, J. H. (1962) Healing following tendon suture and tendon transplants. *Surg., Gynec. and Obst.*, **115**, 467–472.

FLYNN, J. E. & GRAHAM, J. H. (1963) Lyophilized heterologous and autogenous tendon transplants. *Surg., Gynec. and Obst.*, **116**, 345–350.

GARLOCK, J. H. (1927) The repair processes in wounds of tendons, and in tendon grafts. *Ann. Surg.*, **85**, 92–103.

GONZALEZ, R. I. (1949) Experimental tendon repair within the flexor tunnels: use of polethylene tubes for improvement of functional results in the dog. *Surgery*, **26**, 181–198.

GONZALEZ, R. I. Experimental use of teflon in tendon surgery. *Plast. and Reconstruct. Surg.*, **23**, 535–539.

GRANT, GORDON (1953) The effect of cortisone on healing of tendons in rabbits. In Proceedings of the American Society for Surgery of the Hand. *J. Bone and Joint Surg.*, **35A**, 525.

HAUCK, GUSTAV (1924) Ueber Sehnenverletzungen, Sehnenregeneration und Sehnennaht. *Arch. f. Klin. Chir.*, **128**, 568–585.

HOCHSTRASSER, A. D., BROADBENT, T. R. & WOOLF, ROBERT (1960) Sheath replacement in tendon repair. *Rocky Mountain Med. J.*, **57**, 30–33.

HUECK, HERMAN (1923) Ueber Sehnenregeneration innerhalb echter Sehnenscheiden. *Arch. f. Klin. Chir.*, **127**, 137–164.

ISELIN, M., DE LA PLAZA, R. & FLORES, A. (1963) Surgical use of homologous tendon grafts preserved in cialit. *Plast. and Reconstruct. Surg.*, **32**, 401–413.

KAPLAN, E. B. (1963) Discussion summarized in Proceedings of The American Society for Surgery of the Hand. *J. Bone and Joint Surg.*, **45A**, 885.

KREUZ, F. P., HYATT, G. W., TURNER, T. C. & BASSETT, (1951) The preservation and clinical use of freeze-dried bone. *J. Bone and Joint Surg.*, **33A**, 863–872.

LINDSAY, W. K. & MacDOUGALL, E. P. (1961) Digital flexor tendons: An experimental study. Part III. The fate of autogenous digital flexor tendon grafts. *Brit. J. Plast. Surg.*, **13**, 293–304.

LINDSAY, W. K. & THOMSON, H. G. (1960) Digital flexor tendons: An experimental study. Part I. The significance of each component of the flexor mechanism in tendon healing. *Brit. J. Plast. Surg.*, **12**, 289–316.

MASON, M. L. (1957) Primary versus secondary tendon repair. *Quart. Bull. N.W. Med. School*, **31(2)**, 120–123.

MASON, M. L. (1959) Primary tendon repair. *J. Bone and Joint Surg.*, **41A**, 575–577.

MASON, M. L. & ALLEN, H. S. (1941) The rate of healing of tendons. An experimental study of tensile strength. *Ann. Surg.*, **113**, 424–459.

MASON, M. L. & SHEARON, C. G. (1932) The process of tendon repair. An experimental study of tendon suture and tendon graft. *Arch. Surg.*, **25**, 615–692.

McKEE, G. K. (1945) Metal anastomosis tubes in tendon suture. *Lancet*, **1**, 659–660.

NEUBERGER, A. & SLACK, H. G. B. (1953) The metabolism of collagen from liver, bone, skin and tendon in the normal rat. *Biochem. J.*, **53**, 47–52.

PEACOCK, E. E., JR (1959) Morphology of homologous and heterologous tendon grafts. *Surg., Gynec., and Obst.*, **109**, 735–742.

PEACOCK, E. E. (1959) Some problems in flexor tendon healing. *Surgery*, **45**, 415–423.

PEER, L. A. (1955) *Transplantation of Tissues. Cartilage, Bone, Fascia, Tendon and Muscle.* Vol. I, pp. 277–295. Baltimore: The Williams and Wilkins Co.

POTENZA, A. D. (1962A) Tendon healing within the flexor digital sheath in the dog. *J. Bone and Joint Surg.*, **44A**, 49–64.

POTENZA, A. D. (1962B) Effect of associated trauma on healing of divided tendons. *J. Trauma*, **2**, 175–184.

POTENZA, A. D. (1963) Critical evaluation of flexor-tendon healing and adhesion formation within artificial digital sheaths. *J. Bone and Joint Surg.*, **45A**, 1217–1233.

POTENZA, A. D. (1964) Prevention of adhesions to healing digital flexor tendons. *J.A.M.A.*, **187**, 187–191.

SKOOG, TORD & PERSSON, B. H. (1954) An experimental study of the early healing of tendons. *Plast. and Reconstruct. Surg.*, **13**, 384–399.

SCHWARZ, EGBERT. (1962) Ueber die anatomischen Vorgänge bei der Sehnenregeneration und dem plastischen Ersatz von Sehnendefekten durch Sehne, Fascie und Bindegewebe. *Zeitschr. f. Chir.*, **173**, 301–385.

WHEELDON, THOMAS (1939) The use of cellophane as a permanent tendon sheath. *J. Bone and Joint Surg.*, **21**, 393–396.

WRENN, R. N., GOLDNER, J. L. & MARKEE, J. L. (1954) An experimental study of the effect of cortisone on the healing processes and tensile strength of tendons. *J. Bone and Joint Surg.*, **36A**, 588–601.

SURGERY OF THE FLEXOR TENDONS

8. Reparative Surgery of Flexor Tendons in the Digits

C. Verdan

SECTION SYNDROME

The diagnosis of sectioned flexor tendons is not as easy as it may seem. Misinterpretation often occurs because the patient remains capable of metacarpophalangeal flexion. It must be remembered that this articulation can be completely flexed by the interossei and lumbricals. The examiner must maintain the proximal phalanx in extension (protecting the wound if needed with a sterile compress) and ask the patient to flex the middle phalanx to indicate an intact flexor digitorum superficialis. Then, the middle phalanx maintained in extension, the patient must flex the distal phalanx. The same procedure applies to the thumb, with the knowledge that the metacarpophalangeal articulation is flexed by the thenar muscles, the flexor pollicis longus acting primarily on the distal phalanx.

If, in the long finger, both flexor tendons are sectioned, the middle and distal phalanges cannot be flexed. If only the flexor digitorum profundus is damaged, the middle phalanx can still flex actively. Interpretation becomes difficult when only the flexor superficialis is severed, because the flexor digitorum profundus is capable alone of flexing all the articulations. The impression is that the function of the finger is normal, but with diminished strength. In such a case, the examiner holds the other three fingers in complete extension which extends the common muscular mass of the flexor profundus and impedes its contraction. The flexor digitorum profundus cannot be contracted in the damaged finger, and the flexion must be accomplished by the flexor superficialis. If the latter is severed (or adherent), no flexion can be accomplished.

Partial section of tendons may go unnoticed at the initial clinical examination. If the wound has opened the sheath, one must suspect a partial section and examine the tendons along an adequate length, since the lesion may have occurred in flexion or extension of the finger, provoking tendon damage at a fair distance from that of the skin and sheath. Repair of these partial lesions prevents possible secondary rupture, and the occurrence of trigger-fingers.

In the little finger, the flexor superficialis can be very thin and, with isolated section of the flexor profundus, active flexion of the middle phalanx can be limited.

Finally, at the level of the wrist, the intertendinous connections of the flexor profundus in Zones VII and even VI, especially for the three last fingers, Fig. 8.16 and cf. Fig. 18.1, can replace the function of a sectioned tendon and mask the severity of the wound (see chapter by Fahrer).

SURGICAL EXPOSURE

Among the patients sent to us for secondary repair of flexor tendons, we are struck by the great number of unfortunate incisions performed at previous interventions. Apart from the disastrous median longitudinal volar incision, we see often equally retractile scars, because the medio-lateral incision has been done too far anteriorly. These scars are necessarily retractile since they cross the interphalangial creases; what is more, they follow the path of the volar vasculo-nervous bundle and make secondary repair extremely difficult. Incisions should be made on the *dorso*-medio-lateral aspect of the digit (cf. Fig. 8.3a).

'Bayonette' incisions must be totally abandoned; the angles scar poorly, the transverse incision in the PIP or DIP creases threatens the vasculo-nervous bundle which is very superficial at this level, and there are many cases of its iatrogenous section. Secondary intervention is made difficult by the pre-existing scar on both sides of the finger at a place that should serve as the base of a cutaneous flap.

In general, the basic principles of plastic surgery must be followed, and especially so for the hand.

The directives are:
1. Avoid straight longitudinal incisions that cross creases.
2. Cross with care any poorly vascularized zones such as the palmar triangle, respecting the small vessels.
3. Support, prehensile and tactile surfaces should stay free of scars.
4. The incision should be at some distance from the place where the tendon is to be repaired, since their super-position provokes fibrous adherences which compromise the subsequent gliding of the repaired tendon.
5. The incision must be large enough to allow an adequate view of the surgical field.
6. Fresh wounds may be used as access routes, after excision of their edges, when they are enlarged; this is where most mistakes are made, for example by placing a straight longitudinal incision at the centre of a transverse wound. The 'T' scar is exactly on the path of the repaired tendons and their movements are necessarily impeded; also the angles often necrose and are a source of infection and subsequent adhesions.
7. An accidental wound is only enlarged at its extremities (Fig. 8.1) using curved or angular incisions. It is sometimes possible to by-pass a small wound using a lateral incision in the form of a flap.
8. For secondary repair it is best not to re-enter the accidental wound, but to avoid it by a sinusoidal incision. Excision of the scar results in a new suture on the same plane as the repaired tendon and constitution of a fibrous diaphragm which limits sliding.

In any case, careful planning of incisions in ink is advisable! Transverse ink marks aid in aligning the skin for the final suture.

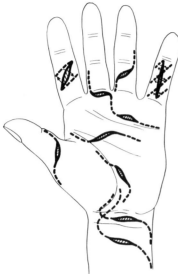

Figure 8.1
Methods of enlarging accidental wounds to allow their exploration. If necessary other transverse incisions can be made to find the retracted tendons. Wounds crossing a cutaneous crease are 'transversalized' using the 'Z' plasty.

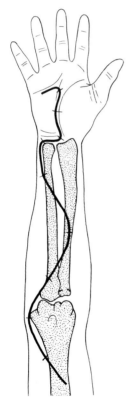

Figure 8.2
A large palmo-antebrachial incision is used for repair of nerves as well as tendons at the wrist and the superior half of the palm. This incision can be used by segments as necessary. It permits the following repairs, in Zone V and VI: repair of flexor tendons, branches of the ulnar nerve, section of the flexor retinaculum; in Zone VII, repair of flexor tendons, median and ulnar nerves, flexor carpi ulnaris tendon, synovectomies and muscular anomalies.

The different incisions that we use are indicated in figures 8.2 to 8.4.

The preparation of the digital canal from the dorso-medio-lateral incision entails exposure of Cleeland's ligament which partitions the finger and protects the neurovascular bundle. Its section allows penetration behind the bundle which is left in the anterior flap, and thus exposure of the flexor sheath. It is resutured at the end of the procedure to avoid the 'swan-neck' recurvatum which occurs when flexor digitorum superficialis has been removed for a tendon graft (see Boyes).

Recent studies of the fine vascularization of flexor tendons (Hunter, 1978) show that a very small artery is running from the collateral artery to the vinculum at the level of the PIP joint. Thus, a surgical approach posteriorly to the pedicle will probably sever this small artery and compromise the vascularization of the tendon in this area. The choice of an anterior approach to the pedicle should be considered and often preferred.

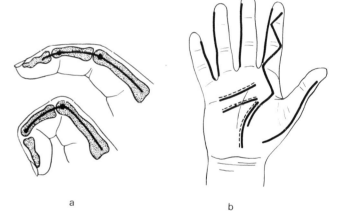

a   b

Figure 8.3
(a) The classical medio-lateral incision should be placed more dorsally than is usually seen, so as to not cross the PIP and DIP creases. It is placed on the side of the finger whose collateral nerve is damaged; if both are intact, the ulnar side of the index, long and ring-fingers and the radial side of the thumb and little finger. (b) Palmar incisions follow as much as possible the cutaneous creases or are placed a few millimetres parallel.

Bruner's 'zig-zag' incision can cover the whole length of the finger and palm, permitting large access and direct view of the flexor sheath. It can be used for primary and secondary operations. The disadvantages are: the tip of the triangle is on the path of the volar neurovascular bundles which must not be cut nor caught in closure of the wound; after repair of noble tissues necessitating flexion of the finger, access to the wound and closure are difficult; after tenolysis which demands immediate active mobilization, the palmar zig-zag can be awkward and its healing impaired. We therefore avoid zig-zag when there are concomitant nerve repairs, tenolysis or scarring of the volar surface of the finger. The same incision can be modified so that the angles are rounded to semi-circles and the diagonal line transformed into a transverse one at the middle of each phalanx (Simonetta). The problems described are for the most part avoided.

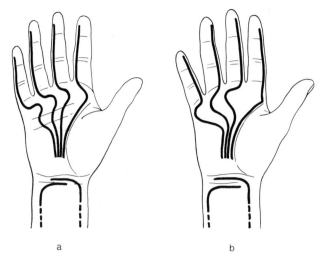

Figure 8.4
Long digito-palmar incisions used in: tenolyses over a long distance; concomitant nerve lesions; tendon grafts where large resections of the sheath are necessary; salvage of complex lesions needing an alloplastic stem to reconstitute a sheath and pulleys and repair nerves etc., and secondarily a tendon graft.

TECHNIQUES OF TENDON SUTURE

The numerous techniques seek to obtain:

1. A correct apposition of tendon ends after they have been trimmed.

2. Sufficient resistance to traction on an organ whose fasciculated longitudinal structure does not hold sutures.

All suture material represents a foreign body and increases the formation of granulation and scar tissue, source of adherences. Concerning the flexors, Lindsay (1960) and Potenza (1975) have shown how trauma to a tendon can be dangerous and cause adherences. Apart from the size of the thread, when tying the thread on tendinous fibres it necessarily happens that bundles are caught in the knot and become ischaemic, then necrotic, and hence increase the scar reaction.

For the flexors it is extremely important to remember that a principal source of nutrition enters by the vincula which must be treated with great care by avoiding exteriorization of the tendons when it is not essential. The tendons can be pushed back gently along their sheath by massage of the muscular mass and flexion of the wrist to make them accessible through the wound. They can be temporarily blocked by a small transverse Kirschner wire, placed proximally (Verdan, 1952, 1960) (cf. also Kleinert and Weiland's chapter).

Since the vessels run mostly along the dorsal surface, it is best to suture on the volar side of the tendon.

As for the suture itself, the principal aims are:

1. Use of fine but strong *material* which is physico-chemically inert and remains so in the tissues and does not provoke scar reaction.

2. Adopt a *technique* of suture that respects the nutritional conditions, hence the repair of the tendon.

3. Try to bury the zone of suture in an undamaged sheath by appropriate modification of the digital position.

Great progress has been made in this area over the last 20 years. Bunnell has shown the advantage of stainless steel wire, over cotton, linen, silk and all other materials used at that time. Mounted on a needle, these wires cause minimal tissue trauma, but they should not be used where tendons change direction, especially in curving over a hard surface, since ultimately they fragment and provoke irritation.

Currently synthetic materials notably nylon, are preferred as tissue tolerance has been shown to be comparable or even superior to stainless steel. The multi-strand fibres are fine, easily handled and very resistant to rupture. Mounted on needles they are completely satisfactory. In hand surgery calibres greater than 4–0 are rarely used, and for tendons in the digital canal, 5–0 for principal sutures and 6–0 for the closure of the epitendon, or small running sutures, allow remarkably precise anastomoses without excessive trauma to the tendon ends.

SUTURE TECHNIQUES

In the hope of avoiding adhesions endosynovial tendon sutures are isolated from the surrounding tissues. Lindsay and Potenza have discussed this problem at length. It is not my intention to repeat the different techniques, but to note the most pertinent sutures used:

1. In *endosynovial zones 1, 2 and 3*, the length of the digital canal of the fingers and thumb, Bunnell's pull-out technique (Figs. 8.5 and 8.6) is used when the lesion is close to the distal extremity; or a blocked suture (Fig. 8.7) (Verdan, 1960 or Kleinert's 1967 method is carried out.

2. In *extrasynovial regions* and *zones of rather free gliding* (topographical surgical zones 4, 5 and 7) sutures illustrated in figures 8.8. to 8.12 are most satisfactory.

At the wrist we, in Lausanne, have often used a suture adapted from Wilms' technique. Small lateral loops catch some tendinous bundles with a single thread knotted between the tendon ends and buried. Before tightening the third loop, one must assure proper contact between the two ends. The procedure is dependable, rapid and does not compromise the vascularisation of too many fibres. It can be completed by a few fine epitendinous stitches (Fig. 8.11).

Koch and Mason's simplified suture (Fig. 8.12) uses two threads knotted between the tendon ends. Precise apposition can also be completed by a few fine epitendinous stitches or a fine running suture.

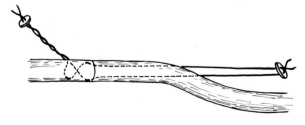

Figure 8.5
Pull-out wire of Bunnell.

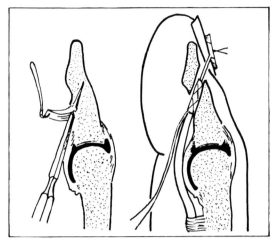

Figure 8.6
Intraosseous insertion into the distal phalanx by means of a stainless steel pull-out wire.

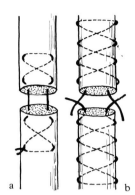

Figure 8.8
Shoe lace suture after Bunnell. (a) with one thread. (b) with two threads, tied with a knot between tendon ends.

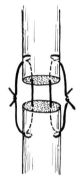

Figure 8.9
Two stitches firmly anchored around lateral fascicles, after Wilms and Sievers.

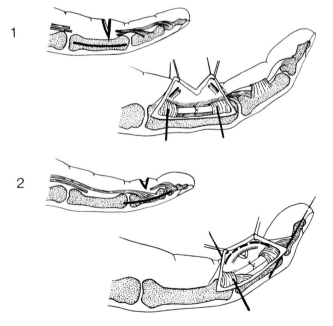

Figure 8.7
(1 & 2) Personal method of blocked suture. Verdan I: with two transverse pins; Verdan II: with one transverse proximal pin and a second placed longitudinally through the DIP joint (short distal end of tendon).

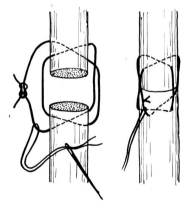

Figure 8.10
Double right angle stitch, after Bunnell; can be done quickly. In spite of its inaccuracy, it is helpful in cases where many tendons have to be repaired and the operation rapidly carried out.

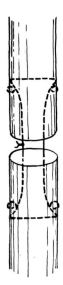

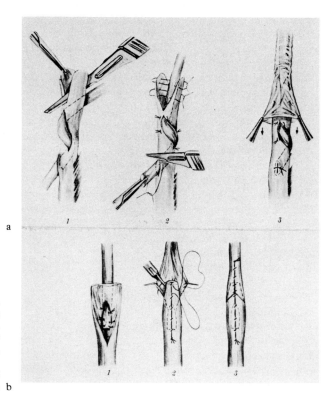

a

b

Figure 8.11
'Home stitch' utilized in Lausanne: lateral anchorage with small loops. One single thread knotted between tendon ends. Before tightening the third loop, make sure that the two tendon ends are in good contact. Safe procedure, rather quick, compromising the vascularization only of a few fibres. Can be completed by very fine adjustment stitches.

Finally, when two tendons of different calibre are joined, a method of interlacing (Pulvertaft) through two or three perforations (Fig. 8.13a) is used. The fine extremity is introduced into a slit of the thicker one. The thicker extremity whose centre has been excised in order to diminish its volume, is slit to form two flaps which are fixed by transverse 'U'-stitches. This procedure is particularly useful for grafting or transferring tendons. Brand's procedure (Fig. 8.13b) entails folding in of smaller into larger extremity.

But the best tolerated material is no material! The 'pull-out-wire' of Bunnell (Figs. 8.5 and 8.6) is based on this principle, as well as variations such as Jenning's 'barbed-wire' (Fig. 8.14) which is recommended in France by Allieu for certain extensor levels as well as for the distal reinsertion of the flexors.

Figure 8.13
(a) (1) and (2) Interlacing suture of two tendons of different calibres, ending with covering of the two tendons (3) with a sleeve of local para-tenon (e.g. palmaris longus). (b) (1) (2) and (3): intratendinous anasto-mosis after Brand.

Techniques of *lengthening* and *shortening* of tendons are based on general orthopaedic surgery procedures and will not be discussed here.

POST-OPERATIVE CARE

Whatever the material, the aim of tendon suture is not only restoration of a strong mechanical union but also *functional sliding of the tendon*. Thus the question has always been after what delay active mobilization can be allowed or encouraged. If immobilization allows fibroblasts to invade the tendinous

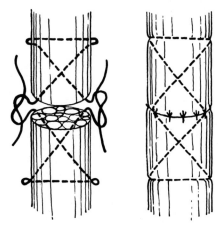

Figure 8.12
Simplified shoe-lace stitch, with two threads knotted between the tendon edges (Koch and Mason).

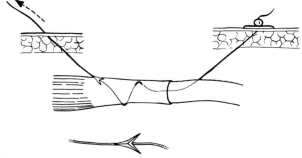

Figure 8.14
Instead of two stainless steel wires, one to make fast and another for pulling out, there is here only one thread with a barbed-wire (after Jennings).

extremities and form a scar mass, its prolongation leads to adhesions, loss of normal sliding and dystrophic problems related to poor peripheral circulation, and stiffening of the joints. This is especially true in elderly patients.

On the other hand, one can admit that early passive or active mobilization, even if only over a short distance, may distend the adherences and transform them into a kind of mesotenon, assuring a better sliding function; contrary to Mason and Allen's findings in 1941 based on experiments with dogs.

Recent experimental work by Urbaniak, Cahill and Mortenson, (1975) measured traction resistance of different types of tendon anastomoses. Stainless steel wire 4–0, Ethylon (nylon), Tevdek (braided polyester impregnated with teflon) and Mersilene (dacron) were compared using eight suture techniques:

1. Four interrupted simple stitches
2. Nicoladoni's intratendinous stitch
3. Side-to-side anastomosis
4. Mason and Allen's stitch
5. Bunnell's lace
6. Pulvertaft's interlacing fish mouth
7. Terminal enlacing
8. Wilm's lateral fixation stitch modified by Kessler.

The flexor tendons of dogs were chosen, all of the same calibre, sutured and immobilized in flexion. The animals were sacrificed at five-day intervals up to the 20th day.

The weakest sutures (*group 1*) were naturally those acting parallel to the collagenous fibres such as the interrupted stitches, Nicoladoni's stitch and the latero-lateral stitch.

In *group 2*, longitudinal tension is transformed into an oblique or transverse force on the tendon ends: in this group are Bunnell's lace, the Wilms-Kessler and Mason and Allen stitches. The two latter were stronger than the Bunnell lace.

Finally, *group 3* sutures including Pulvertaft's anastomosis show that there is no traction directly on the suture but rather perpendicular to the collagenous fibres of the tendon and the force exerted on them. Thus finer material can be used.

From Mason and Allen's work (1941) it is known that the force of resistance to rupture (equal to that of the thread) declines during the first 10 days due to softening of the tendon and lack of fixation of the thread. In the above experiment it was shown that after five days the resistance force of a Bunnell suture was a third that of a Kessler, whereas after 10 days there was no noticeable difference in the methods.

Stainless steel wire and Mersilene obtained similar early scarring results and all ruptures were due to stitches which tore out of the tendon and not the breaking of the thread.

Clinical problems make these experimental findings only partially relevant. Even though interlacing anastomoses are most resistant, they can only be used in loose tissue, surrounded by muscle or areolar connective tissue that permit them to slide. Mason and Allen's, Bunnell's and Wilms-Kessler's stitches are less resistant but allow more precise alignment of the ends when less space is available. Kleinert chose a simplified Bunnell's lace for his endosynovial sutures, reinforced by an epitendinous running stitch or a few fine 'U'-stitches. Our method (Fig. 8.7.) is based on total removal of traction forces by transverse blockage using a 0.7 mm diameter

pin passing through skin, soft tissue, sheath and tendon; a few epitendinous stitches using 6–0 then suffice. But these pins must remain in place for three weeks, and the immobilization of the finger causes other problems with which all are familiar.

This is also true for the anchoring of the flexors at the wrist according to Alnot and Duparc's (1974) technique, except that since the pin fixing the tendon does not traumatize the digital canal, adherences are less important. They occur at the suture line and at the wrist level where gliding is easier.

EVOLUTION OF IDEAS ON REPAIR OF FLEXOR TENDONS

Repair of flexor tendons in the digital canal has always been an absorbing problem. Other difficult subjects of tendon repair, such as that of the delicate extensor system do exist, but poor results in this area do not have such serious consequences; a failure in flexor repair can result in amputation of a finger.

Bunnell and his followers noted that primary suture of flexors in the digital canal nearly always resulted in failure and indicated the following directives:

1. If both tendons are sectioned in 'No man's land' (Fig. 8.15), i.e. in the region extending from the distal palmar crease to the proximal third of the middle phalanx:
   (a) close the skin
   (b) wait for the wound to heal
   (c) three weeks after the accident perform a major secondary intervention consisting of:
   i. resection of the two tendons
   ii. excision of the proximal end of the superficialis (or use it as a graft)
   iii. graft only the profundus (using palmaris longus, plantaris or a toe extensor) from the palm at the level of the lumbrical to the end of the finger, so as to

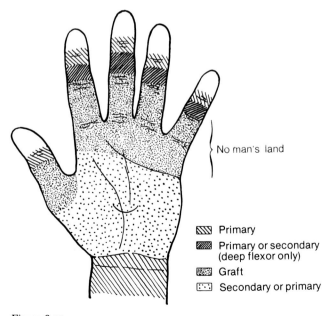

> No man's land

▨ Primary
▨ Primary or secondary (deep flexor only)
▨ Graft
▨ Secondary or primary

Figure 8.15
The 'No-man's land' of Bunnell.

avoid formation of a tendinous scar mass in the digital theca—a narrow inextensible canal in which the tendon must slide freely like a piston in a cylinder (cf. chapter by Boyes and Stark).

(d) or, if the proximal stump of profundus is not mobile enough, use the superficialis as moving element going from the wrist to the fingertip if need be.

2. If only profundus is damaged, never sacrifice superficialis for grafting profundus. Perform a simple *tenodesis* of the distal end (or a distal interphalangial arthrodesis) to avoid instability and hyperextension of the distal phalanx.

3. Finally, if profundus is sectioned near its peripheral insertion (up to 1.5 cm) reinsert it by resection of the distal end and insertion of the proximal end into the bone using a steel wire 'pull-out' technique.

Following these directives carefully in my early career, some results were good, others poor, and I could not predict the outcome. As a general rule we can say that the concomitant section of two neurovascular bundles is a cause of failure because of the serious dystrophic and vascular problems that result. Associated lesions such as fractured phalanges, opening of an articulation, wounds complicated by damage to the extensor system, crushed or bruised skin and all causes of articular stiffness and reduced passive flexibility of the finger can be causes for failure.

It must be recalled that fine, cutting, linear, clean wounds are quite different from lacerations and crush wounds and necessitate different therapeutic measures; a tendon wound must be treated as a part of the total trauma of which it is a result.

Over 25 years ago (Verdan, 1952) I first thought it possible to perform primary sutures of flexor tendons inside the digital theca. Bunnell's term 'No man's land' thus became abusive. My first attempts date back to 1950, the first communication being presented in 1959 in Chicago (Verdan, 1960). At the French orthopaedic congress of 1961 in Paris, Verdan and Michon proposed that the term 'No man's land' be abandoned in favour of a system of 7 topographical surgical zones, 'No man's land' corresponding to Zone II. (Verdan and Michon, 1961) (Figs. 8.15 and 8.16). The suture technique was that described in Fig. 8.7. Let us see under which circumstances this new attitude could be defended:

1. Firstly, my experience was obtained under particular conditions, i.e. an emergency service receiving patients shortly after the accident.

2. The wounds were mostly tidy ones, clean cut and not bruised; this is probably due to Lausanne's lack of heavy industry.

3. Others who adopted our point of view early: Michon in Nancy (1961), Duparc and Alnot in Paris (1974), M. Iselin and F. Iselin (1967), Bolton in England (1975) and Kleinert in the USA (1967) all worked under analogous conditions.

4. The results showed that primary suture correctly performed can give equally good or better results than a graft and at a lesser cost: time saved for the patient, less work incapacity and reduction or absence of hospitalization (Verdan and Crawford, 1971).

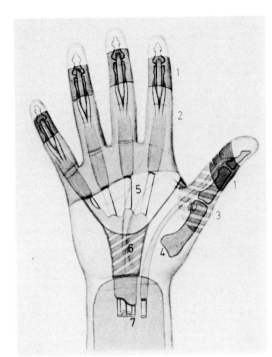

Figure 8.16
Our seven surgical topographic zones of flexor tendons.

5. However, *if the operation is not correctly performed the outcome is gravely compromised.*

The conditions *sine qua non* that such surgery can succeed are: perfect knowledge of anatomy, good anaesthesia, appropriate instrumentation and material, good atraumatic technique such that lining up the two ends is as precise as needed for nerve suture, good haemostasis and adequate bandages. Post-operative care and rehabilitation are also very important. Precise control of the suture is aided by use of a magnifying glass or microscope.

BASIC PRINCIPLES

1. Traction resistant sutures are not enough; a tendon is intended to slide!

2. Often so-called successful sutures are in reality tenodesis.

3. Remember a tendon is a living organ and not a simple cord, as its pearly white aspect may suggest.

4. For its nutrition a tendon has a very interesting delicate vascularization system (Fig. 8.18) which is elastic enough to allow it to follow the movements of the tendon (4 cm at the base of the fingers, 8 cm at the wrist!) in a cylinder closely adjusted to its piston. This nutritional system is assured by the mesotenons and vincula, whose rupture will cause an infarct of the tendon.

5. Note that arterial and venous vascularization is quite poor in the adult, whereas the lymphatic network is highly developed as we have shown with Setti (1972) (Fig. 8.17). This may explain the maintenance of a low cellular metabolic rate for the rare tenocytes.

6. Peacock (1959) has shown that the mesonutritional network is much more important than that which passes by the

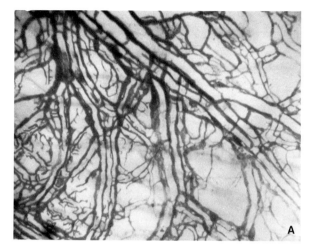

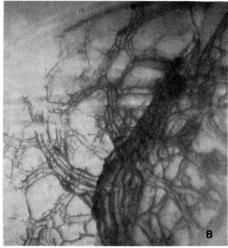

Figure 8.17
The lymphatic network, (A) Plexiform lymphatic system at the surface of tendon and sheath. (B) Lymphatic net inside a tendon. The lymphatics are accompanying blood vessels.

musculo-tendinous and osteotendinous junctions. Recent anatomical study by Caplan, Hunter and Merklin on seven to nine months old foetuses (1975) confirms the existence of two nutritional systems: paratendinous in the palm and mesotendinous in the digital canal. This explains why when a flexor tendon is deprived of its vascularization over a certain length, it can only survive through the invading conjunctive-vascular tissue which is full of neoformed capillaries; this tissue has its origin in the sheath and the wound, where we find 'vessel carrying' adhesions.

This is also true for scar formation which, in the digital canal, can only form from surrounding tissues and probably not from the tendinous ends. The very interesting recent experimental studies of Lundborg (1977) on rabbits (see Verdan, Chapter 1) are not for the moment able to modify our present understanding based on clinical experience and human anatomical findings. In other words, the 'unsatisfied' fibres do not emerge out from the ends, but on the contrary penetrate into them. Capillary buds try to anastomose with the intratendinous capillary and lymphatic networks in two ways:

1. by the mesotendons: this is the ideal way, shown experimentally by Potenza in his work on dogs; in this case sliding of the tendon is assured;

2. or by growing in a mass through the epitendon over a large surface. This produces 'vessel carrying' adhesions, which block sliding completely.

The tendon either dies or is completely immobilized. So we have to accept the inevitable adhesions, while attempting to create physical conditions conducive to final liberation of the tendon. We have three possibilities:

1. close the sheath after tendon suture (when possible), in order to diminish the surface of adhesions and create better nutritional conditions. If not possible:

2. excise primarily part of the fibrous sheath, which forces the adherences to grow on a soft environment which will permit detachment little by little of the adhesions by repeated exercise;

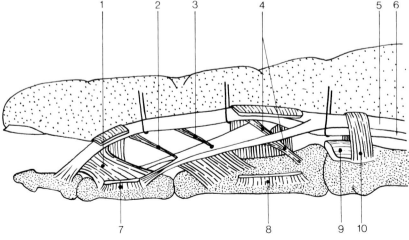

Figure 8.18
Schematic drawing of mesotenons and vincula: (1) Mesotenon; (2) (3) and (4) Vincula; (5) Fl. superficialis; (6) Fl. profundus; (7) Third pulley on middle phalanx; (8) Second pulley on proximal phalanx; (9) Volar plate of MP joint; (10) First pulley: fibrous annulus inserting on MP volar plate.

3. proceed with exterior liberation, a secondary tenolysis which can be an efficient measure as we showed at Stanford in 1970 (Verdan, 1971) (see also Verdan, chapter 18). This is true for sutures and for grafts as well with a few exceptions.

From the therapeutic point of view, mobilization at three weeks post-suture is a critical point. The recent adhesions must be carefully broken by active flexion and extension of the finger which the examiner holds lightly by the proximal phalanx. The middle and distal phalanges may then be passively extended, gently so as to detach or stretch the adhesions. Sometimes a slight cracking is audible. Little by little mobilization increases: during two weeks, most adhesions should be broken and at five to six weeks post suture resumption of work constitutes the best ergotherapy. This re-education is as important as the suture technique.

Kleinert has perfected an operational procedure and mobilization method which allow gentle mobilization during the first post-operative days based on two elements:

1. excellent modern suture material (notably Polydeck 4– 5– and 6–0);

2. immobilization of the wrist in flexion, with the finger held in moderate flexion by an elastic band fixed between the nail and the cast.

The suture is accomplished as a simplified shoe-lace completed by fine running stitches of the epitendon and removal of the steel pins, freeing the tendon immediately after suture (cf. chapter by Kleinert and Weiland).

Caplan, Hunter and Merklin (1975) showed that since the main vessels run longitudinally along the dorsal surface of the flexor digitorum profundus, stitches should be placed more on the volar than on the dorsal surface.

Tsuge (1975) proposed a suture hiding intratendinous sutures which also gave good results.

Immediate mobilization, contested by Mason and Allen (1942) has proved useful when performed on a very short distance under controlled conditions as shown by Kleinert (1967). Very careful daily passive mobilization, as advocated by Duran and Houser (1975) also seems to give good results.

Be it active or passive, the movements would seem to produce stretching of vessel-carrying adhesions, mostly on the dorsal face of the tendon. This distension seems to produce new mesos on the most useful strategic line. A post-mortem study would be necessary to prove this point.

We should also take into account techniques of tenolysis which respect some posterior loose adhesions, when their section is not necessary to obtain a total liberation of gliding.

Another aspect of the problem: when both flexor tendons are cut in Zone II it has been usually accepted that the superficialis be resected and the profundus sutured.

However, the vincula vascularizing the profundus pass through the superficialis where it becomes deep (Fig. 8.18). Resection of the superficialis would mean section of these precious vincula. So it is best to suture both tendons. We have done this since 1969, and the results in 1971 were very good, since 92 per cent achieved flexion 2.5 cm from the distal palmar crease (Verdan, Crawford and Martini, 1971).

In conclusion, our policy is to repair immediately all sectioned structures; tendons, nerves and even collateral arteries if possible—by means of microsurgical techniques—to avoid problems of trophicity.

In cases of bruised untidy wounds, seen under poor general and local conditions, they made us settle for debridement and closure of the skin using plastic surgery procedures. When the wound is quiet we will proceed to a secondary salvaging operation consisting first of formation of a new sheath. (Geldmacher, 1969). The sheath will be created around a Silastic stem or Hunter's rod, introduced in a first intervention during which nerves and destroyed pulleys must also be repaired. Sometimes this may be carried out as a primary procedure. Two to three months later after passive mobilization, a final tendon graft replaces the plastic rod.

This new procedure does not give miraculous results. It is simply a useful contribution in particularly difficult cases (Chamay, Verdan, Simonetta, 1975). The results are however encouraging us to proceed on that way.

As for the source of graft material, an exciting idea (Peacock, 1960 Hueston, 1967) proposed use of a total flexor system graft (both flexors in their sheath removed from a cadaver) to a patient whose flexors have been excised. The remarkable functional results show that the collagenous mass is capable of revascularization and recellularization.

Iselin uses a method of homoplastic tendon grafts ('tendon bank') preserved in Cialit 1/5000, a mercurial solution (Seiffert, 1966). They are in fact collagen fibres grouped into a tendinous structure totally lacking cells. The dead graft must be revascularized and recellularized just like Peacock's graft. Will it not have even more difficulty to glide than an autograft? We do not know.

REFERENCES

ALNOT, J.-Y. & DUPARC, J. (1974) Plaies rècentes des deux tendons fléchisseurs au doigt. *Rev. Chir. orthop.*, **60**, 531.

BOLTON, H. (1975) Primary tendon repair. In: *Proceedings of the Second Hand Club.* 5th meeting April 1958. London: British Society for Surgery of the Hand.

BUNNELL, St. (1956) *Surgery of the Hand.* 3rd edn. London: Pitman Med.

BUNNELL, St. & BOYES, J.-H. (1964) *Bunnell's surgery of the Hand.* 4th edn. Montreal: Pitman Med.

CAPLAN, H.-S., HUNTER, J.-M., & MERKLIN, R.-J. (1975) Intrinsic vascularization of flexor tendons. In: *Amer. Acad. Orthop. Surgeons. Symposium on Tendon Surgery in the Hand.* Saint-Louis: C.V. Mosby.

CHAMAY, A., VERDAN, Cl., & SIMONETTA, C. (1975) Les greffes de tendons fléchisseurs après implantation provisoire d'une tige en silicone. Etude et résultats de 32 cas. *Rev. Chir. Orthop.*, **61**, 599.

DURAN, R.-J., & HOUSER, R.-G. (1975) Controlled passive motion following flexor tendon repair. In: *Amer. Acad. Orthop. Surgeons. Symposium on Tendon Surgery in the Hand.* Saint-Louis: C. V. Mosby.

GELDMACHER, J. (1969) Die Zweizeitige freie Beugesehnentransplantation, *Handchirurgie*, **1**, 109.

HUESTON, J.-T. (1967) Cadaver homografts of the digital flexor tendon system. *Aust. N.Z. J. Surg.*, **36**, 184.

ISELIN, Fr. (1975) Preliminary observations on the use of chemically stored tendinous allografts in hand surgery. *Amer. Acad. Orthop. Surgeons. Symposium on Tendon Surgery in the Hand*. Saint-Louis: C. V. Mosby.

ISELIN, M. & ISELIN, Fr. (1967) *Traité de Chirurgie de la Main*. Paris: Méd. Flammarion.

KLEINERT, H.-E. *et al*. (1967) Primary repair of lacerated flexor tendons in No-man's land. *J. Bone Jt Surg.*, **49A**, 577.

KLEINERT, H.-E. & WEILAND, A.-J. (1976) La réparation primaire des plaies des tendons fléchisseurs en zone II. In: *Chirurgie des Tendons de la Main*. Monographie du GEM. Paris: Expansion Scientifique.

LINDSAY, W.-K. & THOMPSEN, H.-G. (1960) Digital flexor tendons: An experimental study. Part 1. The significance of each component of the flexor mechanism in tendon healing. *Brit. J. plast Surg.*, **12**, 289.

MASON, M.-L. & ALLEN, H.-S. (1941) Rate of healing of tendons; experimental study of tensile strength. *Ann. Surg.*, **113**, 424.

NICOLADONI, C. (1880) Ein Vorschlag zur Sehnennaht. *Wien. klin. Wschr*, **52**, 1413–1417.

PEACOCK, E.-E. (1959) A study of the circulation in normal tendons and healing grafts. *Ann. Surg.*, **3**, 149.

PEACOCK, E.-E. (1960) Homologous composite tissues grafts of the digital flexor mechanism in human beings. *Transplant. Bull.*, **7**, 418.

POTENZA, A.-D. (1975) Concepts of tendon healing and repair. *Amer. Acad. Orthop. Surgeons. Symposium on Tendon Surgery in the Hand*. Saint-Louis: C. V. Mosby Co.

POTENZA, A. (1976) Mécanisme de guérison des plaies tendineuses et des greffes des tendons fléchisseurs. Etude expérimentale. In: *Chirugie des Tendons de la Main*. Monographie du GEM. Paris: Expansion Scientifique. ed. Verdan.

SEIFFERT, K. (1966) *Biologische Grundlagen der homologen Transplantation Konservierter Bindegewebe*. Frankfurt: Habilitationsschrift vorgelegt medizinische Fakultät J. W. Goethe Universität.

SETTI, G.-C. & VERDAN, Cl. (1972) A study of the lymphatic circulation in flexor tendons. *Proceedings 12th Congress of the SICOT, Tel Aviv 1972*. Amsterdam: Excerpta Medica.

TSUGE, K. (1975) *Communication au VIe Congrès international de chirurgie plastique et reconstructive*. Paris.

URBANIAK, J., CAHILL, J. & MORTENSON, R. (1975) Tendon suturing methods: analysis of tensile strengths. *Amer Acad. orthop. Surgeons Symposium on Tendon Surgery in the Hand*. Saint-Louis: C. V. Mosby Co.

VERDAN, Cl. (1952) *Chirurgie réparatrice et fonctionnelle des tendons de la Main*. Paris: Expansion Scientifique Française.

VERDAN, Cl. (1960) Primary repair of flexor tendons. *J. Bone Jt Surg.*, **42A**, 647–657.

VERDAN, Cl. (1972) Die Eingriffe an Muskeln, Sehnen und Sehnenscheiden. In: *Allgemeine und Spezielle Chirurgische Operationslehre*. ed. Wachsmuth, W. & Wilhelm, A. Band X, Teil III. Heidelberg: Springer Verlag.

VERDAN, Cl., & CRAWFORD, G. (1971) *Transactions of the 5th Congress International Plastic and Reconstructive Surgery*. Melbourne: Butterworth.

VERDAN, Cl., CRAWFORD, G. & MARTINI, Y. (1971) Tenolysis in traumatic hand surgery. *Educational Foundation of the American Society of Plastic and Reconstructive Surgeons*. Vol. 3, *Symposium of the Hand*. Saint-Louis: C. V. Mosby Co.

VERDAN, Cl., & MICHON, J. (1961) Le traitement des plaies des tendons fléchisseurs des doigts. *Rev. Chir. orthop.*, **47**, 285.

9. *Flexor Tendon Suture in the Digital Canal*

C. Verdan G. P. Crawford

Despite the recent advances in our understanding of tendon physiology and its reparative processes, the therapeutic approach to severance of both flexor tendons in the digital canal remains controversial. The suggested solutions include primary or secondary suture with or without tenolysis, primary or secondary tendon graft (autograft or homograft), grafting of a homologous complete flexor mechanism, transfer of an adjacent sublimis, prosthetic tendon inserts, tenodesis and arthrodesis. In more extensive injuries with both nerves and arteries sectioned in a single digit, amputation is often advised. When the question of excising or repairing the sublimis in combination with some of the above procedures is added, the number of proposed alternative treatment regimens becomes enormous.

A fresh severance of the flexor digitorum profundus between its distal insertion and the junction between the proximal and the middle third of the middle phalanx (Verdan's Zone I cf. Fig. 8.16)—is generally best repaired by primary suture, with or without tendon advancement. In secondary repairs best treatment is not so obvious. Although the results of secondary suture are not as good as by primary suture, the authors prefer suture to a graft, tenodesis or arthrodesis, if local conditions are adequate.

The area of the greatest controversy is Bunnell's 'No man's land' (Verdan's Zone II). The commonest solution among trained hand surgeons—when both tendons are divided—is a secondary graft, attached to the profundus, combined with sublimis excision. This procedure may follow the injury from several weeks to several months. As reported by Fetrow (1967), a secondary tenolysis is required in 16 per cent of grafts (60 tenolyses out of 374 grafts performed by Pulvertaft) and the period of disability will range from three to six months or more. Good results from grafting (Boyes, 1950 and Pulvertaft, 1956, 1960) are not easily obtained. Such a treatment however remains the best when trained hand surgeons are not available at the time of initial care or where the wound is dirty.

But in fresh, clean wounds a direct tendon suture in the digital canal is possible. The sutures we have performed since 1951, using primary or secondary repair, even if it requires a secondary tenolysis (Verdan, Crawford and Martini, 1970), gives equal or better results than tendon grafting and shortens the period of disability.

PRESENT INVESTIGATION

During a five year period from January 1965 to January 1970, we operated on 76 patients for primary or secondary suture of the flexor tendons in the digital canal. Sixty-six of these patients were reviewed. Thirty-two of them had isolated profundus lesions in Zone I. The 34 remaining patients with 36 involved fingers, were Zone II injuries, 'No man's land', and the analysis of this group is the subject of this paper. We used Boyes's system (1955) to compare our results with those of the tendon grafts.

We included the digits which extend within 40 degrees (computed by adding the extension deficits of all joints) for the index and middle, and within 60 degrees of extension for the ring and little fingers. The distance between the tip and the distal palmar crease (DPC) for the middle, ring and little fingers, and the distal portion of the mid palmar crease for the index were recorded. We recognize the defect of this method in that a digit which touches the palm 1 cm from the distal palmar crease is obviously better than a digit which does not touch, even if it is 1 cm vertically off the crease (1961).

TECHNIQUE

The tendon repair is usually done through a classical dorso-lateral incision with little regard to the wound. The nerves, if damaged, are repaired at the end of the operation.

The tendon sheath is excised so that the site of the sutured tendon can freely glide without contacting the sheath. A knowledge of the tendon gliding amplitude at each level is necessary. The sheath excision is approximately 3 cm. The tendon is sutured with four epitendinous simple or U-shaped sutures using 5-0 or 6-0 siliconized silk. Such a weak suture is sufficient, once the proximal portion of the profundus has been proximally transfixed (blocked) by a fine transverse stainless steel pin through the adjacent skin and the sheath. Occasionally, when this pin is not used, the digit is held in flexion by a suture through the tip to the palmar skin. Three weeks later, the immobilization is removed, the pin is taken away and gentle active motion exercises begin.

RESULTS

This series included 34 patients with 36 fingers with Zone II injuries. Two patients had two fingers injured. The average age was 23 years with the range from 2–54 (Fig. 9.1). There were 20 males and 14 females. Sixteen of these patients had digital nerve lacerations, and of these, five had both digital nerves sectioned.

Of these 36 fingers, 31 had sufficient extension to be included in the Boyes evaluation system.

Among the five excluded cases, three were excluded because of extension deficits. One digit required amputation (following

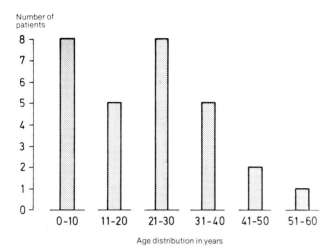

Figure 9.1
Age of the 29 patients (31 fingers)

a desperate attempt to save an index finger in a hand with a previous thumb amputation—the index damage included severance of both tendons, arteries and nerves). One patient underwent a secondary tendon graft following a poor result from primary repair and the final result was excellent. It is interesting to note that among the five excluded fingers three had both digital nerves sectioned.

Of the 31 included fingers, 15 were primarily treated and 16 secondarily, 12 digits required secondary tenolysis to give a better result. Three possibilities existed: both tendons were sutured, the profundus was sutured and the sublimis excised, the profundus alone had been severed and was repaired (Fig. 9.2).

SUTURE OF THE PROFUNDUS AND THE SUBLIMIS

This double suture of severed tendons in 'No man's land' has been only performed recently with encouraging results. It is an obvious improvement when compared with other known techniques. Its adoption was prompted by a desire to preserve the vascular tendon supply through the vincula or mesotenons. These vessels are usually injured during sublimis resection.

Fourteen fingers in 14 patients had surgical repair of both tendons in Zone II. Ten of these were repaired as the primary treatment and four secondarily. The age average in this group

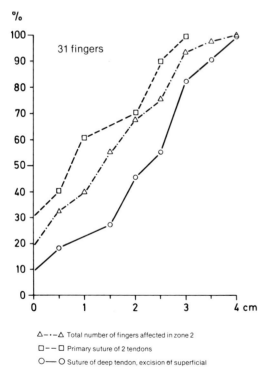

Figure 9.2
This table compares the flexion ability of 31 fingers with 10 fingers having primary suture of both tendons, and 11 fingers with sublimis excision.

Triangles: total of severed fingers in Zone II
Squares: primary suture of both tendons
Circles: suture of profundus, excision of sublimis.

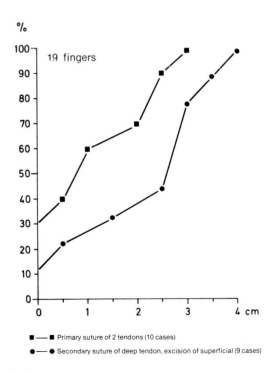

Figure 9.3
This table eliminates the two cases of primary profundus repair with sublimis excision. In this way the primary and secondary factors may clearly appear.

Squares: primary suture of both tendons (10)
Circles: secondary suture of profundus, excision of sublimis (9)

was 24 years; five were children of whom the eldest was nine years old.

Five of these fingers had one digital nerve and two had both nerves injured.

As noted on Fig. 9.2, 90 per cent were able to flex to within 2.5 cm (1 inch) from the distal palmar crease.

SUTURE OF THE PROFUNDUS WITH SUBLIMIS EXCISION

In 11 digits, the sublimis was excised when the profundus was repaired, two primarily and nine secondarily. In five cases, there was also one collateral nerve division, and in one case both nerves were severed.

In this group only 55 per cent (Fig. 9.3) were able to flex to within 2.5 cm of the distal palmar crease.

SUTURE OF THE PROFUNDUS

Six digits involved only profundus severance although the anatomical site of the lesion was in Zone II. Two cases were seen initially and primary repairs were performed. One case had an associated nerve lesion. All six digits were able to flex to within 2.5 cm from the distal palmar crease.

COMPARISON OF PRIMARY AND SECONDARY REPAIR

As seen on the figures, fresh clean lacerations of both tendons were usually treated by both tendons repair.

In secondary repairs the sublimis was usually excised.

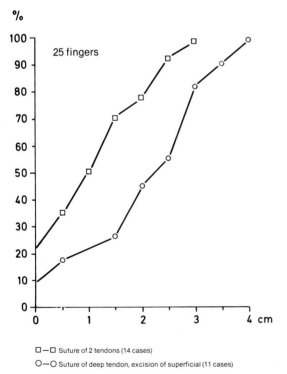

Figure 9.4
Compares the results of 25 fingers with both tendons severed, regardless whether primary or secondary suture was performed.

Squares: suture of both tendons
Circles: suture of the profundus with sublimis excision

Fig. 9.5 compares the results of our Zone II repairs regarding primary or secondary treatment. Sixty-eight per cent of secondarily sutured cases could flex to at least within 2.5 cm from the distal palmar crease, while 95 per cent of primarily repaired cases could flex at least within 2.5 cm.

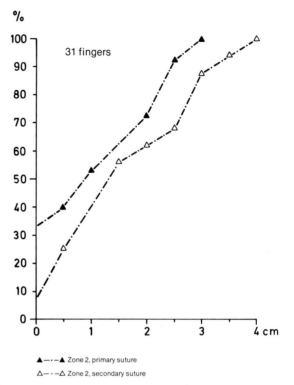

Figure 9.5
Compares all 31 cases taking into account only primary and secondary treatment.

Black triangle: primary suture (Zone II)
White triangle: secondary suture (Zone II)

DISCUSSION

As we advocated long ago (Verdan, 1952, 1958, 1960), flexor tendon suture in almost any region, when performed by trained hand surgeons, gives excellent results. We believe that primary tendon repair in clean cut wounds in the canal will yield equal or better results than tendon grafting. This point of view has been confirmed by other authors. Of course, such results are achieved faster than with secondary grafts, thereby shortening the period of unemployment and lowering the associated medical costs.

The previous reliance in tendon grafts is certainly too rigid. We know that good results may be reached with secondary suture, but the results with primary suture are obviously better. In primary repair both tendons may be sutured, but 30–40 per cent will require a secondary tenolysis. In our series only four cases had secondary repair of both tendons, and the results of these were not different from the primary group; but the number of secondary cases is too small for definitive statements. It should be noticed that the results of profundus suture with sublimis excision were inferior and that these cases were done secondarily (nine out of 11 fingers).

Fig. 9.4 compares the digits with both tendons severed, regardless of whether primary or secondary suture was performed.

Suture of sublimis and profundus (14 cases) give usually a better result than suture of the profundus alone with sublimis excision.

The immediate suture of both tendons allow a better pre-servation of tendon vascularization through vincula and lowers adhesions between surrounding tissues and suture. This may be the reason for our good results. And Fig. 9.5 comparing primarily and secondarily repair shows that immediate suture gives better results.

So primary suture of the sublimis also seems to be an improvement in flexor tendon repair and has to be taken into consideration.

REFERENCES

BOLTON, J. (1970) Primary tendon repair-The hand. *J. Brit. Soc. Surg. of the Hand*, **2**, No. 1.

BOYES, J.-H. (1950) Flexor tendon grafts in the fingers and thumb. An evaluation of end results. *J. Bone Jt Surg.*, **32-A**, 489.

BOYES, J.-H. (1955) *6th International Congress of Sicot in Berne, Switzerland, 1954.* Bruxelles: Imprimerie Lielens.

FETROW, K.-O. (1967) Tenolysis in the hand and wrist. *J. Bone Jt Surg.*, **49-A**, 667.

KLEINERT, H.-E., KUTZ J.-E., ASHBELL, S.-T., & MARTINEZ, E. (1967) Primary repair of lacerated flexor tendons in no man's land. *J. Bone Jt Surg.*, **49-A**, 577.

MADSEN, E. (1970) Delayed primary suture of flexor tendons cut in the digital sheath. *J. Bone Jt Surg.*, **52-B**, No. 2.

McCASH, C.-R. (1961) The immediate repair of flexor tendons. *Brit. J. plast. Surg.*, **14**.

PULVERTAFT, R.-G. (1956) Tendon grafts for flexor tendon injuries in the fingers and thumb. *J. Bone Jt Surg.*, **38-B**, 175–194.

PULVERTAFT, R.-G. (1960) The treatment of profundus division by free tendon graft. *J. Bone Jt Surg.*, **42-A**, 1363.

VERDAN, Cl. (1952) *Chirurgie réparatrice et fonctionnelle des tendons de la main.* Paris: Expansion Scientifique française.

VERDAN, Cl. (1958) La réparation immédiate des tendons fléchisseurs dans le canal digital. *Acta orthop. Belg.*, **24**, suppl. 3.

VERDAN, Cl. (1960) Primary repair of flexor tendons. *J. Bone Jt Surg.*, **42-A**, 647.

VERDAN, Cl. & MICHON J. (1961) Le traitement des plaies des tendons fléchisseurs des doigts. *Rev. Chir. orthop.*, **47**, 285.

VERDAN, Cl. (1966) Primary and secondary repair of flexor and extensor tendon injuries. In: *Hand-surgery.* ed. Flynn, J. E. Baltimore: Williams and Wilkins Co.

VERDAN, Cl., CRAWFORD, G.-P. & MARTINI-BENKED DACHE, Y. (1970) Tenolysis in traumatic hand surgery. *Stanford Univ.*, Saint-Louis: C. V. Mosby.

10. *Primary Repair of Flexor Tendon Lacerations in Zone II*

H. E. Kleinert A. J. Weiland

Primary repair of flexor tendon injuries within the flexor digital sheath has been one of the most difficult problems in hand surgery. The poor results of tendon repair within the pulley area caused Bunnell (1947) to coin the phrase 'No man's land'. Verdan subsequently described this region as Zone II (Fig. 10.1). Anatomically it consists of that portion of the fibro-osseous canal between the first annular pulley and the flexor digitorum superficialis insertion.

Improved techniques have recently permitted successful primary repair of flexor tendons within the fibro-osseous tunnel but at the same time have aroused controversy. Successful primary repair should be our goal (Kleinert *et al.*, 1973). It has several advantages:

1. The injury is taken care of immediately and there is less time off work.

2. Most patients can be treated on an outpatient basis with less expense to the patient and the community.

3. Less surgical dissection is necessary and since no donor tendon is required, there is less discomfort to the patient.

4. There is only one operative procedure.

The likelihood of the inexperienced or unqualified surgeon attempting primary tenorrhaphy is the greatest disadvantage in encouraging the use of this technique. Such ill-advised attempts end in a scarred, contracted finger that may be impossible to restore with a secondary grafting procedure.

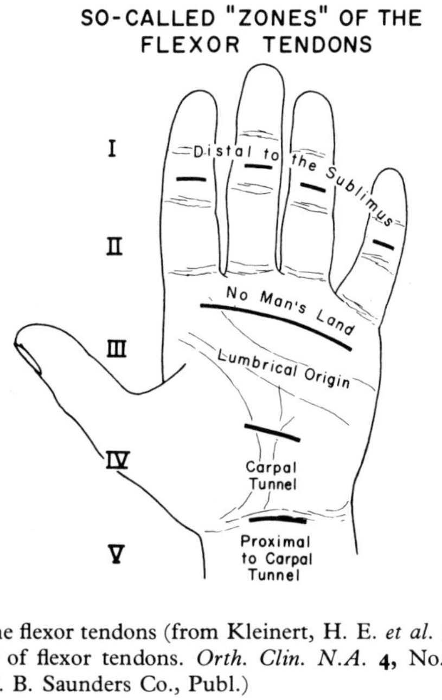

Figure 10.1
'Zones' of the flexor tendons (from Kleinert, H. E. *et al.* (1973) Primary repair of flexor tendons. *Orth. Clin. N.A.* **4**, No. 4, 866. Courtesy W. B. Saunders Co., Publ.)

ANATOMY

Within this region the flexor digitorum superficialis and flexor digitorum profundus lie juxtaposed as they pass through the fibro-osseous canal separated from each other and the surrounding canal by only a film of synovial fluid. The fibro-osseous canal is a closely applied semi-rigid tunnel through which the tendons pass. The fibrous portion of the canal is comprised of three annular pulleys (Fig. 10.2). The first is at the metacarpophalangeal joint level. It attaches to the junction of the volar plate and the deep transverse intermetacarpal ligament. The second and third pulleys are at the mid portions of the proximal and middle phalanges. They attach firmly to the volar lateral ridges of the phalanges. Between each annular pulley is a cruciform portion which is more filmy, flexible and overlies each joint. The second and third pulleys are the most important elements of the system. The floor of the fibro-osseous canal is the volar aspect of the phalanges and volar plates of the metacarpals and proximal interphalangeal joints.

The flexor digitorum superficialis enters the fibro-osseous canal volar to the profundus and splits just beyond the first pulley. Each slip rotates 180 degrees as it passes lateral and then dorsal to the profundus. Once dorsal to the profundus, the two slips rejoin and decussate forming Camper's chiasm before passing distally to insert at the mid middle phalanx. This creates a sloping ring aperture through which the profundus passes to become superficial to the decussation. The flexor digitorum profundus has an excursion between 2.7 and 3 cm while the flexor digitorum superficialis moves 0.5 to 0.75 cm less (Kaplan, 1959). The capacity for synchronous full range of motion requires smooth gliding of the tendons against the fibro-osseous canal and upon its mate. The close approximation of the tendons to each other and to the surrounding sheath and the lack of any surrounding loose areolar tissue provide little leeway for scar formation. The smallest cicatrix will tend to be rigid and limit motion.

The tendon blood supply is limited. Arteries pass through four folds of mesotenon termed vincula. The short vinculum of the profundus arises at the neck of the middle phalanx. It attaches to the profundus as a short flat sheet just proximal to its insertion. The short vinculum of the superficialis arises at the level of the neck of the proximal phalanx and enters the superficialis either in the centre of the chiasm or as two branches entering each slip separately. The arterial supply to these vincula comes through transverse branches of the digital arteries. The long vincula of the profundus arise from the decussation of superficialis and enter the profundus more proximally than the short vincula. The intratendinous blood supply has been

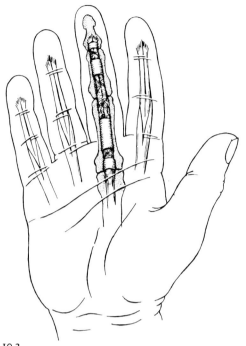

Figure 10.2
The fibro-osseous canal in Zone II is comprised of three annular and two cruciform pulleys. (From Kleinert, H. E. *et al.* (1975) *Primary Repair of Zone II Flexor Tendon Lacerations. Symposium on Hand Tendon Surgery*, Chapter 11. Courtesy C. V. Mosby Co., Saint Louis.)

shown to be primarily dorsal arising from the musculotendinous junction proximally and the insertion distally (Kaplan *et al.*, 1975).

TECHNIQUE

All repairs are carried out under axillary block using 1 per cent Carbocaine which is effective for three to four hours or if a longer block is required 0.5 per cent Marcaine provides 12 to 18 hours of anaesthesia. The hand is prepared, finger nails cleaned and trimmed, and the injured part is washed for 10 minutes. All patients are given prophylactic antibiotics. The arm is draped and irrigation of the wound is performed with Ringers lactate followed by $\frac{1}{4}$ per cent Neomycin solution. If the wound is contaminated several litres of Ringers lactate may be delivered using a surgical jet lavage. The arm is elevated and exsanguinated and the pneumatic tourniquet inflated. Loupe magnification of 2.5 × is routinely used.

It is important to note the position of the hand at the time of injury. If the finger is cut in flexion the distal end will be distal to the wound, while if lacerated in extension the distal end will be found at the level of the skin wound (Fig. 10.3).

Extension of the wound using a volar zig-zag or dorsolateral incision should be in a distal direction if necessary to adequately expose the distal cut tendon.

The dissection proceeds carefully to avoid further damage to the fibro-osseous canal. All questionably viable tissue and

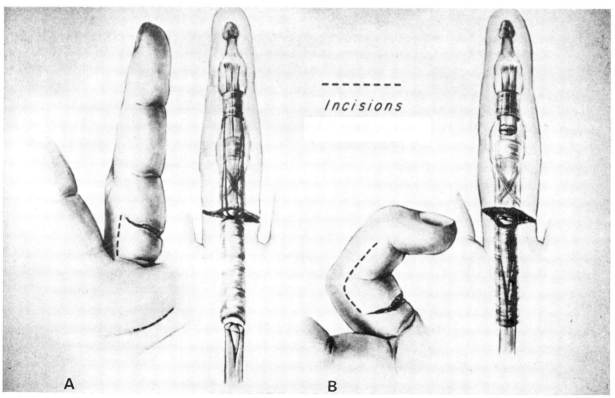

Figure 10.3 A, B
Exposure is important for atraumatic repair. Note distal location of severed tendon when finger is lacerated in flexion. (from Kleinert, H.

E. *et al* (1973) Primary Repair of Flexor Tendons. *Orth. Clinics N.A.* **4,** 866. Courtesy W. B. Saunders Co.)

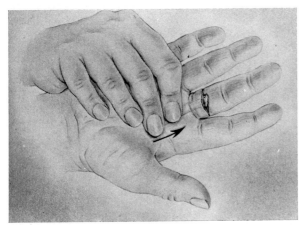

Figure 10.4
Wrist and finger flexion coupled with milking the forearm and hand will usually bring the proximal tendon stump into the wound. (from Kleinert, H. E. *et al.* (1975) *Primary Repair of Zone II Flexor Tendon Lacerations. Symposium on Hand Tendon Surgery*, Chapter 11. Courtesy C. V. Mosby Co., Saint-Louis.)

foreign material are debrided. Only sufficient overlying tendon sheath is windowed to permit adequate exposure for repair. Preservation of the pulley is necessary to prevent bowstringing of the tendon. In addition wherever sheath or pulley is excised, the tendon is exposed to a large area of raw fibrous tissue and extensive adhesions may occur.

The proximal tendon is often tethered by the vincula and prevented from withdrawal into the palm. Wrist and finger flexion coupled with milking the forearm and hand will usually bring the proximal tendon stump into the wound (Fig. 10.4). If the tendon has retracted into the palm proximal to the pulley a palmar incision is often required to pass the tendon into the canal. The tendon ends are brought into the wound and handled only by the cut surface. A temporary block with a

small Keith needle through the proximal tendon relieves suture line tension during the repair.

In a clean, sharply incised laceration no tendon debridement is required. If the tendon cut surface is ragged it may be recut with a straight razor blade. A criss-cross 4–0 Mersilene stay suture is placed. The cross limbs are placed at least 1 cm from the cut end of the tendon. The suture. is placed in the volar one half of the tendon to avoid additional vascular compromise. The suture is tied so there is no puckering or an accordian effect. A 6–0 or 7–0 running suture started opposite the knot of the 4–0 suture with a temporary long end provides no touch control of the tendon. This circumferential suture is placed co-apting only the epitenon in 1 mm bites. After the volar running suture is completed the tendon is reversed in a fashion similar to vessel repair and the dorsal epitenon is approximated. All loose ends are satisfied leaving a smooth suture line (Fig. 10.5). The flap or window in the fibro-osseous sheath, necessary to gain exposure, may be replaced and tacked with interrupted 5–0 Mersilene to reconstruct an intact sheath.

The tourniquet is released, pressure is held until the arterial flush has passed and complete haemostasis is obtained with either ligatures of 6–0 dexon or bipolar bovie to prevent haematoma formation. The skin is closed with multiple fine interrupted 6–0 nylon sutures. A double loop of 5–0 nylon is passed through the nail and knotted. A rubber band is attached. A thin, nonconstrictive dressing is applied to the wound. A dorsal plaster splint is constructed with the wrist flexed approximately 30 degrees short of full flexion, and blocking full extension of the metacarpophalangeal and interphalangeal joints. The position is obtained by holding the arm pronated, elbow extended and supported under the distal humerus. The splint extends beyond the involved finger tips to the high forearm and has bilateral side supports for strength. In children it is essential to apply a long arm plaster to prevent loosening of this splint and dressing. A loosely applied ace elastic bandage

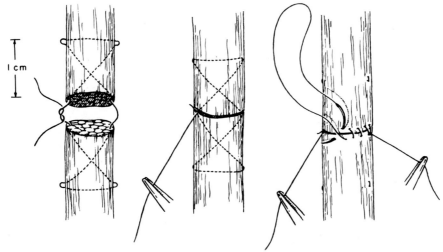

Figure 10.5
Technique of primary tendon repair. The tendon ends are approximated by a single criss-cross stay suture. Accurate smooth tendon anastomosis by circumferential suture completes the repair. (from Kleinert, H. E. *et al.* (1975) *Primary Repair of Zone II Flexor Tendon Lacerations. Symposium on Hand Tendon Surgery*, Chapter 11. Courtesy C. V. Mosby Co., Saint-Louis.

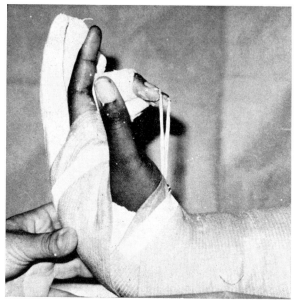

Figure 10.6
The repaired digit is immobilized in a dorsal plaster splint to maintain the finger and wrist in moderate flexion. (From Kleinert, H. E. *et al.* (1975) *Primary Repair of Zone II Flexor Tendon Lacerations. Symposium on Hand Tendon Surgery*. Chapter 11. Courtesy C. V. Mosby Co. Saint-Louis.

is used for an overwrap. The rubber band is placed on traction and a safety pin fastened proximal to the wrist and taped to hold position (Fig. 10.6).

The dynamic rubber band traction applied to the finger nail holds the finger in flexion but permits active extension to zero degrees. During finger extension the flexor muscle relaxes by

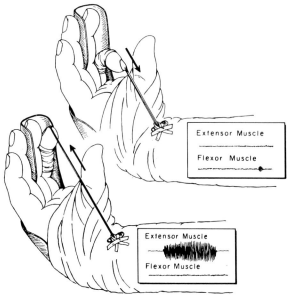

Figure 10.7
Synergistic relaxation of extrinsic flexor muscles using rubber-band splinting. (From Kleinert, H. E. *et al.* (1975) *Primary Repair of Zone II Flexor Tendon Lacerations. Symposium on Hand Tendon Surgery*. Chapter 11. Courtesy C. V. Mosby Co. Saint-Louis.

synergistic reaction. On attempted flexion the rubber band immediately flexes the finger, removes tension on the tendon juncture, and lessens the likelihood of rupture as the flexor muscle contracts (Fig. 10.7).

After three weeks the splint is removed and active exercises begun. The patient is instructed not to use his hand for any power function and no passive extension is allowed. At six weeks assistive extension and dynamic and static splinting may be used to increase extension if indicated. The patient is followed closely during the interval

Results

We have performed over 400 primary digital tenorrhaphies within the flexor digital sheath. A combination of gradings by White (1956) and Boyes (1947) was used to evaluate these cases.

Excellent: Flex within 1 cm of distal palmar crease with less than 15 degrees loss of extension.

Good: Flex within 1.5 cm of distal palmar crease with less than 30 degrees loss of extension.

Fair: Flex within 2 to 3 cm of distal palmar crease with more than 30 degrees loss of extension but less than 50 degrees.

Poor: Greater value of distance to distal palmar crease, or extension or both.

More than 75 per cent of the patients have obtained good or excellent function. There were four types of repair: repair of the superficialis with intact profundus, repair of the profundus with intact superficialis, repair of both superficialis and profundus, and excision of the superficialis and repair of the profundus only.

As expected, all digits with laceration and repair of the superficialis only had excellent function postoperatively. Over 82 per cent of the patients had good or excellent function when both superficialis and profundus were cut and both were repaired. Less than 70 per cent obtained good results after excision of the cut superficialis and repair of the profundus. Practically all cases of primary repair rupture were in this group and this accounted for most of the poor results. When the profundus only was cut and repaired a good to excellent result was achieved in 79 per cent of the cases. Surprisingly, nearly 70 per cent good or excellent results were obtained in crushing injuries many with associated fractures (Kleinert, *et al.*, 1973). Age of the patients ranged from 1 to 92 years, and as would be expected, the best results were obtained in patients age 10 or less. Tenolysis is done when required (18 per cent of the cases) but not until six months after repair and then only if function fails to show continued improvement.

A more recent study of 79 tendon injuries occurring in Zone II revealed 75 per cent excellent or good results compared to 84.4 per cent excellent or good results in other zones. However, when both tendons in Zone II were repaired 85.7 per cent of the patients had good or excellent results compared to 42.9 per cent when only the profundus was repaired and the sublimis excised. The results in Zone II were as good as the results in

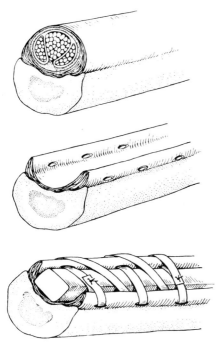

Figure 10.8
Weilby digital pulley reconstruction using the fibrous rim of the previous pulley and a free tendon graft.

other zones when both tendons were repaired (Lister, personal communication).

We feel that the sublimis should be repaired because it provides a gliding bed for the profundus in addition to preserving an intact blood supply to the profundus. The intact sublimis also functions as a check ligament of the proximal interphalangeal joint, allows for greater individual finger motion and increases finger power. It also lessens chance of rupture of the repair.

When pulley reconstruction is required we employ the technique described by Dr Andreas Weilby of Copenhagen using a woven tendon graft through the remains of the fibro-osseous canal to restore a strong pulley that will permit immediate motion (Weilby, personal communication). The strength of this reconstructed pulley is derived from its attachment to the fibrous rims of the fibro-osseous canal that remains even when the original pulley sheath is destroyed.

A free tendon graft is obtained in the usual manner from available donor sites and is split to allow a graft of approximately 4 cm in length and 0.25 cm in width. The border or rim of the fibro-osseous tunnel is carefully identified over the proximal phalanx and middle portion of the middle phalanx. Multiple perforations are made through the fibro-osseous rim. The split tendon graft is then passed through these perforations over the tip of the flexor tendon with the use of a small pointed haemostat in a weave fashion. The weave is anchored to the rim with a nonabsorbable suture with each weave and tension is adjusted to allow tendon excursion beneath the graft with minimal resistance to motion (Fig. 10.8).

SUMMARY

Primary repair of flexor tendon injuries within the fibro-osseous tunnel is a controversial subject. In the past flexor tendon graft was the established and accepted method for treating these injuries. Improved techniques in primary tenorrhaphy within the flexor digital sheath has produced results at least equal to those with flexor tendon graft. Review of our cases shows that the results in Zone II were as good as those obtained in other zones when both the sublimis and profundus tendons were repaired.

The likelihood of the inexperienced or unqualified surgeon attempting primary tenorrhaphy is the greatest disadvantage in encouraging the use of this technique. Such ill-advised attempts at primary tenorrhaphy end in a scarred, contracted finger that may be impossible to restore with a staged tendon graft procedure.

REFERENCES

Boyes, J. H. (1947) Immediate versus delayed repair of the digital flexor tendons. *Ann. West. Med. Surg.* **1**, 145–152.

Bunnell, S. (1918) Repair of tendons in the fingers and description of two new instruments. *Surg. Gyn. & Obst.* **26**, 103.

Caplan, H. S., Hunter, J. M. & Merklin, R. J. (1975) Intrinsic vascularization of flexor tendons in the human. Presented at *Amer. Soc. Surg. of the Hand*, San Francisco.

Kaplan, E. (1959) The structural and functional anatomy of the hand. 2nd edn. Philadelphia: Lippincott.

Kleinert, H. E., Kutz, J. E., Atasoy, E. & Stormo, A. (1973) Primary repair of flexor tendons. *Orth. Clin. N.A.* **4**, No. 4, 865–876.

Verdan, C. (1960) Primary repair of flexor tendons. *J. Bone Jt. Surg.* **42-A**, 647–657.

White, W. L. (1956) Secondary restoration of finger flexion by digital tendon grafts: an evaluation of seventy-six cases. *Amer. J. Surg.* **91**, 662.

11. *The Intact Sublimis*

E. A. Nalebuff

The restoration of active digital flexion in patients who have injured both flexor tendons is one of the most perplexing problems of hand surgery. It is a problem that is not yet fully solved. The difficulty in achieving full mobility following flexor tendon repairs within the digital sheath is well recognized. However, one aspect of flexor tendon surgery which deserves separate consideration is the treatment of those patients who have lost the profundus action but have an intact sublimis. These patients differ in several important ways from patients who have had both tendons cut: the functional loss is less, the prognosis is better, and the diagnosis is more subtle. Because of the anatomical relationship of the flexor digitorum profundus to the other flexor tendons, it becomes vulnerable to an external wound over the distal portion of the middle phalanx where it passes through the bifurcation of the superficial flexor. It is from this point distally that it can be divided without an injury to the superficial flexor. However, isolated damage of the flexor digitorum profundus can occur in other ways. For example, an isolated rupture of the deep flexor can result from an excessive strain applied to its terminal attachment. Certain disease processes such as rheumatoid arthritis can weaken its substance and cause spontaneous rupture by attrition either at the wrist or within the palm.

In this chapter I shall discuss our approach with patients who have an intact sublimis, an approach that minimizes the risk of further impairment of digital function and is usually successful in improving the remaining function. Many forms of treatment have been advocated for patients with an intact sublimis. These include *primary or secondary repair or advancement, fusions, tenodesis,* and even the insertion of *flexor tendon grafts.* Little wonder that confusion exists regarding the proper management of this condition. I shall try to clarify the situation by describing our indications for each surgical procedure.

DIAGNOSIS

The diagnosis of a flexor digitorum profundus rupture is often missed initially. With the presence of an intact, fully functioning sublimis, the remaining digital function is good. When one compares this to the circumstances of a traumatic rupture, it is easy to understand how this occurs. For example, a typical patient may be a football player who injured his finger attempting a tackle. The momentary discomfort is shrugged off by both the player and the trainer as a sprain. Usually, he continues to play and it is only later that the loss of distal joint flexion is noted. Another example is the patient with rheumatoid arthritis, who lives with intermittent or constant discomfort. The slight alteration in digital flexion is first looked upon

as a temporary nuisance. A complete evaluation and diagnosis may not be made until the hand is examined as a result of other more significant changes. Another example is patients with small lacerations on the volar aspect of the finger who are usually given a cursory examination to determine the presence of sensation and the ability to flex the finger. The loss of profundus action is overlooked in the excitement of the injury and the emergency care. Later, the patient notices a lack or weakness of terminal flexion and re-examination by a more experienced doctor clarifies the diagnosis.

Actually, the diagnosis of the isolated profundus lesion should be easy. It requires suspicion or awareness plus a thorough clinical examination. As a general rule, one may assume that *all longitudinal structures passing the site of laceration are divided until proven otherwise.* With this in mind one is unlikely to overlook the divided flexor digitorum profundus. It is not necessary to inspect the depth of the wound in order to make the diagnosis. An altered digital posture should alert the examiner. The distal joint of the involved finger stays in less flexion than the adjacent digits. An individual testing of the range and strength of active flexion of the terminal joint should confirm the diagnosis. Once the diagnosis has been made, either initially in the emergency ward or at some later date, one must then further evaluate the situation. Three factors that need to be determined are:

1. *the level of tendon injury*
2. *the degree of tendon retraction* and
3. *the functional capacity of the remaining superficial flexor.*

Certainly the patient's age and occupation as well as the over-all functional loss should also be considered. All else being equal, the three aforementioned factors are the most useful in determining the proper treatment for each individual case.

The level of skin laceration does not necessarily indicate the level of tendon division. This relationship depends upon the position of the finger at the time of injury. If the digit was in acute flexion, then the cut tendon will be distal to the skin injury. For example, the patient might have a skin laceration over the proximal phalanx, yet the tendon division could be beyond the sublimis bifurcation in an area where repair could be considered. The reverse, of course, it true. A distal skin cut over the middle phalanx might have occurred in extension leaving the cut flexor tendon ends more proximal within the flexor tendon sheath deep to the superficial flexor.

A factor closely related to the level of tendon injury is that of tendon retraction. If the laceration is distal to the vinculum, the tendon may not retract significantly. The gap between the cut tendon and distal attachment is small. Attempts at spontaneous healing may restore some limited active motion to the distal joint which adds to the difficulty of making a diagnosis in a late case. The vincula are particularly helpful in keeping the flexor digitorum profundus within the digit in a traumatic tendon rupture. Sometimes X-rays are helpful when a small bone fragment is pulled off the distal phalanx and can be seen in the soft tissues over the middle phalanx. With division more proximal the tendon retracts into the tendon sheath over the proximal phalanx or into the palm where it adheres to the surrounding structures. These adhesions may cause a tenosynovitis and adhesions which subsequently reduce sublimis function. The location of the proximal tendon is an important fact in determining the proper treatment. Palpation of the digit is helpful in making this determination. The lack of fullness distally in the presence of a tender swelling in the palm indicates proximal retraction. In this position the tendon thickens and ultimately shortens making attempts at later repair or advancement futile.

The most significant function to determine as part of the evaluation is the extent of the remaining superficial flexor function. Ideally, the sublimis should be functioning normally. In those patients who have normal digital extension as well as flexion of the finger to the palm, the functional loss may be slight. The need for treatment then depends upon the patient's occupation, age, and which digit is involved. A patient who has some terminal joint stability might not require any treatment. In this situation a diagnosis and explanation to the patient usually are all that is necessary. In other patients with significant functional loss, surgery should be undertaken to improve over-all digital function.

TREATMENT

Although the operative procedures advocated for this condition are many, and the timing of treatment is controversial, there are essentially only three main objectives regardless which surgical procedure is chosen. These are:

1. *to restore the profundus,*
2. *to provide terminal stability* and
3. *to improve over-all digital flexion.*

The choice of surgical procedure depends upon the factors previously discussed (level of tendon injury, degree of tendon retraction, and extent of superficial flexor function). Diverse surgical approaches such as tendon repairs, advancement, tenodesis, flexor tendon grafts and flexor tenolysis should be considered in the light of these many factors in order to obtain a rational approach to treatment.

(Chart 1)
RESTORE PRE-EXISTING PROFUNDUS

The first group of operations I will discuss attempt to restore the pre-existing flexor digitorum profundus, by tendon advancement or repair. This approach is only indicated in distal lesions. These patients typically have good superficial flexor function. This approach of repair or advancement of the flexor digitorum profundus is not indicated in proximal lesions. In this situation it is best to close the skin and provide terminal

joint stability at a later date. Tendon repair or advancement can, of course, be carried out either primarily or at a later stage. If a patient is seen within a few hours of injury and the proper diagnosis is made of either a traumatic rupture or a very distal laceration, the best treatment is tendon advancement. In this technique the tendon end is reattached to the base of the distal phalanx with a pull out wire. The suture line is, therefore, brought beyond the terminal joint minimizing the risk of restricted terminal flexion. Again by bringing the suture line distally one minimizes the risk of interfering with the superficial flexor. If wound conditions are good, the primary approach is indicated. However, this procedure can be done several weeks or several months later with an excellent prognosis if the tendon has not retracted proximally (Fig. 11.1). This may be determined by clinical palpation. Complications of flexor tendon advancement result from carrying out the advancement over too great a distance. This is not a problem in spontaneous tendon ruptures in which no length is actually lost. If the advancement is carried out more than one-half centimetre, the patient may develop a flexion contracture of the terminal joint. If this occurs, it is not necessary to release the flexor tendon unless the adjacent fingers have been affected. All that is necessary is to arthrodese the distal joint in a less flexed position (Fig. 11.2). Tendon repair, either primary or secondary, can be carried out in those patients who have a more proximal tendon lesion, but one that is still beyond the superficial bifurcation. These cases are usually done late because the diagnosis that the tendon lesion is distal enough may not be obvious clinically and, in fact, may not be discovered until surgery. With this technique, one exposes the tendon sheath over the middle phalanx. The deep flexor is often found adherent at this point and can be freed from surrounding tissues. With excision of the surrounding tendon sheath it is then possible to carry out an end-to-end repair using very fine suture material. Tension is taken off the repair with a transfixing wire using the Verdan technique (Fig. 11.3). The most significant feature in this repair is that it is carried out beyond the proximal interphalangeal joint so that sublimis function is not compromised. If one carries out a secondary repair over the middle phalanx and the tendon becomes adherent at this point, one has essentially provided a tenodesis with stability of the terminal joint.

PROVIDE DISTAL JOINT STABILITY

The second approach in the management of these injuries provides joint stability by fusion or tenodesis. These procedures do not increase finger flexion and are, therefore, not indicated as the sole consideration for those patients who have only fair superficial flexor function. If there is no doubt about the proximal level of tendon injury and the patient has maintained good sublimis function, one can proceed to fusion via a dorsal approach without any volar surgery (Fig. 11.4). However, if there is some doubt as to the level of deep flexor, one can carry out an exploration over the middle phalanx. If the lesion is found to be proximal, then it is possible to carry out a tenodesis with the terminal tendon stump suturing it either to the middle phalanx or to the flexor tendon sheath. In order to protect the tenodesis a Kirschner wire should be passed

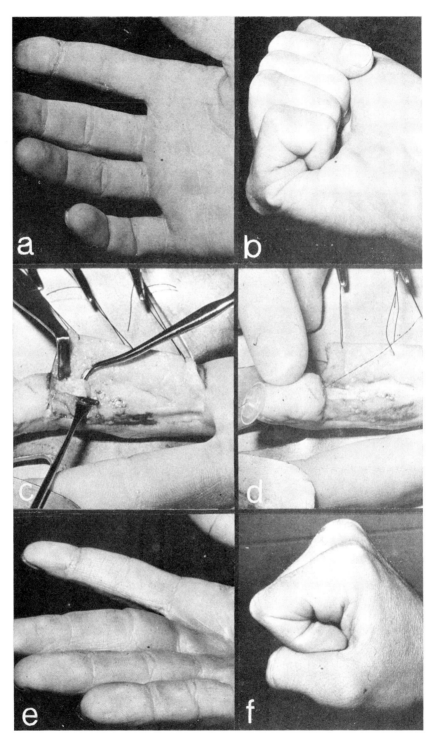

Figure 11.1
An example of secondary advancement of the flexor digitorum pro-   flexion. (c) Appearance of tendon at surgery. (d) Advancement per-
fundus. (a) Note the healed distal laceration of the index finger. (b)   formed with pull out wire technique (e) (f) Shows post-operative func-
The patient has excellent sublimis function but lacks terminal joint   tion with restoration of terminal joint flexion.

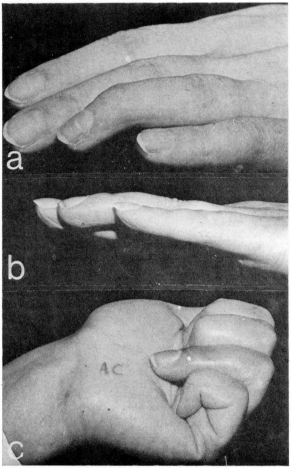

Figure 11.2
A complication of primary advancement. (a) Note flexion contracture of distal joint of the ring finger. (b) Distal joint deformity corrected by fusion (c) Patient demonstrates full sublimis function.

across the distal joint for six weeks. It should be emphasized that fusion or tenodesis is not indicated unless the patient has good sublimis function.

IMPROVEMENT OF DIGITAL FLEXION

Those patients who have cut the deep flexors and have limited superficial flexor function require the third approach: an improvement of over-all active digital flexion. Fusion or tenodesis to stabilize the distal joint is not enough when the patient cannot flex the finger close to the palm. There are basically two ways to improve active digital flexion. One is by the insertion of a free flexor tendon graft through the intact sublimis and the other is by removal of the adherent deep flexor with tenolysis of the superficial flexor to restore its normal excursion. Flexor tendon grafts have been advocated by many; all agree that removal of an intact sublimis is never indicated. Those surgeons who attempt to restore profundus function with a tendon graft try not to disturb the sublimis. They usually take the thin plantaris tendon as the graft of choice. The technique of inserting the flexor tendon graft has been adequately described elsewhere and will not therefore be repeated here. However, special risks are involved especially when sublimis function is already good. In this situation one risks losing over-all digital motion to gain active control of the distal joint (Fig. 11.5). This is a risk not to be taken lightly. For this reason, I prefer to restore superficial flexor tendon function and stabilize the distal joint. A volar zig-zag incision is made in the distal palm. The profundus tendon is usually found to be shortened and adherent to the sublimis tendon and tendon sheath. It is separated and divided near the lumbrical attachment. Traction on the superficial flexor should fully flex the proximal interphalangeal joint. If this does not occur, the incision is carried distally and a more extensive tenolysis performed. Once traction on the superficial flexor achieves full flexion, attention should be directed to the distal joint if additional stability is needed. An example of tenolysis and fusion is shown in Figure 11.6. This approach usually restores good digital motion with satisfactory strength except in the small finger where the sublimis may be quite small and weak. Faced with an intact but weak sublimis, we suture the profundus tendon to the superficial flexor in the palm to add its strength in flexion (Fig. 11.7).

CONCLUSION

In this chapter I have presented the various surgical procedures for patients with an intact sublimis tendon emphasizing those factors to be considered before choosing the most appropriate approach for improving function with minimal risk.

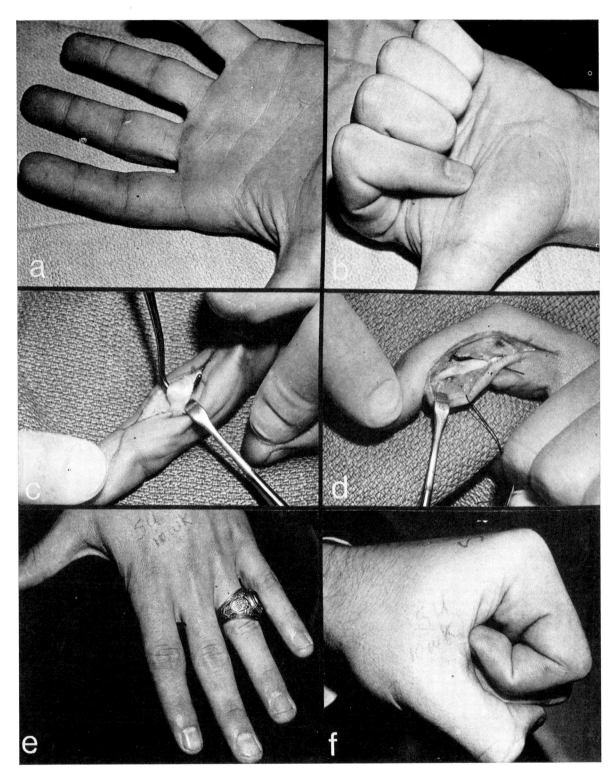

Figure 11.3
An example of secondary repair of the flexor digitorum profundus using the Verdan technique. (a) Note healed laceration at the base of the middle phalanx of the index finger. (b) Patient demonstrates full proximal interphalangeal joint flexion, but lacks distal joint flexion.

(c) Appearance at surgery. Deep flexor tendon found adherent over the middle phalanx. (d) Shows tendon repair. Note proximal transfixing pin. (e) (f) Shows the patient's post-operative flexion and extension.

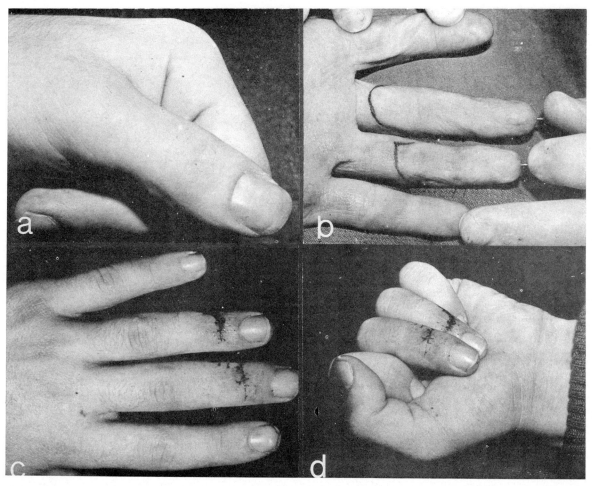

Figure 11.4
Restoration of terminal joint stability by fusion. (a) Patient demonstrates pre-operative flexion. (b) Note proximal level of injury. Fusion
performed without exploring flexor tendons. (c) (d) Post-operative
function shows excellent sublimis function.

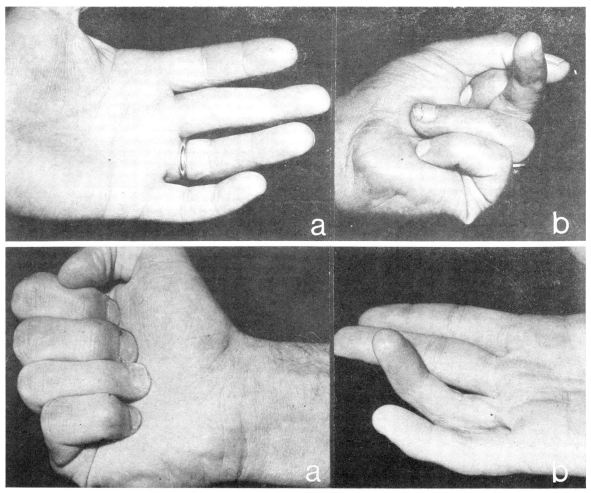

Figure 11.5
Two complications of flexor tendon grafting with intact sublimis. Top—(a) (b) This patient has full extension but reduced ability to flex the mid finger following graft. Bottom—(a) (b) This patient regained terminal joint flexion of the ring finger, but developed a significant residual flexion contracture of the interphalangeal joints.

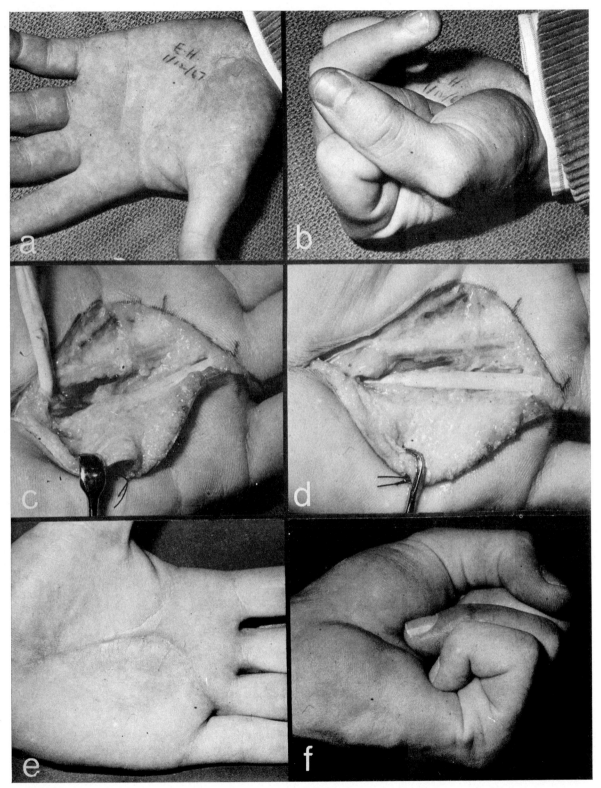

Figure 11.6
The use of tenolysis to improve digital motion. (a) (b) This patient has only partial sublimis function which is not sufficient to flex the ring finger to palm. (c) Shows profundus tendon being removed from the palm. (d) Appearance of sublimis tendon following tenolysis and removal of profundus. (e) (f) Shows improved post-operative function. Note fusion of distal joint.

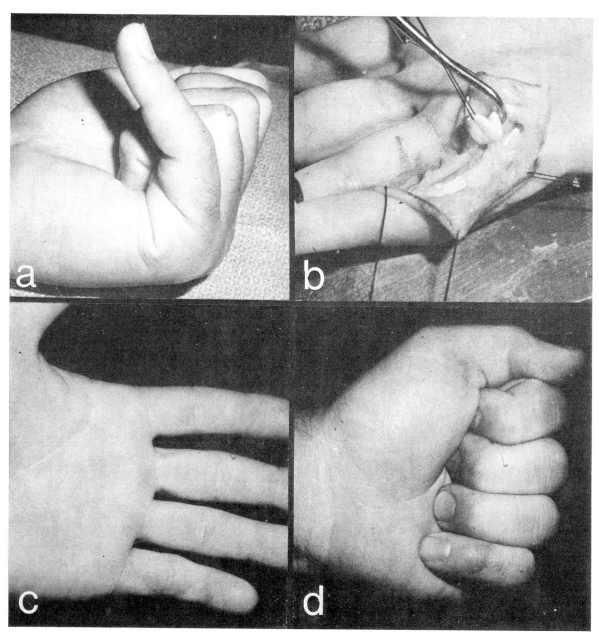

Figure 11.7
The use of tenolysis and transfer in a patient with intact sublimis in the small finger. (a) Patient has weak, insufficient digital flexion. (b) Note intact sublimis and short deep flexor which was sutured to the sublimis in the palm. (c) (d) Improved post-operative function shown. Distal joint fused to provide stability.

J. H. Boyes H. H. Stark

PRELIMINARIES

As in all reconstructive operations on tendons, the soft tissues should be in good condition and the joints of the digits should be freely movable. Time is necessary to allow the induration from the original trauma to subside, and the skin and subcutaneous tissues to become soft and supple. Even when the original injury appears relatively minor, it is important to delay the tendon grafting for several weeks. If there is scarring or stiff joints because some preliminary operation has been done, the final tendon reconstruction should be delayed until the optimal conditions are present.

Mobilization of stiffened interphalangeal joints should be carried out until all possible passive motion has been obtained. We cannot expect a tendon graft placed in a finger with limited joint motion to function to such a degree that the joint range will increase. Experience has shown that the final range of motion in such a joint is always less. Dynamic splinting to increase the range of flexion is more valuable than intermittent passive motion, and forcible manipulations and stretching may increase the stiffness and prolong the waiting time before the final operation.

Damage to the digital nerves alters the results of tendon grafts, though there is little difference when only one nerve has been severed. Damage to both nerves means that both neuro-vascular bundles are injured and some trophic changes are to be expected. In the past it was thought advisable to repair the nerves first as a separate procedure, thus hoping to restore the sensibility and improve the condition of the digit. Such a plan meant that two operative procedures were required, resulting in additional scarring and many months were wasted before the expected sensory recovery had any effect. Except in unusual circumstances, it is probably better to attempt the whole reconstruction of tendons and nerves in one operative stage.

There is one other factor not under the control of the surgeon that influences the result of our operation. Unless the patient is willing to cooperate and work diligently when active use and exercise are essential, and unless the patient maintains this co-operation throughout the whole rehabilitation period, the results will fall far short of our expectations.

PREOPERATIVE PREPARATION

In planning the operation, one must consider the possibility of using donor tendons other than the palmaris longus, which is our first choice. One should be prepared, if necessary, to use the tendons of the foot or to provide some gliding substance, such as paratenon material.

The usual preoperative preparation consists of shaving of the forearm, thorough cleansing with soap and water, and at the time of operation, skin preparation with one of the iodine compounds.

Local anaesthesia is not advisable for a procedure of this magnitude, but block anaesthesia is satisfactory. Brachial or axillary block can be used. The peripheral nerves, the ulnar at the elbow and median and radial at the wrist can be easily blocked.

OPERATION

A tourniquet is used to provide a bloodless field. The arm is exsanguinated by elevation and by wrapping it snugly with a rubber bandage. A pneumatic tourniquet is then applied to the upper arm and inflated to approximately 300 mm of mercury. This is maintained throughout the operative procedure and can safely be left in place for a period of one and a half hours.

Exposure of the area of tendon damage in the finger is through a midlateral incision passing dorsal to the neurovascular bundles (Fig. 12.1). This incision is preferred as it allows

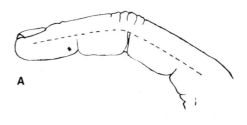

A

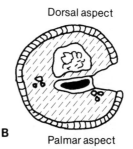

Dorsal aspect

B

Palmar aspect

Figure 12.1
(A) The finger incision is made in the midlateral line. It is important to make the incision dorsal to the flexion creases.
(B) The neurovascular bundle remains with the volar skin flap.

adequate exposure for the tendon reconstruction as well as repair, if necessary, of both digital nerves. The incision extends the full length of the finger, from the tip, allowing complete exposure of the insertion of the profundus tendon to the proximal flexion crease, that is, the level of the web (Boyes, 1953). If one of the digital nerves has been severed, the incision is usually made on that side of the finger; otherwise, we prefer to enter the radial side of the index, middle, and ring fingers, and the ulnar side of the little finger. The incision is not extended in the palm except in unusual circumstances, and then only if the index or little fingers are involved and the site of injury is over the metacarpophalangeal joint (Fig. 12.2). In the middle and ring fingers, rather than make a continuous incision, we prefer a separate incision in the distal palm. When opening a finger in the midlateral line, it is necessary to traverse the layer of digital fascia which surrounds the finger. This layer is thick and discrete at the PIP joint level and the cut edges should be isolated and identified. In the final closure of the wounds, as will be described later, restoration of this structure is important and acts to prevent a late recurvatum deformity of the digit (Boyes and Stark, 1971). Through the midlateral incision, the flexor tendons can be exposed throughout their length. All tendon remaining in the finger is removed. A thorough excision of scar is done and all the thickened synovial sheath is removed. The pulleys, or fibrous sheaths, are preserved if possible and if not involved in the damaged area, may be narrowed by excising a portion, but there is no advantage in doing this to such a degree as to leave only a narrow strand. The mechanical effect of a pulley is essential to the proper functioning of the tendon and the location and size in the normal finger are not accidental occurrences.

All parts of both flexor tendons are removed. There is no advantage in leaving the 'Chiasm of Camper' of the superfi-

cialis tendon but rather the entire tendon should be removed, including the studs of the insertion into the middle phalanx where they lie beneath the middle segment pulley. These are carefully and thoroughly removed. When this is done, the finger is free of scar and only the fibrous pulleys remain. The area of insertion will now be prepared by exposing the base of the terminal phalanx, removing all the remnants of the profundus tendon, and turning up an osteoperiosteal flap. A drill hole is made through the nail, diagonally to exit in this opening in the terminal phalanx, and through it is passed a loop of wire to act as a guide (Fig. 12.3).

If there is evidence of damage to one of the digital nerves, exposure of the nerve is carried out and the ends carefully freed; however, the neuroma is not excised but left until the final stage of the operation when the nerve repair is accomplished.

Incisions in the palm are made paralleling the distal flexion crease and placed proximal to the digit involved. Through this incision, one exposes the flexor profundus tendon at the lumbrical origin and carefully frees it from all surrounding scar tissue

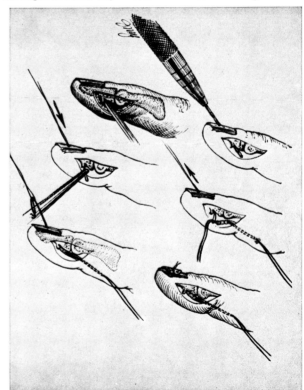

Figure 12.3
The steps in proper attachment of flexor tendon to distal phalanx, using the pull-out wire technic. (Top) A flap of cortex is elevated at the site of proposed insertion, and the drill is aimed from the dorsum of the midportion of the nail to the exposed bone. (Centre) A loop of wire is passed through nail and phalanx as a guide wire. Both ends of the tendon suture wire are passed through the loop of the guide wire. (Bottom) The raw cut end of the tendon is brought snugly up against the raw surface of the bone, and the suture is tied over a button on the nail. The pull-out loop is passed through the skin of the volar surface in the midline and at such a point proximally that the entire suture course is a straight line. (Bunnell, 5th edn. Lippincott)

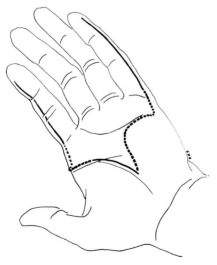

Figure 12.2
In the index and little fingers, a continuous incision is permissible, but separate incisions are ordinarily used. Separate incisions in the finger and palm are always advisable in the middle and ring fingers.

and excises the thickened paratenon. The superficialis is likewise freed and both tendons are withdrawn from the finger. The superficialis will be removed later through a transverse incision at the wrist and will be divided at its musculotendinous junction. If the superficialis is to be used for the graft in the digit, care is taken in handling of the surface of the tendon. The profundus tendon is freed and an adequate amplitude of motion of the profundus is demonstrated by removing any adherence of this tendon at the level of the lumbrical origin.

Since the site of insertion of the graft has already been prepared, one now can remove the palmaris longus if it is to be used for the graft. The tendon is then sutured into the terminal phalanx of the finger, using the pull-out wire suture of Bunnell (1944). Following the insertion of the suture into the end of the tendon, the two ends are passed through the guide loop and by means of this, the suture in the tendon is brought out through the nail bed and over the nail. Here, it is tied over a button, drawing the raw end of the tendon snugly up against the raw surface of the bone. The proximal end of the tendon is then passed through the pulleys and into the palm where it will later be sutured to the cut end of the profundus tendon. After the tendon graft is passed into the palm, traction on it will flex the finger and demonstrate the importance of the pulleys. However, the skin and subcutaneous tissues are not closed until the deep fascia of the finger is sutured. Two nonabsorbable sutures are placed diagonally from proximal and dorsal to distal and volar in such a way that, when tied, the finger will fall into about 20° of flexion at the PIP joint. This must be done before the proximal suture of the graft to the profundus has been done, or the closure of the fascia will restrict extension later. When the fascial layer is closed, nerve repair is carried out and the skin of the finger closed.

The suture of graft to profundus should be as far proximal as possible so that the tendon juncture lies at the lumbrical origin or just slightly distal to it and when completed, the lumbrical muscle will overly the suture line. If, for some reason, the suture line is not completely buried by the overlying lumbrical, we have found it useful to fasten the lumbrical muscle to the tendon with a few interrupted catgut sutures. This is done by carefully drawing the lumbrical muscle distally before attaching it around the tendon junction. If the lumbrical is pulled proximally, then one can expect at a later date to find the so-called 'lumbrical positive' or 'extensor habitus' sign in the finger. Bunnell pointed out many years ago that when attaching the lumbrical to the profundus, that it should be pulled distally on the involved tendon (Bunnell, 1944).

To determine the length of the graft, or in other words, the tension on the transplant, we have found that if the wrist is placed in a neutral position; that is, straight with the forearm and the normal fingers allowed to flex, the length of the tendon graft is such that the involved digit will be in the same degree of flexion as the digit in the normal hand.

Mayer's rule for tendon transfer called for approximation of tendons without tension when the origin and insertion of the muscle tendon unit were approximated. This, however, we have found to be somewhat tight for tendon grafts and therefore have utilized the wrist at the neutral position in order to measure the length of the graft.

Most errors are made in making the graft too long and therefore, particularly on the ulnar side of the hand where the fingers tend to be in more flexion than they do on the radial side, it is perhaps better to err on the side of having the grafts slightly shorter. This should not be done at the expense of making the junction in the palm more distal, but by making the graft long enough so that the proximal junction can be made at the lumbrical origin.

The proximal suture is of stainless steel wire, utilizing the Bunnell method of suture. This wire suture will remain buried in the tendon and has caused no difficulty (Boyes, 1953; Bunnell, 1944).

Closure of the skin is by mattress sutures in the palm and continuous sutures in the digit. A compression dressing is applied and the hand is placed with the wrist in palmar flexion, the forearm in supination, and a dorsal plaster splint is applied to prevent extension of the fingers. There should not be a splint, however, on the volar surface for any involuntary activity of the muscles would pull the digit against a fixed point and thus put stress on the suture lines in the tendon. The plaster splint extends almost to the elbow and continuous splinting is used for a minimum of three weeks.

There are some possible variations in the surgical technique. For donor tendons, one may use the superficialis of the same digit, providing the surface has not been traumatized and it is of adequate length. There is no advantage in using tendons of small calibre, and we have found the use of the plantaris and the use of the superficialis of the little finger to be a disadvantage (Boyes and Stark, 1971). Our results show that ruptures have occurred when small calibre tendons have been used for grafts. We have therefore, as our first preference, used the palmaris longus; our second choice would be the superficialis of the involved digit, and our third choice would be the long extensor tendons of the toes.

One other variation would be in a finger in which such severe damage is apparent at the time of operation that the insertion of a graft in a scarred bed would not function adequately. For such a problem, it would be better to plan a two-stage operation. First reconstruct the pulley mechanisms, (Fig. 12.4) repair the nerves, and excise all the possible scar, and insert a silastic rod. This should be of relatively small calibre, approximately 4–5 mm in size, and should extend proximal to

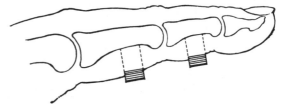

Figure 12.4

Diagram to show the optimal location for pulleys in the digital flexor mechanism. In reconstruction, two pulleys provide adequate fulcrums for the one reconstructed flexor tendon. (Adapted from Barton, N. J. (1969) *Plast. Reconstr. Surg.*, **43**, 125.) (Bunnell, 5th edn. Lippincott)

the lumbrical origin in the palm. It can be attached to the terminal tendon at the distal phalanx. After a few months, the silastic is removed and the tendon graft is placed in the finger.

POSTOPERATIVE CARE

The first dressing three or four days after operation is a simple inspection of the wounds to be sure that a haematoma is not present. Removal of skin sutures is done on the ninth to twelfth day, and the dorsal splint is maintained for a period of three weeks. At this time, the pull-out wire suture is removed from the tendon graft insertion and gentle, active motion of the finger is started. Some restriction of wrist motion should be carried out for an additional week, and the splint can be used for this, but the patient is allowed to remove it occasionally for gentle washing of the hand but with guarded motion to prevent extreme dorsiflexion of the wrist. Voluntary motion is encouraged and in the fourth week, further force is put upon the tendon. At this time, the proximal segment of the finger is held with the metacarpophalangeal joint in extension and the wrist in neutral position. With the examiner's hand passively flexing the finger, the patient is asked to flex the digit voluntarily (Fig. 12.5). This avoids extreme strain upon the tendon insertion and tends to promote better gliding of the tendon. The finger is then passively flexed completely into the palm and held so by the examiner and with the wrist in neutral position, not in dorsiflexion, the patient is asked to make a strong, powerful grip. When he does this, all force is applied to the tendon, causing it to slip through the digit.

If at this time the finger is in a flexion contracture and extension is limited, a spring-type splint can be applied to the dorsum of the finger, to be worn for a period of two or three hours a day or night. This helps the finger to extend gradually. If, however, at the end of the fourth week passive extension is still limited, then with the wrist in neutral position and the metacarpophalangeal joint sharply flexed, the examiner pass-

ively extends the middle joint of the finger. At this time, the patient does not take any voluntary effort to flex. Sometimes in this manner, the tendon can be slipped through the tissues and a greater range of motion can be obtained.

Careful measurements are made of the limitation of extension and of the amount of flexion at each visit, and a record made so that complete control is maintained.

Exercises and specific instructions and personal contact with the patient are carried out at weekly intervals during the next three weeks, at which time the patient can be allowed to use his hand actively to the degree of tolerance. Formal physiotherapy is useless and personally directed exercises to an intelligent patient will suffice. If extension of the interphalangeal joint is limited at six weeks, this can be overcome by splinting the finger several hours each day (Fig. 12.6).

Motions will improve over a period of several months so that at the end of six months, one can estimate the result of the operation, although there may be further slight improvement over a period of at least another year.

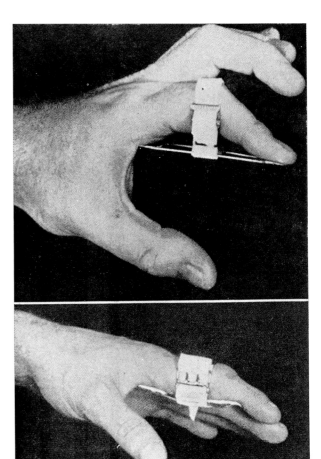

Figure 12.6
Splinting of finger for several hours each day will improve extension in many fingers after grafting. (Bunnell, 5th edn. Lippincott)

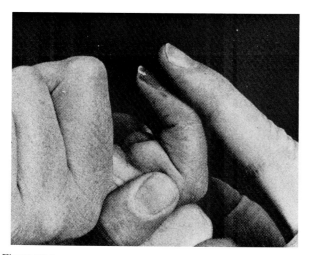

Figure 12.5
Manoeuvre that often helps overcome minor adhesions to the tendon grafts. The examiner holds the metacarpophalangeal joint in extension and the proximal interphalangeal joint in flexion, while the patient makes a strong attempt to flex the terminal joint.

SECONDARY OPERATIONS

Tenolysis following the tendon graft has been carried out in very few instances. We have found that a tenolysis, to be successful, requires a radical excision of scar from the tendon graft throughout its entire length. It is not simply the release of one or two adhesions but an operation of the same magnitude as the original tendon graft. If the finger is limited in extension, this type of operation may result in some improvement in the range of extension; however, it has been our experience that if the tendon graft is not functioning adequately to flex the digit, that tenolysis is of little use. One should be prepared to remove the tendon graft and reinsert a new graft or a silastic rod as a preliminary to another procedure. Our experience with tenolysis to improve flexion following a tendon graft has not been satisfactory.

SUMMARY

One might summarize the operative technic of flexor tendon grafts by saying that the principle is to first have a digit which is freely movable and the soft tissues in good condition. Second, to excise the scar as well as all the thickened synovial sheath, and particularly the paratenon in the palm. Third, to insert the graft into the bone in the terminal phalanx and as far proximal in the palm as possible at the level of the lumbrical origin. The lumbrical muscle should surround this proximal suture line. Fourth, pulleys should be maintained or should be reconstructed if necessary. Fifth, the first three weeks following the operation, there should be no attempt to move the tendon in its bed. A tendon graft requires a blood supply which must come from the surrounding tissues and, therefore, there must be adhesions. Sixth, the postoperative care, after the first three weeks, should be under the personal direction of the surgeon, with strict control of the amount of activity and prompt identification and correction of the complications which may jeopardize the final results.

FACTORS INFLUENCING RESULTS OF TENDON GRAFTS

This technique, with only minor variations, has been used since 1954 (Boyes & Stark, 1971). Thus, as many variables as possible have been eliminated and a study of 700 consecutive grafts allows us to determine the other factors, not under our control, which may affect the results.

Of the 700 grafts, 607 were in fingers and 93 were in thumbs. All the grafts in the fingers were done because of division of *both* flexor tendons. Ninety-seven point four per cent of all patients were last examined four months or more after grafting (Table 12.1). In 19 instances (16 fingers and three thumbs) the result was unknown because the final examination was less than four months after operation.

At each examination, the motion of each joint was measured and recorded, and for the fingers, we also recorded the distance the pulp lacked of flexing to the distal palmar crease (Fig. 12.7). The last recorded motion was considered the final result for each finger. We have found that finger motion usually improves for at least eight months after grafting, and often maximum motion is not regained until 12 months after grafting. Since 15 per cent of our patients were last examined four months after grafting, and another 15 per cent were last examined six months after grafting, the overall results would have been better if all patients could have been followed for a longer time. By contrast, failures are evident within three months after grafting and grafts that disrupt at their proximal or distal attachment do so within two months after surgery.

We use a cumulative method of reporting finger flexion. We believe this is more descriptive than any arbitrary grading of results as good, fair, or poor. Slight loss of finger extension is not a particular handicap, but when extension is so limited that the finger cannot open for grasp, the result is a failure, even though the finger flexes to the palm.

PREOPERATIVE CLASSIFICATION OF FINGER

Since the previous study showed that the preoperative condition of a finger had a great influence on the result after grafting, five preoperative classifications were defined, and each finger was placed in one of these five classifications:

1. Good: All fingers classed as good were originally cut by a sharp object such as a knife, broken glass, or a piece of metal. Furthermore, initial treatment consisted of wound closure *without* tendon repair, skin healing occurred without infection, the bones were uninjured, and the joints were supple. In other words, these fingers had minimal injury and were minimally scarred. Trophic changes were absent, but one or both digital nerves might have been severed.

TABLE 12.1   Length of follow-up (fingers)

Class	Not Followed	4 Months	4–6 Months	6–8 Months	8–12 Months	More than 12 Months	Total
Good	6	42	35	30	48	45	206
Scar	7	28	22	27	39	49	172
Joint	2	7	7	14	12	24	66
Multiple	0	10	21	15	34	51	131
Salvage	1	6	6	4	5	10	32
Total	16	93	91	90	138	179	607

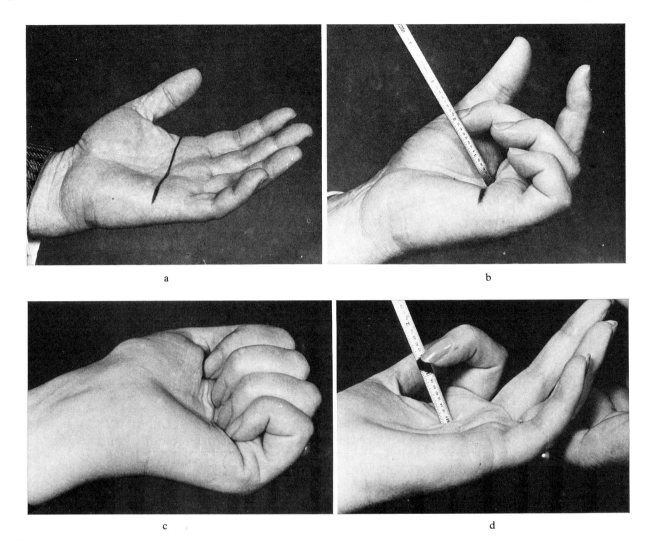

a   b

c   d

Figure 12.7
(a) Composite finger flexion is described as measuring the distance the finger pulp, not the nail, lacks of flexing to the distal palmar crease. This crease is directly over the metacarpophalangeal joints of all fingers.
(b) A finger may flex to touch the palm, but still lack a considerable distance of flexing to the distal palmar crease. In this instance, the pulp of the middle finger lacks more than 3 cm of reaching the crease but it touches the thenar eminence of the palm.
(c) This little finger flexes to the distal palmar crease.
(d) The index finger lacks 2.8 cm of flexing to the distal palmar crease.

Two hundred and six fingers were placed in this category, and 200 of these were last examined at least four months after grafting. Twenty-three per cent of these fingers flexed to the distal palmar crease, 64 per cent to within 1.2 cm, and 85 per cent to within 2.5 cm of the distal crease of the palm (Fig. 12.8).

2. Scarred: A finger was classed as scarred for one of three reasons.

    (a) Injury had been caused by a crushing or tearing laceration, such as occurs when it is struck by a saw or grinding machine. Many of these wounds became superficially infected, skin healing was delayed, and the finger was scarred internally;

    (b) primary tendon surgery had been attempted and failed;

    (c) a tendon graft had been placed in the finger and had failed.

One hundred and seventy-two fingers were placed in this category. Of these, 45 were placed there because of the type of injury they sustained. In 37 fingers, after treatment of the wound, a *previous* tendon graft had been inserted in the finger and that graft had failed. Ninety fingers were classified as scarred because the flexor tendon had been repaired primarily and the repair had failed. That is, these 90 fingers would have been classified 'good' if a primary tendon repair had not been performed.

In the scarred group, seven of the fingers were followed less than four months, leaving 165 for study. Only 9 per cent of these scarred fingers flexed to the distal palmar crease after grafting. Twenty-seven per cent flexed to within 1.2 cm, and 58 per cent to within 2.5 cm of the distal palm (Fig. 12.8).

At the time of grafting, passive flexion was limited in 41 of the 172 fingers but the finger scar, rather than joint injury, was

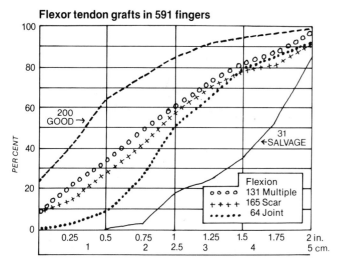

Flexor tendon grafts in 591 fingers

Figure 12.8
A cumulative graph shows that the result after grafting varies with the preoperative condition of the finger. Because of poor flexion, there were 16 failures in 607 flexor tendon grafts. These 16 failures are not plotted on the graph, and the results in 591 fingers are given.
(A) Tissues in a good condition (200)
(B) Multiple lesions (131)
(C) Scarred tissues (168)
(D) Joint lesions (64)
(E) Unhealed lesions (1)
(J. H. Boyes and H. H. Stark (1971) *J. Bone and Jt Surg.*, **53A**)

the primary cause of the limited passive flexion. Before grafting, 32 of the 41 fingers lacked 1.25 cm, and nine lacked more than 1.25 cm of complete passive flexion. After grafting, only four of the 32 fingers flexed to within 1.25 cm of the distal palmar crease, and only one of the other nine flexed to within 2.5 cm of this crease. *Without exception, joints with limited passive flexion before grafting will have just as much, and usually more, limitation of voluntary flexion after grafting.*

3. Joint: Fingers that were minimally scarred but that had less than normal passive motion of an interphalangeal joint were classified as having a joint problem. Joint stiffness results from one of the following causes:

(a) direct damage to the volar capsule at the time of injury;
(b) prolonged disuse following injury; or
(c) direct damage to one or both of the articular surfaces of the proximal interphalangeal joint.

Sixty-six fingers were placed in this category, and 64 of these were last examined four months or more post grafting. After weeks, or even months, of preoperative passive exercise and diligent use of a web strap and other assistive devices, only one-third of these fingers could be passively flexed so the tip touched the distal palmar crease. On the other hand, even after persistent efforts to improve passive motion, two-thirds of the fingers in this group still lacked passive flexion. At the time of grafting, 21 fingers in this 'joint' category could be flexed to the distal palmar crease passively, but nine lacked .63 cm, 22 lacked 1.25 cm, 14 lacked 1.87 cm, and seven lacked 2.5 cm or more of complete passive flexion.

Thirty-two of the 66 fingers were index fingers. *This suggests*

that an index finger has a great tendency to stiffen after division of its flexor tendons. It is easy for a patient to use the middle finger as a substitute for the index finger and in doing so, he will keep the index finger in extension, and this allows the joints to stiffen.

After grafting, none of the fingers in this preoperative classification flexed to the distal palm. Nine per cent flexed to within 1.25 cm, and 50 per cent flexed to within 2.5 cm of the distal palmar crease (Fig. 12.8).

In every instance where a finger had limited passive flexion before grafting, the limitation of voluntary flexion *after* grafting was at least as great as the preoperative limitation of passive flexion. For example, if a finger lacked 1.25 cm of flexing to the distal palm *passively* before grafting, it would, after grafting, lack *at least* 1.25 cm of flexing to the distal palm voluntarily. *Therefore, it is essential to delay grafting until maximum passive joint motion has been regained.*

4. Salvage: Fingers were placed in this classification when they were so badly damaged that restoration of any motion after grafting was considered beneficial. Usually these hands were damaged by a homemade bomb or some similar blast injury, or they had massive avulsion of multiple tissues from the distal palm. One-third of these patients had a wound infection after their injury, and over 60 per cent had preliminary surgery before tendon grafting. This surgery included free skin grafting to overcome contractures, pedicle flaps to provide better cover and nutrition, joint reconstruction, or a combination of several of these procedures.

Thirty-two fingers were placed in this category, and all but one was examined four months or more after grafting, leaving 31 for follow-up study. Before grafting, only *five* fingers in this group could be flexed to the distal palmar crease passively, while *eight* lacked 1.25 cm, *ten* lacked 1.87 cm, and *nine* lacked 2.5 cm or more of complete passive flexion.

After grafting, none of these fingers flexed to within 1.25 cm of the palm. Eighteen per cent flexed to within 2.5 cm, and only 34 per cent to within 3.8 cm of the distal palmar crease.

5. Multiple: This classification applied when the flexor tendons were injured in more than one digit. Since division of both flexor tendons in more than one finger usually indicated a greater injury to the hand, we assumed that the result after grafting would be less satisfactory than when injury was limited to one finger.

Sixty-two patients with 131 injured fingers were placed in this category (Table 12.2), and all were examined four months or more after grafting.

TABLE 12.2 Distribution of patients with tendon injury in more than one digit

No. Fingers injured	No. Patients	Total Fingers
2	45	90
3	12	36
*1 + thumb	5	5
Total	62	131

* See text

Two fingers were injured in 45 hands, three fingers in 12 hands, and a thumb and one finger in five hands.* After grafting, 9 per cent of all fingers in this classification flexed to the distal palmar crease, while 33 per cent flexed to within 1.25 cm, and 61 per cent to within 2.5 cm of the distal palmar crease. The age of the patient, the level of tendon injury, the source of the graft, and the use of pulleys had no significant effect on the end result in this group.

Since the results in the multiple group were significantly better than the results in the scar and joint group, we reclassified all fingers in the multiple category according to the *preoperative condition of each individual finger* (*Table 12.3*). For

TABLE 12.3   Distribution of 'Multiple' Fingers after Reclassification According to Preoperative Condition of Each Finger

Good	56
Scar	26
Joint	24
Salvage	25
Total	131

example, in a patient with tendon damage in three fingers, one finger might be classified 'good', one 'scarred', and one as 'salvage'. Of the 131 fingers, 25 were reclassified as 'salvage', 50 as either 'scarred' or 'joint', and 56 as 'good'.

After reclassification, the final flexion of these 56 fingers in the 'multiple' group was almost identical with the final flexion of the 200 fingers in the preoperative 'good' classification. In fact, 60 per cent of these 'good' fingers flexed to within 1.25 cm of the distal palmar crease, even though tendon grafts had been placed in more than one finger of each hand. Similarly, each of the other sub-groups of this 'multiple' category (salvage, scar, and joint) had results similar to those obtained in the corresponding preoperative classification. *It is the condition of each digit by itself that is the determining factor in the result, and not the presence of tendon damage in several digits of the same hand.*

SUMMARY OF INFLUENCE OF PREOPERATIVE CLASSIFICATION

The preoperative condition of the digit was probably the most important factor effecting the result of flexor tendon grafting. In the good cases, regardless of age, time since injury, specific digit injured, or tendon used as a graft, 23 per cent of the fingers flexed so the pulp touched the distal palmar crease. Only 9 per cent in the scar and multiple groups could do so, while in the joint and salvage groups, none could flex the tip to the distal palmar crease. The results were similar in both sexes, and the results were the same in private patients and those covered by compensation.

SITE OF TENDON INJURY

Both flexor tendons can be severed in 'no-man's land' if the wound occurs between the distal palmar crease and the middle flexion crease of the finger. We divided this area into three zones (proximal, middle, and distal) (Fig. 12.9) and by eliminating all other variables, we tried to determine whether or not the specific level of tendon injury within 'no-man's land' influenced the result after grafting Table 12.4.

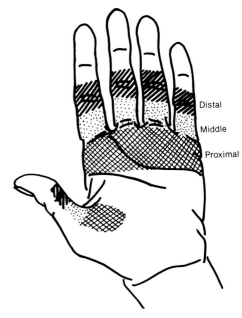

Figure 12.9
'No man's land' was arbitrarily divided into three zones, which are labelled. When all other variables were eliminated, the area of tendon damage had little influence on the result after grafting (J. H. Boyes and H. H. Stark (1971) *J. Bone and Jt Surg.*, **53A**).

TABLE 12.4   Site of tendon severance

Class	Proximal	Middle	Distal	Total
Good	34	92	80	206
Scar	57	64	51	172
Joint	10	26	30	66
Multiple	53	44	34	131
Salvage	20	6	6	32
Total	174 (29%)	232 (38%)	201 (33%)	607

Interesting observations from this analysis were:

1. Only 16 per cent of the fingers classified as 'good' sustained the tendon injury in the proximal zone.

2. Almost half of the fingers classified as 'joint' were injured in the distal zone, which is directly over the proximal interphalangeal joint.

3. In 40 per cent of the 'multiple' group and in 60 per cent of the 'salvage' group, the tendon injury occurred in the distal palm (proximal zone).

4. Flexor tendons in children under five years of age are usually severed in the distal palm (proximal zone). Quite commonly, tendons are divided by striking their open palm on a sharp object when they fall.

5. *All other factors being equal, it did not make any difference on the result after grafting, if the injury was in any specific portion of the area called 'No man's land'.*

INJURY TO THE DIGITAL NERVES

Ordinarily, we repaired damaged digital nerves at the time of grafting. When one nerve was damaged, it was always

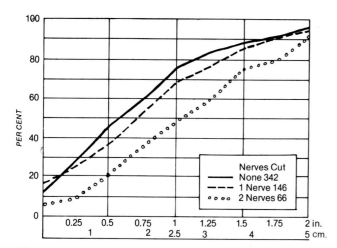

Figure 12.10
In the entire group, damage to one digital nerve had little effect on the results. However, fingers with both nerves damaged had a worse effect.
(A) Fingers without nerve damage (342)
(B) Fingers with one digital nerve damaged (146)
(C) Fingers with both digital nerves damaged (66)

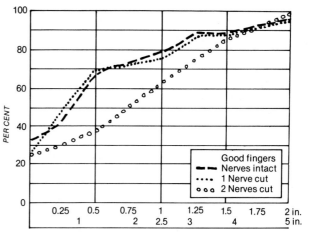

Figure 12.11
Damage to one digital nerve did not impair the result in 'good' fingers, but when both nerves were damaged, the result was compromised.
(A) Fingers without nerve damage.
(B) Fingers with one nerve damaged.
(C) Fingers with both nerves damaged.
(J. H. Boyes and H. H. Stark (1971) *J. Bone and Jt Surg.*, **53A**)

repaired, but if both nerves were severed and circulation to the finger was precarious, we repaired only one. Most of the 'salvage' fingers had both nerves damaged, while in the 'good' fingers, damage was usually limited to one digital nerve (Fig. 12.10).

Division of one nerve in a finger did not effect the result of grafting, but when both nerves were damaged, the resulting flexion was definitely compromised. This was true in all fingers, regardless of their preoperative classification; the influence of nerve damage in the 'good' classification was especially important. Seventy per cent of the 'good' fingers that had both nerves intact, or that had only one nerve divided, flexed to within 1.25 cm of the midpalmar crease after grafting (Fig. 12.11). By contrast, only 38 per cent of fingers with both nerves damaged could flex to within 1.25 cm of the midpalmar crease.

AGE OF PATIENT

The youngest patient was 17 months, and the oldest was 72 years. Ten per cent of the 538 patients were under six years of age, 38 per cent were 16 to 30 years of age, 30 per cent were 31 to 50 years of age, and 6 per cent of the patients were 50 and over (Table 12.5).

The effect of age on the result was studied in all preoperative classifications. In the 'good' group, patients over 30 years of age had worse results than younger patients, and after age 40 only one of 28 grafted fingers flexed completely (Fig. 12.12). An unexpected finding was that children under six years of age had worse results than all other age groups below 40 years (Table 12.6).

TABLE 12.6   Influence of age of patient on result in 'good' fingers

Age	No.	Flexion complete	Flexion to within 1.27 cm of distal palm
0–5	32	[10]%	[51]%
6–10	22	24 %	73 %
11–15	31	42 %	77 %
16–20	24	30 %	66 %
21–30	36	34 %	79 %
31–40	33	17 %	56 %
41+	28	[5]%	[30]%
Total	206		

Specifically, only 10 per cent of the 'good' fingers in children under six years of age flexed completely. The best results occurred in patients between 11 and 15 years of age; 42 per

TABLE 12.5   Age distribution in years (patients)

Class	0–5	6–10	11–15	16–20	21–30	31–40	41–50	51–60	Over 61	Total
Good	32	22	31	24	36	33	31	5	2	206
Scar	13	14	12	15	46	37	22	12	1	172
Joint	4	1	5	6	18	12	13	3	4	66
Multiple	6	3	5	9	15	10	11	2	1	62
Salvage	0	0	2	4	10	10	4	1	1	32
Total	55	40	55	58	125	102	71	23	9	538

cent of the 'good' fingers in this age group flexed completely after grafting. After age 41, only 5 per cent flexed to the distal palmar crease, and only 30 per cent flexed to within 1.27 cm of the distal palm.

In the 'scar' group, only 43 per cent of patients over age 40 flexed to within 2.5 cm of the distal palmar crease after grafting, while 60 per cent of patients younger than 40 could do so.

FINGER INJURED

Regardless of the preoperative classification, the best results were in the little finger and the worst results were in the index finger (Fig. 12.13). In the total group, 25 per cent of the little fingers flexed completely, and 85 per cent flexed to within 2.5 cm of the distal palmar crease. On the other hand, only 4 per cent of the index fingers flexed completely, and only 51 per cent of them flexed to within 2.5 cm of the distal palmar crease. Both the middle and ring fingers had better flexion than index fingers.

A study of the 200 fingers classified as 'good', provided further proof that the finger is important in determining the result (Fig. 12.14). Seventy-five little fingers and 59 index fingers were in this 'good' category. Thirty-seven per cent of the little fingers flexed completely, 88 per cent of them flexed to within 1.2 cm of the palm, and *all* of them flexed to within 3.1 cm of the distal palmar crease. By contrast, only 7 per cent of the index fingers flexed completely, while 36 per cent of them flexed to within 1.2 cm, and 80 per cent flexed to within 3.1 cm of the mid-palmar crease. If everything else is equal, flexion in a little finger after grafting will be much better than it will be in an index finger. Several factors are probably responsible for this finding. Since the index finger has much more independent function than the other fingers, it is easy

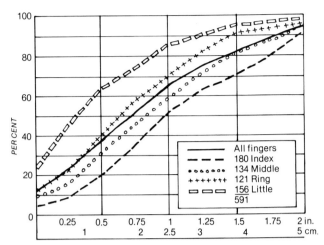

Figure 12.13
In the total group, the little fingers had much better flexion than the index fingers (J. H. Boyes and H. H. Stark, (1971) *J. Bone and Jt Surg.*, **53A**).

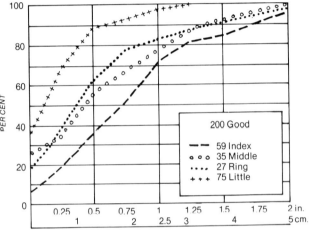

Figure 12.14 see text.

to avoid using the index finger by substituting the middle finger. Therefore, patients must make a deliberate effort to flex the index finger after grafting. On the other hand, when a patient can flex his ring and middle fingers, he will, after grafting, flex the little finger to some degree and this will hasten its recovery. Furthermore, the final 2.5 cm of finger flexion in the index is, from a functional standpoint, of little importance to most patients. Since this motion in a little finger is of great importance to most patients, they will struggle to regain it; (this is also true of the middle and ring fingers), but they have little incentive to exercise their index finger once it flexes enough to use it for pinch.

TIME FROM INJURY TO OPERATION

There is a mistaken idea that tendon grafting must be done soon after injury. Our results show that if joints remain supple, there is remarkably little effect caused by a time lapse between injury and operation. It is sensible to delay reconstruction due to school requirements of the patient, or to allow the soft tissues

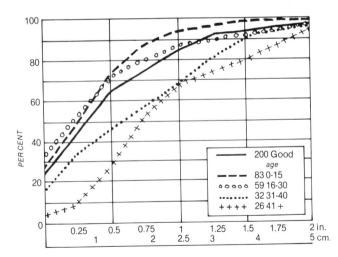

Figure 12.12
In the good preoperative classification, the percentage of fingers flexing to the distal palmar crease diminished after age 30, and after 40 years, only 4 per cent flexed to the palmar crease and only 28 per cent flexed to within 1.2 cm of the crease (J. H. Boyes and H. H. Stark (1971) *J. Bone and Jt Surg.*, **53A**).

to become more supple and the joints to be mobilized. Since several months elapsed between injury and grafting for the fingers that were classified as 'scarred', 'joint', or 'salvage', time between injury and grafting could not be studied as a single variable in these groups. This study was possible in the 200 fingers classified as 'good', for in this group many were grafted within a few weeks after injury, while others were grafted months, or even years, after injury. Forty-one of the 200 'good' fingers were grafted within two months after injury. The result in these 41 fingers was identical with the result of the fingers in the 'good' group which were grafted four months, six months, and twelve months after injury. Of the 200 'good' cases, 16 were grafted from two to twenty-four years after tendon injury. The original profundus tendon was used as a motor in each instance, and these fingers had results comparable to those fingers that were grafted within three months, six months, or one year after injury.

Restoration of useful finger flexion by grafting can be accomplished years after the tendon injury, providing the joints have remained limber and the fingers have adequate sensibility to justify reconstruction.

It is usually possible to use the original profundus tendon as a motor, but it is important that it be free of scar in the palm and wrist, and that it have a good excursion. Time spent mobilizing the profundus tendon is worthwhile, for when the profundus is too badly scarred and a superficialis tendon must be used to power the graft, a less favourable result can be anticipated.

EFFECT OF FAILED PRIMARY TENDON REPAIR ON TENDON RECONSTRUCTION

Ninety fingers were placed in the 'scar' category because of a failed primary tendon repair. Since the tendons in these fingers were cut by a sharp object and the fingers were without bone, joint or significant soft tissue injury, we can assume that these 90 fingers should have obtained the same result after grafting as the 200 that were classified as 'good', had not the tendon been repaired primarily. These 90 fingers had a less favourable result than the 200 'good' fingers (Fig. 12.15). Thirty-eight per cent of them flexed to within 1.2 cm of the distal palmar crease, while 64 per cent of the 'good' group did so. *The additional scar caused by a failed primary tendon repair compromised the results of secondary tendon grafting.*

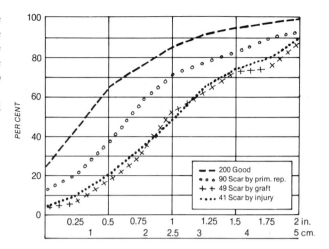

Figure 12.15
Ninety fingers classified as 'scarred' following the failure of a primary tendon repair which produced a clearly inferior result after the graft than did 200 fingers which had been treated solely by closure of the wound and secondary grafting.

Scarring from a failed primary tendon repair did not compromise the result as much as did scarring caused by the injury (41 fingers) or scarring following a failed tendon graft (49 fingers). At least one previous tendon graft had been placed in 49 fingers before our first treatment, and this graft had failed. A new graft provided useful motion to most of these fingers. Very few of them flexed completely, but 53 per cent flexed to within 2.5 cm of the distal palmar crease.

SOURCE OF GRAFTS

Table 12.7 shows the source of the tendon graft used in the 607 fingers. We used the palmaris longus with its paratenon in a few of the badly scarred fingers, but this experience is too limited to determine the value of a graft surrounded by paratenon. It is our current practice to use a silastic rod or ribbon in severely scarred fingers which we formerly treated with a paratenon graft. Even though the superficialis tendon of the middle and ring finger is of a larger calibre, we did not hesitate to use these tendons as a graft in children. In addition, we used one of these superficialis tendons as a graft when grafting two or more fingers at the same operation (multiple group).

When all other variables are eliminated, the source of the

TABLE 12.7 SOURCE OF GRAFT

Class	Palmaris	Palmaris with Paratenon	Flexor Superficialis	Plantaris	Toe Extensor	Other	Total
Good	159		34	6	6	1	206
Scar	129	5	23	4	10	1	172
Joint	44	4	14	3	1		66
Multiple	61		52	5	11	2	131
Salvage	20	2	5	3	1	1	32
Total	413	11	128	21	29	5	607

graft was not a significant factor in the end result. This conclusion was suggested by a study published in 1954, and the findings in this current and larger study reconfirmed that conclusion. In the 'good' group, a superficialis tendon was used as a graft in 34 fingers. The index finger superficialis was used as a graft in the index finger ten times, the middle finger superficialis was used in the middle finger nine times, the ring finger superficialis in the ring finger seven times, and the little finger superficialis in the little finger eight times. The palmaris longus without paratenon was used in 159 fingers and a plantaris tendon or a toe extensor tendon was used in the other 13 fingers.

Though the source of the graft had no effect on the result, in two of the eight fingers where the superficialis of the little finger was used as a graft, the graft disrupted in the palm.

PULLEYS

If possible, pulleys should be preserved in each finger, one in the middle segment, and one in the proximal segment near the web. If pulleys cannot be salvaged, then they should be reconstructed by free grafts. Fifty-three of the 607 fingers, or 7 per cent, had a pulley graft placed in the finger at the time of tendon grafting.

TABLE 12.8

Class	No. of Fingers	Pulleys
Good	206	8
Scar	172	22
Joint	66	3
Multiple	131	7
Salvage	32	13
Total	606	53

Two pulleys were placed in four fingers, one near the proximal interphalangeal joint and the other in the distal palm. As might be expected, pulley grafts were most often necessary in the 'scarred' and 'salvage' fingers (Table 12.8). When all other variables were eliminated, the 53 fingers with pulley grafts had results that were comparable to those in fingers where adequate pulleys were preserved from the fibrous sheath. We were surprised at this finding, but we must conclude that a *free pulley graft can be placed in a finger at the time of tendon grafting without compromising the result.*

COMPLICATIONS

Although we did not have a postoperative infection, a complication occurred in 47 of the 607 fingers. A postoperative haematoma occurred in six hands. In three of these the graft failed because the palmar tendon juncture separated. The other three grafts were salvaged by a secondary tenolysis, although these fingers had limited motion. *When a haematoma occurs postoperatively, the graft will, in all probability, either stick or disrupt and even if the graft is salvaged and the finger regains some useful motion, the result will be compromised.*

A graft can pull loose from its insertion into the distal phalanx, or it can separate at the palmar tendon juncture. Disruptions occur between the second and fifth week after grafting, but many of these grafts can be salvaged by re-operation. Of the 15 grafts that disrupted in the palm, eight were resutured to the profundus tendon immediately. Six of these fingers regained useful flexion and two were failures. Seven were not resutured because the patient refused surgery or because he was considered a poor candidate for further reconstruction. Seven of the tendon grafts that disrupted in the palm were of small calibre; that is, they were either a small superficialis of a little finger, or a plantaris tendon. These small grafts were used in less than 10 per cent of the fingers, yet almost 50 per cent of the disruptions occurred when small calibre grafts were used. *A small calibre tendon graft has a greater tendency to rupture or to pull loose from an attachment; the use of a tendon such as a superficialis of the little finger or a plantaris increases the likelihood of this complication.*

Six grafts ruptured at their insertion. All were reattached and five of these fingers regained useful function, while one was a failure.

Since we began closing the digital fascia with nonabsorbable sutures, less than 2 per cent of the fingers have developed a recurvatum deformity of the proximal interphalangeal joint. 'Good' fingers are apt to develop this deformity; fingers in the 'joint', 'scar', and 'salvage' categories usually have residual joint stiffness which precludes this complication. *For limber fingers, a meticulous closure of the digital fascia is an important part of the surgical technique.*

Other unusual complications included discomfort in the palm due to the wire tendon suture (two patients), trophic ulcer of a finger tip because of damage to both digital nerves (two patients), graft rupture caused by the patient breaking or removing his cast within two weeks after grafting (two patients), and an aneurysm of the common digital artery that was later resected (one patient). The two patients who ruptured their grafts were failures, but the other five patients had a useful finger after treatment of the complication.

SALVAGE PROCEDURES

Most of the fingers with a complication were salvaged by further surgery (Table 12.9).

Fourteen of the graft disruptions were resutured immediately and eleven obtained a satisfactory result. The distal

TABLE 12.9   Further surgery

	Number	Salvaged
Resuture of graft	14	11
Distal joint fusion	6	6
Tenolysis	14	8
Amputation of finger	3	0
New graft	3	0
Other	6	5
Total	46	30

joint of a finger was fused six times because of a severe flexion contracture. The graft was providing good motion to the proximal interphalangeal joint in these three fingers and after fusion of the distal joint, the finger was quite useful. Tenolysis was performed 14 times and motion was improved in eight of the 14 fingers. Tenolysis improved finger extension providing the graft was gliding, and providing it flexed the finger *before* tenolysis. If, however, the graft was adherent and did not flex the finger, tenolysis did not improve flexion. We perform a tenolysis to improve extension if a finger has good flexion, *but when a finger fails to flex well after a tendon graft, it is better to perform a new tendon graft than to try to restore flexion by tenolysis.*

FAILURE BECAUSE OF LIMITED FLEXION

Thirty-two grafts in 607 fingers, or 5 per cent, were considered complete failures due to lack of flexion (Table 12.10).

TABLE 12.10   Cause of failures due to lack of finger flexion

Separation of graft	9
Palmar hematoma and separation of graft	3
Uncooperative patient	5
Graft didn't slide	14
Other	1
Total	32

These failures were due to disruption of the graft or to failure of the finger to flex to within 5 cm of the distal palmar crease. The incidence of failure due to lack of flexion was highest in the 'salvage' and lowest in the 'multiple' and 'good' groups. Nine failures were due to rupture of the junction between the graft and the profundus tendon in the palm, and three ruptured in the palm because of a palmar haematoma. Five failures occurred in uncooperative patients who removed or damaged their splints during the immediate postoperative period. Fourteen failures were due to cicatrix binding the graft and preventing finger motion. In one patient, the graft necrosed throughout its length, as was demonstrated by later exploration.

FAILURE BECAUSE OF LIMITED EXTENSION

Even though a finger has excellent flexion after grafting, extension may be so limited that the result should be con-

FAILURES

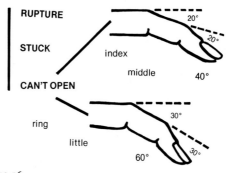

Figure 12.16
If the combined loss of extension in the two interphalangeal joints is greater than illustrated, the finger is a failure *because of limited extension.* Grafts fail because of limited flexion if they disrupt or if they fail to flex the finger tip to within 5 cm of the distal palmar crease.

sidered a failure. Although such fingers may still be useful to the patient because of the flexion provided by the graft, function of the finger is seriously impaired if extension loss is significant. We believe that if the combined extension loss of the two interphalangeal joints is less than 40 degrees in the index and middle fingers, and less than 60 degrees in the ring and little fingers, and if the finger flexes well, that satisfactory function has been restored (Fig. 12.16). Most patients can tolerate this much contracture of the interphalangeal joints. Loss of extension of the metacarpophalangeal joint has not been a problem in our patients, and flexion of this joint is a function of the intrinsic muscles rather than of the extrinsic muscles of the hand. *Regardless of the amount of flexion, we consider the result a failure due to lack of extension when the combined loss of extension of the two interphalangeal joints is greater than that described.* Using this criteria, we had 33 failures because of loss of extension. By combining these 33 fingers with those that failed because of limited flexion, we see that 10.7 per cent of the 607 fingers were called failures, (Table 12.11).

Only 3 per cent (6 fingers) of the fingers in the 'good' preoperative classification failed, three because of limited flexion and three because of extension loss. The percentage of failures was greatest in the index finger and smallest in the ring and little fingers (Table 12.12).

It is highly significant that half of our failures were due to limited

TABLE 12.11

Class	No. of Patients	No. of Grafts Poor Flexion	No. of Grafts Excessive Loss of Extension	Total No.	Per Cent
Good	206	3	3	6	3
Scar	172	15	6	21	12.7
Joint	66	6	3	9	15
Multiple	131	4	12	16	12
Salvage	32	4	9	13	40
Total	607	32	33	65	

TABLE 12.12   Total failures of tendon grafts in 607 fingers

	No. Grafts	Failed Because of Limited Flexion	Failed Because of Limited Extension	Total
Index	189	8%	7%	15%
Middle	137	4%	7%	11%
Ring	123	6%	2%	8%
Little	158	3%	6%	9%
Total	607			

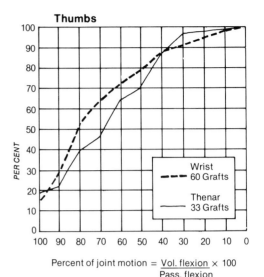

Percent of joint motion = $\dfrac{\text{Vol. flexion}}{\text{Pass. flexion}} \times 100$

Figure 12.17

In the thumb, grafts that extend to the musculotendinous junction above the wrist give better results than the shorter grafts. Percentage of joint motion = active flexion/passive flexion × 100.

extension, and this cannot be determined unless motions of all finger joints are actually measured with a goniometer and the motion recorded. A comparison of the results obtained by other methods of treatment will be meaningful only when a uniform but simple method of reporting results is adopted.

TENDON GRAFTS IN THE THUMB

Since 1954, tendon grafts were placed in 93 thumbs. In 70 per cent of these thumbs, the original wound was treated by primary closure. The palmaris longus tendon was used as a graft in 79 of the 93 thumbs, a pulley graft was placed in three, and the end result was known in 90 of the 93 thumbs. There were two failures, both in uncooperative patients. The result was not influenced by the location of the wound of injury, by the time lag between injury and operation, or by adding a pulley graft to the operation. The amount of preoperative scarring had little effect on the final result.

Final function was recorded by measuring in degrees the voluntary flexion of the interphalangeal joint after grafting. This figure was used as the numerator. The preoperative passive flexion of the same joint was used as the denominator, and the fraction reduced to a percentage. Young patients had better results than older patients. Sixty per cent of patients under 31 years of age regained 70 per cent of their preoperative flexion after grafting. Although the damage to both volar nerves of the thumb had an adverse effect on the result, the effect of nerve damage was much less than it was in fingers. This probably indicates that a person will use a thumb even though it has poor sensibility, while he will bypass a numb finger and use an adjacent finger that has better sensibility, if it is possible to do so.

A previous study suggested that a graft extending from the distal phalanx of the thumb to the musculotendinous junction at the wrist (a long graft) gave better results than grafts extending from the distal phalanx to the thenar eminence (a short graft). This present study afforded an opportunity to test the validity of that assumption. Slightly better results were obtained in the 66 thumbs treated by a long graft, although the difference in the result was not as great as anticipated (Fig. 12.17). However, all badly scarred thumbs were treated with

a long graft, while those with minimal scar received a short graft. None of the 66 patients had median nerve irritation because of use of the longer graft.

Five patients had a significant loss of extension after surgery. Patients who lost more than 25 degrees of extension of the metacarpophalangeal joint were dissatisfied, even though the interphalangeal joint extended normally. This circumstance occurred in three of the five patients. Two other patients were unhappy because they lost 45 degrees or more of combined extension of the metacarpophalangeal and interphalangeal joint, even though their thumbs had 80 per cent of normal flexion. If stability and useful flexion of the interphalangeal joint flexion is restored by the graft, and if metacarpophalangeal joint flexion is not reduced by more than 25 degrees, patients will consider the result of surgery worthwhile, even though interphalangeal joint extension is limited by as much as 40 degrees.

GENERAL CONCLUSION

This study shows the result that can be expected from reconstruction of a flexor tendon in fingers when both flexors have been cut, and the influence of factors such as scarring, joint stiffness, age, and donor tendon, on the result. This study also suggests that primary repair of flexor tendons might be justified in patients under six years of age and over 40 years, for the results after grafting in patients of this age group are less gratifying than in patients between the age of six and 40 years.

REFERENCES

BOYES, J. H. (1950) Flexor-tendon grafts in the fingers and thumb. An evaluation of end results. *J. Bone and Jt Surg.*, **32-A,** 489–499.

BOYES J. H. (1955) Evaluation of results of digital flexor tendon grafts. *Am. J. Surg.*, **89,** 1116–1119.

BOYES, J. H. (1953) Operative technique of flexor tendon grafts. In *Instructional Course Lectures, American Academy of Orthopaedic Surgeons*. vol. 10. Ed. Pease C. N., Ann Arbor, Michigan: J. W. Edwards.

BOYES, J. H., & STARK, H. H. (1971) Flexor-tendon grafts in the fingers and thumb. A study of factors influencing results in 1000 cases. *J. Bone and Jt Surg.*, **53-A,** 1332–1342.

BUNNELL, Sterling (1944) *Surgery of the Hand.* 1st edn. Philadelphia: J. B. Lippincott.

13. Two Stage Flexor Tendon Reconstruction: A Technique Using a Tendon Prosthesis Prior to Tendon Grafting

James M. Hunter

INTRODUCTION

In 1965, evidence was presented that a new tendon bed and sheath would form in response to a gliding tendon prosthesis and that a free tendon graft could be inserted in the new sheath and remain functional (Hunter, 1965; Hunter, 1967). Since the presentation of these findings, our progressively improving clinical results (Hunter and Salisbury, 1971) in the salvage of fingers with severe tendon injuries has led us to believe that a reliable tendon prosthesis inserted as one stage in tendon reconstruction is the additional step needed to improve the results of flexor-tendon reconstructive surgery.

The method has been applied in more than 150 tendon reconstructions of various types. It is the purpose of this report to describe the presently used two-stage technique for flexor-tendon reconstruction in hands in which the conditions are less than optimum and to report the results in seventy-four of eighty-six consecutive cases in which this method has been employed.

THE PROSTHESIS

With the cooperation of the Holter Company a division of Extracorporeal Medical Specialties, Inc., the Philadelphia College of Textiles and Science, and the Orthopaedic Research Laboratories at Jefferson Medical College, a free-gliding prosthesis was developed. The prosthesis is constructed of a woven Dacron core (Fig. 13.1) which is moulded into radio-opaque silicone rubber. The surface finish is smooth and the cross-sectional design is ovoid to aid optimal tendon sheath development. The prosthesis has the necessary combination of firmness and flexibility, as well as the smooth glistening surface required to ensure ease of insertion and free passive gliding throughout the finger, palm, and forearm.

The prosthesis is currently available through distributors* in four sizes: 3 mm × 23 cm, 4 mm × 23 cm, 5 mm × 25 cm, and 6 mm × 25 cm. At the time of insertion, the prosthesis may be trimmed for proper length with a scalpel.

Currently, new yarns and cables, made of stainless steel, Titanium, and a combination of tantalum and platinum are being tested in the hope that, with proper design and fabrication of the yarn and the addition of end devices, an active tendon prosthesis can be developed which may be used for extended periods before a second-stage procedure for tendon grafting is required.

INDICATIONS FOR USE

There is sufficient evidence to suggest that the surgeon trained in hand surgery should consider using a tendon prosthesis in selected primary injuries where the tendon gliding

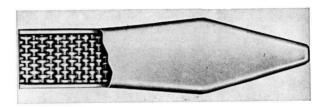

Figure 13.1
Appearance of the tendon prosthesis, made up of a nucleus of Dacron tissue moulded in a radio opaque siliconed india-rubber. The surface is smooth and the outline transverse ovoid.

bed has been severely damaged. The results also indicate that a failed primary suture in 'no man's land' need not compromise the secondary flexor tendon graft if this two-stage technique is used.

Staged tendon reconstruction using the tendon prosthesis prior to tendon grafting is indicated in most instances where the tendon gliding bed has been damaged. In fact, all patients to be tendon grafted are potential candidates for this procedure since only at surgery can the true extent of damage to the tendon bed be determined.

TECHNIQUE

Patients selected for the two-stage tendon reconstruction are put on a programme designed to mobilize stiff joints and to improve the condition of the soft tissues as much as possible before the first stage.

STAGE I

The damaged flexor tendons and their scarred sheath are exposed. In the finger, this is done through a zig-zag incision (Fig. 13.5) as popularized by Bruner (1967). In the palm, exposure is accomplished through a transverse incision or through a proximal continuation of Bruner's zig-zag incision. In the forearm, an ulnarly curved volar incision (Fig. 13.3) is made to expose the proximal portions of the flexor tendons and their musculotendinous junctions. A stump of the profundus tendon (Fig. 13.2), one centimetre in length, is left attached to the distal phalanx. Scarred tendons, sheath, and retinaculum are then excised. If the excision is stopped in the palm at the lumbrical level, the contracted and scarred lumbrical muscle is excised. Contracted or scarred lumbricals should always be excised (Hunter and Salisbury, 1970). This is done to prevent the paradoxical motion of the lumbrical which is seen after some tendon grafts (Parkes, 1971). This motion causes the finger to extend rather than flex as the patient attempts to flex the finger completely.

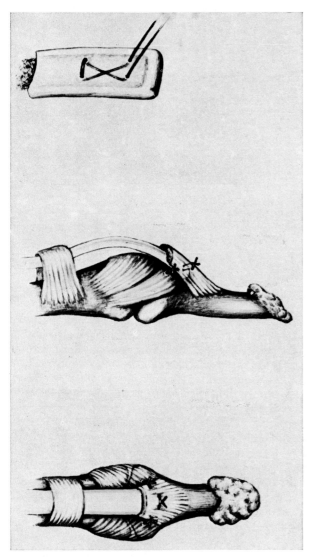

Figure 13.2
The distal extremity of the prosthesis is sutured to the tendinous stump by a figure of eight stitch and made fast laterally by lateral stitches passed through the adjaent fibrous tissues.

Undamaged portions of the flexor fibro-osseous retinaculum (pulley system) which are not contracted are retained. Any portion of the retinaculum that can be dilated instrumentally with a hemostat is also preserved. The rest is excised. The retinacular pulley system (Fig. 13.2) should be preserved or reconstructed proximal to the axis of motion of each joint, otherwise normal gliding of the tendon will not be restored. Four pulleys are preferred: one proximal to each of the three finger joints and one at the base of the proximal phalanx.

New pulleys may be fashioned from available tendon material to be discarded. The tendon graft should be fixed laterally to the fibro-osseous remnant of the old pulley. The pulley diameter should be of ample size to permit easy gliding of the prosthesis.

Meticulous care of the prosthesis is most important. The prosthesis is normally supplied sterile; if however, it should become contaminated the manufacturer's instructions regarding cleaning and sterilizing should be followed exactly. After sterilization, the prosthesis should be kept in a lint free receptacle. When handled at operation, gloves should be freshly moistened with sterile saline or Ringer's solution before contact with the implant, or sponges wet with sterile saline or Ringer's solution should be used to hold the device. A large tendon prosthesis (5 mm) is preferred. It is first placed on sponges moistened with sterile saline or Ringer's solution on the volar aspect of the forearm, and then a tendon passer, with a diameter slightly larger than that of the prosthesis, is passed proximally from the palm through the carpal tunnel into the forearm. The distal end of the prosthesis is secured to this and pulled into the palm, whence it can be pushed through the retinaculum and pulleys to the distal end of the finger—a process facilitated by moistening the prosthesis with sterile saline or Ringer's solution. An alternate method is to insert the prosthesis in a proximal direction by seeking a free plane in the carpal canal by blunt instrumentation. The superficialis and profundus tendons may be transected either proximal or distal to the carpal canal. If proximal, the tendon is sutured to the fascia beneath the flexion crease of the wrist. The purpose of this suture is (1) to prevent the muscle (a potential motor for the free tendon graft to be inserted during Stage II) from shortening: (2) to provide for some isometric function of the muscle during the interval between Stage I and II, and (3) to facilitate identification of the muscle during Stage II and hence to reduce the amount of dissection required.

The distal end of the prosthesis is sutured beneath the stump of the profundus tendon after resecting all but the most distally attached fibres of the tendon (Fig. 13.2). A figure-of-eight suture of No. 32 or 34 monofilament stainless steel wire on an atraumatic taper-cut needle is used. In addition, medial and lateral sutures of No. 35 multifilament wire are usually put through the tendon, the prosthesis, and the fibroperiosteum for further fixation. Any excess of profundus tendon is resected. Traction is then applied on the proximal end of the prosthesis in the forearm, to be sure that the attachment of the prosthesis is distal to the distal interphalangeal joint and its volar plate and that there is no binding of the tendon during flexion and extension. The prosthesis is also observed during passive flexion and extension of the finger (Fig. 13.3), to make sure that it glides freely with no binding or buckling distal to some part of the pulley system which is too tight. If any portion of the system is tight, it must be removed and replaced with a new pulley constructed from a free tendon graft.

The proximal end of the prosthesis should also be observed during passive flexion and extension to make sure that it glides properly. Preferably, this end of the prosthesis should be in the forearm so that the newly-formed sheath will extend to the region of the musculotendinous junction of the motor muscle. The prosthesis may be placed superficial or deep to the antebrachial fascia or deep in one of the intermuscular planes. The bed for the prosthesis can be fashioned by separating tendon mesenteries with the moistened gloved finger. If such a bed cannot be established by spreading and adjustment of the

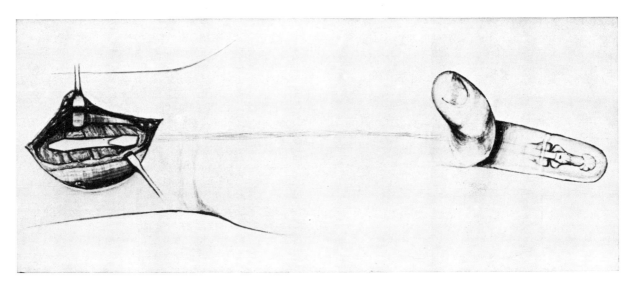

Figure 13.3
Flexion and extension of the digit show the gliding amplitude of the prosthesis.

tissues, the prosthesis should be shortened so that, when the finger is fully extended, the proximal end of the prosthesis lies just proximal to the flexion crease at the wrist.

When multiple prostheses are threaded through the carpal canal, the superficialis tendons are generally removed from the canal. To date, carpal tunnel syndrome has not been observed with one or more prostheses traversing the canal.

Finally, before the wound is closed, traction should again be applied to the prosthesis and the amount of active finger motion determined and recorded. If this manoeuvre does not produce full flexion it may be necessary to modify the pulley system. This is a most important point and is a unique feature of this technique.

POSTOPERATIVE TECHNIQUE—STAGE I

Following skin closure, a standard post-operative hand dressing is applied, with the wrist and metacarpophalangeal joints in moderate flexion (40 to 50 degrees) and the interphalangeal joints in slight flexion (20 to 30 degrees). Where there were joint contractures prior to insertion of the prosthesis, intermittent dynamic splinting may be required to prevent recurrence of the contracture. Intermittent elastic finger traction may be started during the first postoperative week. Gentle passive motion of all joints is started gradually during the second to the fourth week. Regular passive stretching, under the supervision of a hand therapist, is begun in the fifth week and the patient is taught at this time to flex the finger whenever possible, using an adjacent finger hooked over the damaged one. Usually, by the sixth week, there is a functional range of passive motion. During this time the hand should be examined regularly for evidence of synovitis in the new sheath. If this has not developed within the first six weeks, it is not likely to occur and the patient may resume normal activities, including going back to work, until he is ready for the second stage.

A small amount of barium sulphate is impregnated in the prosthesis so that its function can be checked roentgenographically at six weeks and again just before insertion of the tendon graft (Fig. 13.4). Anteroposterior and lateral roentgenograms of the hand and distal one-half of the forearm are made with the fingers and wrist in full extension and full flexion. These roentgenograms will demonstrate how much the proximal end of the prosthesis moves with respect to the distal end of the radius. If there is a full range of motion of the wrist and all finger joints, an excursion of 5–7 cms is not unusual. These roentgenograms will also show any evidence of buckling. Slight or intermittent buckling may cause no difficulty. However, if there is appreciable buckling, synovitis is likely to occur and the patient should be followed carefully. If synovitis develops, the finger should be immobilized promptly and if the synovitis persists, the second-stage procedure should be done sooner before chronic fibrosis develops.

The interval between Stage I and Stage II should be two to six months, or long enough to permit maturation of the tendon bed to the point where it can nourish and lubricate the gliding tendon graft. In fingers in which fixed flexion contractures of many months' duration are mobilized for the first time at the Stage I procedure, Stage II should be delayed until maximum softening of the tissues and mobilization of the stiff joints have been achieved. Each case must be individualized and the decision to do the second-stage procedure must be made by the surgeon on the basis of the findings in the hand.

STAGE II

When Stage II is begun, the limits of extension and flexion of the finger must first be accurately measured and recorded. A short mid-lateral or Bruner zig-zag incision is then made to locate the distal end of the prosthesis where it is attached to the distal phalanx (Fig. 13.5). This attachment is left intact and a second ulnarly curved volar incision is made in the forearm through the original Stage I incision to expose the proxi-

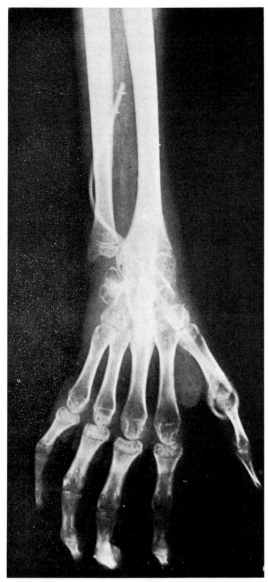

Figure 13.4
An X-ray shows clearly the passage of the endoprosthesis.

(Fig. 13.5). Leaving the distal end of the prosthesis attached to the distal phalanx, the rest of the prosthesis, with the attached tendon graft, is pulled distally, thereby threading the graft through the new sheath. The prosthesis is then removed and discarded. Free motion of the graft in the sheath can now be confirmed by grasping each end of the graft with a haemostat and pulling it proximally and distally.

The tendon graft is secured to the distal phalanx using a Bunnell button-pull-out wire suture, with the button on the fingernail. Medial and lateral reinforcing sutures through the profundus tendon stump are placed. Traction is now applied to the proximal end of the graft and the predicted range of active flexion, measured as the distance of the finger pulp from the distal palmar crease, is determined. After this manoeuvre, the attachment of the graft to the distal phalanx is inspected, to check on the security of the fixation.

The condition of the tissues at the site of the proximal anastomosis is critical. Atraumatic technique should be used during the dissection. Scar tissue and thickened antebrachial fascia are excised to minimize motion-restricting adhesions. When the firm fascia is carefully dissected away from the newly-formed tendon sheath, the sheath is found to be soft, with loose mesentery-like attachments to the surrounding tissues (Fig. 13.5). If the sheath is thickened or scarred as the result of synovitis, it is resected far enough distally so that there will be no scar in the region of the tendon suture. If the anastomosis is small in diameter, the sheath may be placed around it. This is not always possible, however, due to the bulk of the graft-tendon junction. In this event the sheath is either dissected away completely so that there is no contact between the anastomosis and the sheath, or the sheath may be left open so that one side of the anastomosis glides on the sheath.

In most patients in the series reported here, the proximal anastomosis was in the forearm. For the index finger when either the superficialis or the profundus muscle was available as a motor, the graft was anastomosed to the proximal segment of the motor tendon according to the method of Pulvertaft. For the long, ring, and little fingers, on the other hand, the graft was woven through oblique stab incisions in the common profundus tendon securing the different tendons together as one tendon unit. In a few instances in which the palm was not involved, a palmaris longus graft was used and the proximal end of the graft was sutured to the profundus tendon at the origin of the lumbrical muscle. If the proximal anastomosis is done in the palm, the superficialis or profundus of the injured finger or the superficialis of an adjacent finger may be used as the motor. If the forearm is the site of the anastomosis, the same three options are available.

It is essential to adjust the length of the graft accurately. The excursion of the tendon graft should now be checked by pulling on the graft, starting with the finger in full extension (Fig. 13.6). Having determined the excursion necessary to produce a full range of flexion, the excursions of the available motors are then determined and the one is selected which has the requisite excursion. Obviously, if the motor lacks sufficient excursion, active motion will not be complete, even if the anastomosis is exact and the tendon graft glides perfectly.

mal end of the prosthesis and the musculotendinous junction of the superficialis or profundus tendon, whichever is to be used as a motor for the tendon graft.

While the prosthesis is still in place, the excursion of the proximal end of the prosthesis should also be measured as an additional check on the amount of excursion that the motor muscle must have to provide full finger motion.

A long tendon graft is then obtained from one leg—the plantaris preferably—but if this is missing a long toe extensor tendon may be used. If a toe extensor must be employed, the graft is obtained using a modified Brand tendon stripper and two or more incisions, so that the portion of the tendon proximal to the ankle retinaculum is obtained. Any attached fat or muscle is removed and one end of the graft is sutured to the proximal end of the prosthesis with a catgut or polyester suture

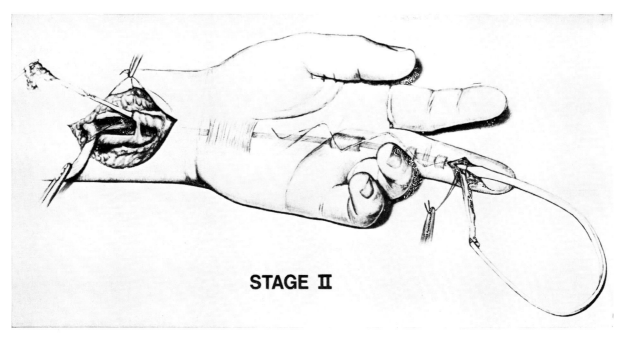

Figure 13.5
The graft sutured to the prosthetic shaft is drawn up distally across the new sheath. Note the new growth connecting the sheath to the surrounding tissues, easily visible in the forearm.

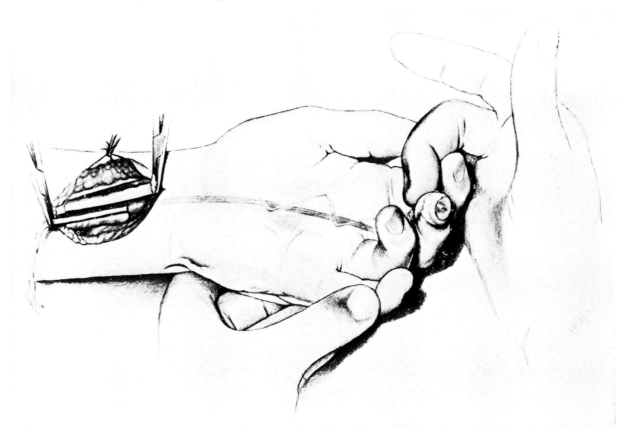

Figure 13.6
Before carrying out the proximal anastomosis, the course of the graft must be measured and choice made of a motor muscle which follows the same course as that of the graft.

The tension of the graft is adjusted so that, with the wrist in neutral, the involved finger rests in slightly more flexion than that of the adjacent fingers. When the anastomosis has been completed, the tension is checked with the wrist in both flexion and extension to assess the tenodesis effect and to make sure that the tension of the graft is correct. Currently all uncomplicated Stage II procedures are done under local anaesthesia, supplemented with a sedative analgesic drug (Innovar). A pneumatic arm tourniquet is used intermittently during the procedure. After the distal anastomosis is completed and the distal wound is closed, the graft is sutured tentatively to the motor tendon; and, after the tourniquet has been deflated for ten to fifteen minutes, the patient is asked to flex and extend the finger. If the predicted amount of active flexion is not achieved, the tension of the graft is readjusted or a motor tendon with a better excursion is selected. When the patient can accomplish the predicted amount of flexion the anastomosis is completed and the wound is closed and dressed.

This procedure eliminates the guess work in establishing optimum tension in the graft and the results to date have been very encouraging. Removal of the tendon graft from the leg under this type of anaesthesia has not caused difficulty. If a tendon stripper is used the patient may have some, but not excessive, discomfort. No patient has complained that the procedure was unduly uncomfortable.

When the proximal anastomosis is completed, the peritenon may be pulled distally and sutured to the proximal end of the newly formed sheath or to the surrounding tissues as far distally as possible. The wound is irrigated with sterile saline solution and then closed, and the final dressing is applied, with a plaster splint to maintain the wrist and metacarpophalangeal joints in moderate flexion and the interphalangeal joints in slight flexion.

POST OPERATIVE TECHNIQUE—STAGE II

Early protected active flexion of the grafted finger is encouraged while a padded dorsal splint prevents sudden forceful extension. Each patient is instructed at the first postoperative dressing, usually after five to seven days, to splint the metacarpophalangeal joints while the proximal and distal interphalangeal joints are actively flexed and extended. If necessary, intermittent splinting is continued during the fourth week while the pull-out suture and button are still in place. In the fifth week the pull-out wire is removed and light passive stretching exercises may be started if necessary. Some vigorous patients with full excursion of the graft may require intermittent splinting during the fourth week to protect the proximal anastomosis from excessive stress. If stubborn contractures were present prior to tendon grafting, a supervised programme of passive stretching and splinting may be required after the fifth week. Patients should achieve a full range of active motion during the sixth to twelfth week. Intensive training in active exercises personally supervised by the operating surgeon during this period are essential.

COMPLICATIONS

The complications related to the Stage I and Stage II operations were analysed separately.

STAGE I

The complication of synovitis is characterized by the following (singly or in combination): pain in the finger tip, swelling along the volar surface of the finger, and swelling and erythema at the site of the incision in the forearm. In some of the earlier cases, this complication was caused by soiling of the prosthesis. After the technique was perfected, synovitis occurred only occasionally, caused by excessive motion of the prosthesis too soon after surgery or when there was mechanical obstruction to the gliding of the prosthesis producing buckling. If the synovitis does not respond to five to seven days of immobilization followed by gradual resumption of activity, the Stage II procedure should be performed earlier and the thickened synovium excised in the region of the proximal anastomosis.

STAGE II

There are two complications after Stage II tendon grafting that deserve discussion:

1. Adhesions along the tendon graft or at the proximal anastomosis; and

2. rupture of the anastomosis of the tendon graft.

Restrictive adhesions may occur along the tendon graft, particularly at sites of dense scar and tight pulleys where sheath nutrition is poor, if good freely lubricated movement of the graft is not established early after surgery.

Restrictive adhesions may form around the proximal anastomosis particularly when there has been previous trauma to this area with subsequent scarring. The functional significance of adhesions about the proximal end of the tendon graft cannot be overemphasized. These adhesions, of course, are part of the normal healing reaction but at times they may be the only adhesions preventing good function. Under these circumstances, the adhesions can best be released under direct vision.

If tenolysis is necessary, it is performed three months after Stage II using local anaesthesia, Innovar analgesia, and a tourniquet. Since tourniquet ischaemia rather consistently produces paralysis of the extrinsic muscles after 25 minutes and of the intrinsic muscles after 30 minutes, the tourniquet should be released at 25-minute intervals so that active function of the finger flexors can be tested. Thus during the first 25 minutes active function can be tested with the tourniquet inflated. It then must be deflated and reinflated as need be to test function.

By this means it is possible to visualize the problem while the patient actively flexes and extends his fingers. The region of the proximal anastomosis should be explored first, with attention directed initially to the junction of the new tendon sheath and the tendon graft; next, to the proximal anastomosis; and, lastly, to the tendon graft within the new sheath. Only adhesions which actually restrict motion should be lysed.

After surgery, immediate active motion of the lysed tendon graft is necessary to preserve the increased ranges of motion.

RESULTS

It is difficult to compare the results of tendon repair reported by different authors (Hunter and Salisbury, 1971; Littler, 1947; Tubiana, 1960), because criteria for selection and methods of grading the preoperative status of the hands have varied. However, if these differences are kept in mind, a meaningful comparison of these results with those of Boyes, White, and Pulvertaft seems possible.

The results in the thumb were reported as a percentage—the active flexion divided by the passive flexion. Boyes (1955) reported on 21 cases, 11 of which were in the good categories preoperatively. Ten per cent of his patients achieved 90 per cent motion. Most of them were treated with short grafts with the proximal suture line in the thenar eminence. The two best results in his series were obtained when the proximal anastomosis was placed at the musculotendinous junction in the forearm. Pulvertaft reported on 42 cases in which there were all grades of involvement preoperatively. All of his patients were treated with tendon grafts and 30 per cent of them achieved 90 per cent motion in their thumbs. In our five thumbs, all graded in the poor categories preoperatively and all treated by the two-stage method, 90 per cent motion was achieved.

The fingers reported on by Boyes and by us were selected and graded preoperatively in essentially the same manner.

For the purposes of evaluation, the patients' status at their initial examination was graded according to the following classification, modified from the one proposed by Boyes (1950, 1955).

Grade 1 (good): Good soft tissues, supple joints, and no significant scarring. (No Grade 1 patients were included in this series, since in all of these conventional tendon grafts can be used.)

Grade 2 (scar): Deep cicatrix, resulting from injury or previous surgery, as well as mild soft-tissue contractures which, in a few instances, were severe enough to require preliminary plastic procedures.

Grade 3 (joint): Limitation of passive joint motion, usually in the proximal interphalangeal joint, sufficient to require mobilization by traction and dynamic splinting. (In this series,

all Grade 3 patients had scarring of the tendon bed. Those with extensive scarring were classed Grade 5.)

Grade 4 (nerve): Nerve damage with associated trophic changes in addition to scarring of the tendon bed and joint stiffness. (There were no Grade 4 patients in this series; but, in future studies, patients with injuries to both digital nerves in one finger will be included.)

Grade 5 (multiple): Soft tissue scarring or joint changes in more than one digit, or a combination of injuries in a single digit of such character at Grades 2, 3 and 4 did not apply, and in addition, involvement of the palm in many cases.

The result in each patient was correlated with the preoperative grade.

The results in these two series are compared in Table 13.1, eliminating Boyes cases which were classified good. The incidence of fingers which postoperatively could flex sufficiently to bring the pulp to within 2.5 cm or less of the distal palmar crease is strikingly higher in our series. Although our series is considerably smaller, the comparison, nonetheless, strongly suggests that the procedure described here can produce results better than those attained by conventional methods in less than optimum cases.

White classified his cases as good and less than good preoperatively, and reported that of the 48 patients with less-than-good fingers, 35 per cent could flex the pulp of the involved finger postoperatively to within 2.5 cm of the distal palmar crease. Of our 69 patients, all with a less-than-good rating preoperatively, 80 per cent could flex their finger to within 2.5 cm or less of the distal palmar crease at follow-up. These results represent a considerable improvement over those reported by White.

Pulvertaft grouped all of his tendon grafts together and reported that 70 per cent of his 90 patients achieved pulp-to-crease flexion of 2.5 cm or less. Again our results compare very favourably.

Finally, it is worth noting that, in their good cases, 2.5 cm pulp-to-crease flexion was achieved in 84 per cent by Boyes (Grade 1) and in 79 per cent by White. The percentages in these good cases are essentially the same as the percentages in our cases, all of which were less than good.

TABLE 13.1   Comparison of results in this series with those of Boyes in hands graded 2, 3 and 5*: Preoperative grade versus distance of finger tip pulp from distal palmar crease

	Grades		0 cm	1.3 cm	2.5 cm	3.8 cm	No. of Cases
Hunter and Salisbury, 1970	2 Scar		16 +	57	85	85	12
	3 Joint		31	62	85	85	13
	5 Multiple		25	45	79	79	44
		Total Cases					69%
Boyes, 1955	2 Scar		8	24	49	82	79
	3 Joint		12	30	64	82	33
	5 Multiple		2	6	45	—	64
		Total Cases					176%

* No Grade 1 fingers included in this series.
† Figures are in percentages which are cumulative.

CASE REPORT

M.D., a left-handed female cafeteria worker, had sustained a severe laceration of the left palm on a broken bottle. Primary skin closure was performed, followed one month later by tenorrhaphies in the palm. Six months later, the patient was referred for treatment of her persistent numbness and lack of flexion of the left long, ring, and little fingers.

Four neurorrhaphies were performed and the scarred superficialis tendons of the long and ring fingers were excised. Five months later, after the patient had received intensive physical therapy and had acceptable sensation and active flexion of the long and ring fingers but not in the little finger, a Stage I procedure was performed on the little finger. This included excision of dense scar which extended from the base of the finger proximally for the full extent of the tendon bed in the palm. The tissues in the finger were atrophic, an appearance consistent with what would be expected after absence of function for one year. A medium prosthesis was inserted from the distal phalanx to the forearm and the finger pulleys were preserved or reconstructed. The potential range of motion was then from full extension to full flexion and the finger was assigned Grade 2, since the defect was primarily scarring of the bed.

The postoperative course was uneventful and, five months later, a Stage II procedure was performed. A long toe-extensor tendon was used as the graft. In the forearm, the common tendon of the profundus muscle of the ring and little finger was used as the motor.

Two months later, the pulp of the little finger could be actively flexed to within 0.6 cm of the palmar crease, and one month later, flexion was complete (Figs. 13.7A and 13.7B).

The good result in this patient is believed to be significant because this finger was of the type in which a conventional graft is often attempted with a poor result. Typically the tissues are soft and the joints are mobile but there is extensive scarring of the tendon bed in the finger and in the palm.

The excellent result obtained in this little finger suggests that this procedure has a place in the treatment of borderline injuries which do not belong in the salvage category, yet often do not do well after conventional tendon grafts.

SUMMARY

The two-stage procedure for tendon reconstruction using a gliding silicone Dacron-reinforced prosthesis has important advantages. A new tendon bed and anatomical pulley system, with gliding surfaces, is established prior to the insertion of the graft. At the first stage, it is possible to do multiple procedures, such as digital neurorrhaphy, osteotomy and capsulotomy, (Curtis, 1954, 1966) in addition to resection of scar, construction of the pulley system, and insertion of the prosthesis. By careful preoperative planning it is therefore possible to reduce the number of operations necessary to reconstruct a severely damaged hand. It should be emphasized, however, that fingers which are stiff, as the result of severe injury or repeated unsuccessful operations, cannot be benefited by this

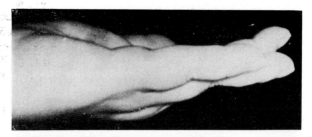
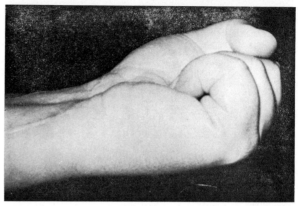

Figure 13.7
(A) and (B) Result of a flexor graft carried out in two stages at the level of the little finger.

procedure. Restoration of a tendon sheath and a gliding tendon will not mobilize a stiff finger.

When there has been extensive damage to the palm, the two-stage procedure, with a long graft and the proximal anastomosis in the forearm, has great advantages and is the procedure of choice. When this is done, the proximal anastomosis may be placed beneath the profundus peritenon, within the superficialis peritenon, or within the newly formed sheath, thereby reducing the formation of restrictive adhesions.

The evidence from our clinical experience suggests that the sheath which forms about the gliding tendon prosthesis after Stage I procedure can provide the nutritional requirements of a free tendon graft with minimum or no adhesions. When the gliding prosthesis is removed, the sheath which has formed around it apparently has both the physiological and the anatomical characteristics necessary to nourish a tendon graft.

Results in the salvage of fingers with severe tendon injuries has led us to believe that a reliable tendon prosthesis inserted as one stage in tendon reconstruction is the additional step needed to improve the results of flexor tendon reconstructive surgery.

Although the results with the passive prosthesis have been distinctly encouraging, it would seem that a reliable active prosthesis would have advantages under certain circumstances. From our earlier experience it would appear that an active tendon prosthesis results in better organization of the tissues in the region of the proximal anastomosis so that at the Stage II procedure there is a good connective tissue mesentery which can be preserved when the graft is inserted. As a result there is an earlier return of function after grafting. In addition, with an active prosthesis the muscle which is to be the motor for the graft continues to function, fewer adhesions form, and functional training after grafting is simplified.

Continuing research with porous synthetic and metal fabrics, metal end devices, indicates the basic direction for further research in the development of active artificial tendons in the future.

The prosthesis, as it is now produced should be used primarily as a passive gliding device with no proximal attachment. However, in carefully selected and closely supervised patients, the prosthesis may be made active by suturing its proximal end to the proximal tendon stump or musculotendinous junction of the motor muscles in the palm or forearm.

GREAT BRITAIN
Charles F. Thackray, Ltd
P.O. Box 171
Park St
Leeds LS 1 1RQ, England
GERMANY
Dr E. Fresenius KG
Gluckensteinweg 5
638 Bad Homburg V.D.H. Germany
FRANCE
Climo S.A.
104, Cours Albert Thomas
69–Lyon (8ᵉ), France

REFERENCES

BOYES, J. H. (1950) Flexor tendon grafts in the fingers and thumb. An evaluation of end results. *J. Bone and J. Surg.*, **32-A,** 489–499.

BOYES, J. H. (1955) Evaluation of results of digital flexor tendon grafts. *Am. J. Surg.*, **89,** 1116–1119.

BRUNER, J. M. (1967) The zig-zag volar-digital incision for flexor-tendon surgery. *Plast. Reconstruct. Surg.*, **40,** 571–574.

CURTIS, R. M. (1966) Joints of the hand. In *Hand Surgery*, Flynn, J. E. pp. 350–375. Baltimore: The Williams and Wilkins Co.

CURTIS, R. M. (1954) Capsulectomy of the interphalangeal joints of the fingers. *J. Bone and J. Surg.*, **36-A,** 1219–1232.

HUNTER, J. M. (1965) Artificial tendons: early development and application. *Am. J. Surg.*, **109,** 325–338.

HUNTER, J. M. (1965) Artificial tendons: Their early development and application. In Proceedings of the American Society for Surgery of the Hand. *J. Bone and J. Surg.*, **47-A,** 631–632.

HUNTER, J. M. & SALISBURY, R. E. (1970) Use of gliding artificial implants to produce tendon sheaths. Techniques and results in children. *Plast. Reconstruct. Surg.*, **45,** 564–572.

HUNTER, J. M. & SALISBURY, R. E. (1971) Flexor-tendon reconstruction in severely damaged hands—A two-stage procedure using a silicone-dacron reinforced gliding prosthesis prior to tendon grafting. *J. Bone and J. Surg.*, **53-A,** 829–858.

LITTLER, J. W. (1947) Free tendon grafts in secondary flexor tendon repair. *Am. J. Surg.*, **74,** 315–321.

LITTLER, J. W. (1964) Principles of reconstructive surgery of the hand. In *Reconstructive Plastic Surgery*, Converse, J. M. Vol. 4, pp. 1612–1674. Philadelphia: W. B. Saunders.

MAYER, LEO, & RANSOHOFF, NICHOLAS (1936) Reconstruction of the digital tendon sheath. A contribution to the physiological method of repair of damaged finger tendons. *J. Bone and J. Surg.*, **18,** 607–616.

PARKES, ATHOL (1971) The 'Lumbrical plus' finger. *J. Bone and J. Surg.*, **53-B,** 236–239.

PULVERTAFT, R. G. (1956) Tendon grafts for flexor tendon injuries in the fingers and thumb. A study of technique and results. *J. Bone and J. Surg.*, **38-B,** 175–194.

TUBIANA, R. (1960) Greffes des tendons fléchisseurs des doigts et du pouce. Technique et résultats. *Rev. Chir. Orthop.*, **46,** 191–214.

VERDAN, C. E. (1966) Primary and secondary repair of flexor and extensor tendon injuries. In *Hand Surgery*, Flynn, J. E. pp. 220–275. Baltimore: The Williams and Wilkins Co.

14. *The Two-Stage Graft: A Salvage Operation for the Flexor Apparatus (A clinical study of 28 cases)*

A. Chamay C. Verdan C. Simonetta

The disabling sequelae left by severe or untidy wounds and by infections of the hand frequently originate in a tendon injury. However, the purpose of this paper is not to study as a whole the problem of the sequelae of lesions to the flexor tendons but to report our experience in reconstructing the flexor apparatus by means of the Hunter technique.

This technique is generally used for cases in which the conditions required for tenolyses or a simple graft are no more suitable. It may be recalled briefly that the conditions for tenolysis are:

1. good vascularization in the tendon,
2. a flexor apparatus sufficiently robust to enable early mobilization,
3. the presence of a continuous tendon with a smooth surface,
4. a good range of joint motion,
5. surrounding tissue of a favourable nature, that is to say without layers of scar tissue,
6. digital nerves repaired or reparable.

As for simple grafts, the clinical work by Boyes demonstrates clearly that the most important reasons for failure are joint stiffness, the presence of scar tissue and trophic disorders.

What can be done with the numerous cases that do not satisfy these criteria? What is to be done when tenolysis fails? Should a well-positioned arthrodesis be suggested? Or an amputation? It is the author's belief that a certain number of cases can be improved by means of a two-stage graft using the Hunter method.

Our series contains 28 digits: two thumbs, eight index fingers, six middle fingers, seven ring fingers and five little fingers.

The average age of our 22 patients was 20 years and there were two women and 20 men. The youngest patient was aged 16, the oldest 51 years. The longest interval since the previous interventions was three years amd the shortest three months.

Localization of the primary tendon lesion: In 23 fingers the lesion was in Bunnell's 'No-man's land' (Zone II). In three it was in the palm (Zone V). In the case of thumbs the lesion was at wrist level in one case (Zone VI) and in the region of the metacarpophalangeal joint in the other (Zone III). In our series of 22 patients there were almost as many tidy wounds as untidy wounds at the outset:

1. 4 caused by broken glass,
2. 6 caused by cutting instruments,
3. 4 untidy injuries caused by machines,
4. 8 untidy injuries due to various causes.

The two-stage grafting was carried out:

1. four times on digits on which there had been no primary attempt to repair the flexor apparatus because of the extent of the damage done by the injury;
2. eight times on digits in which the flexor tendons had simply been sutured;
3. ten times on digits which had undergone two operations (suture and tenolysis of the flexor apparatus or drainage of an abscess or correction of a defective suture);
4. six times on digits which had been operated on three times or more.

In these cases the two-stage grafting operation may well be considered as an attempt to salvage the flexor apparatus, as the last hope of recovering some function.

PREOPERATIVE CLASSIFICATION OF THE LESIONS

On the basis of the classifications of Hunter and Boyes we divided our cases up in the following way:

Group 1: This group comprises digits with no scar tissue and with a complete range of joint motion.

Group 2: This group comprises digits with scarring but with normal passive joint motion.

Group 3: This group comprises scarred digits in which passive interphalangeal motion before the surgical procedure was below normal. The stiffness is due in some cases to tendon adhesions in others to a joint lesion.

Group 4: This group comprises digits in which the two collateral nerves had been sectioned and the lesion was associated with internal scarring and joint stiffness.

Group 5: This group comprises digits forming part of a mutilated hand in which several other fingers have lesions of the flexor apparatus associated with restricted joint motion and internal scars.

Group 1 =	0 digits
Group 2 =	0 digits
Group 3 =	14 digits
Group 4 =	4 digits
Group 5 =	10 digits
Total	28 digits

Fourteen digits have had the two nerves divided. They were comprised in groups 4 and 5. Four patients were given a two-stage graft on two fingers in the same hand and one patient a two-stage graft on three fingers.

RESULTS

Digital function was evaluated as follows:

In the fingers: maximum active flexion was given a mark of two figures. The distance from pulp to palm was measured and the distance separating the pulp from the distal palmar crease in the case of the middle finger, the ring finger and the little finger and from the medial palmar crease in the case of the index finger. Extension defects were evaluated as a whole by means of a single figure in degrees indicating the sum of extension loss in the three finger joints.

In the thumb: the range of voluntary movement of the metacarpophalangeal and interphalangeal joints was measured. This figure was used as numerator and the preoperative passive range of motion as denominator. The ratio thus found is a percentage which give a good idea of the result obtained.

RESULTS OF TWO-STAGE GRAFTS ON THE LONG FINGERS AND THE THUMB

THE THUMB

Two thumbs were operated on with one good result (67%) and one moderately good result (45%). The less good result presented an adhesion of the graft at its distal end, restricting joint motion.

THE FINGERS

To simplify analysis of these results they were put in several categories on the basis of evaluation criteria corresponding to those described by Boyes and Stark:

Excellent: function normal.

Good: moderate deficiency in flexion and extension (less than 45 degrees), the pulp reaches at least to within 2.5 cm of the distal palmar crease while touching the palm.

Fair: the pulp touches the palm more than 2.5 cm from the distal palmar crease and a marked deficiency of flexion or extension persists (over 45 degrees).

Mediocre: a pulp-palm distance of 0.5 cm to 3 cm.

Poor: a pulp-palm distance exceeding 3 cm.

When the final result was compared with the preoperative passive joint motion the digits were classified in three categories (Table 14.1):

1. 'worsened digits' are those whose final functional condition was worse than it had been before the graft;

2. 'improved digits' were those whose final functional condition was better than it had been before the graft, and

3. 'unchanged digits' are those whose final functional condition was little different from what it had been before the graft.

All our cases belonged to Hunter's groups 3, 4 and 5. With such a small series it is impossible to affirm that one group has a better prognosis than another. However, the poor quality of results obtained must be emphasized: only five fingers out of 26 touched the palm on maximum flexion. Two digits were in a worse condition than before. These were two cases in which tenolysis had given a mediocre functional result which it had been wrongly attempted to improve by means of a two-stage graft.

Out of five 'good' and 'fair' results, three had only had a single operation before the two-stage graft, one had had no operation at all and one had had two (tendon suture and tenolysis). All these cases were operated on less than three months after the accident. All five had initially had injuries in Verdan's Zone II.

Among the 11 bad results, six were in Hunter's groups 3 and 4, seven were operated on between six and 12 months after the accident and four more than 12 months afterwards. Eight digits had undergone tenolysis before the graft and two digits underwent tenolysis after the graft without lasting improvement.

REPEATED OPERATIONS BEFORE THE GRAFT

Of 10 fingers given a two-stage graft which had had one or more tenolysis following tendon suture, nine showed 'poor' or 'mediocre' results and one a 'fair' result. It seems therefore that the effect of operating on a digit several times before attempting a two-stage graft may well be an unfavourable factor, since tenolysis increases fibrosis.

TYPE OF IMPLANTS

In the first stage of the operation 14 Silastic cylinders were used and 12 Hunter rods. No statistically significant difference was found in a comparison of the results of the two series.

SOURCES OF TENDON GRAFTS

In the second stage of the operation the tendon grafts used were the palmaris longus tendon in 11 cases, an extensor digitorum longus tendon in three cases and the plantaris tendon in 12 cases. No statistically significant difference was found between the three types of tendons.

LENGTH OF THE GRAFT

In six cases the graft was anastomosed in the palm and in

TABLE 14.1 Distribution of the results (The two thumbs are omitted from the table)

	Number of cases	Excellent	Good	Fair	Mediocre	Bad	Worsened	Improved	Unchanged
Group 3	14	0	1	2	6	5	2	10	2
Group 4	3	0	1	0	1	1	—	3	—
Group 5	9	0	0	1	3	5	—	5	4
Total:	26	0	2	3	10	11	2	18	6

20 cases at wrist level. The results are statistically more favourable when the anastomosis is done in the palm. Among the six short grafts three digits touched the palm whereas among the 20 long grafts only three digits flexed sufficiently to do so. However, it is essential not to draw conclusions too hastily since the short grafts were always done in palms free of adhesions and only for injuries in the digits, whereas the long grafts were often done for lesions that extended into the palm.

MOTOR TENDON

Among our six anastomosis in the palm we used the flexor profundus five times and the flexor superficialis once. Use for the superficialis led to a poor result. Among our 18 anastomoses at wrist level (excluding thumbs), in 10 cases the graft was anastomosed to the superficialis and in eight cases to the profundus. When the anastomosis is made with the flexor profundus the distal part of the tendon and its lumbrical are resected. The proportion of good and poor results is approximately the same in both motor groups when the anastomosis is carried out in the wrist.

COMPLICATIONS

SECONDARY ADHESIONS

In 10 cases secondary adhesions of the graft took place. Six grafts underwent tenolysis. In three cases adhesions fixed the proximal anastomosis in the palm. Two of these cases remained

poor while the third improved from 'poor to fair'. Once, a restrictive adhesion held down the graft at the level of the basal pulley: releasing it improved the result from 'poor to mediocre'. In one case adhesion of the whole new sheath made necessary its excision but the improvement was only moderate. In one case tenolysis had to be done on the proximal anastomosis in the wrist, this improving the result from 'poor to mediocre'.

THE 'INTRINSIC PLUS' PHENOMENON

In three cases a secondary 'swan-neck' deformity occurred in the digit. In two cases the graft had been anastomosed to the flexor superficialis in the wrist, leaving the stump of the flexor profundus and its lumbrical under too much tension in the palm. The third case was a short graft anastomosed to the flexor profundus in the palm (Fig. 14.1).

In two cases an incipient 'swan-neck' deformity was produced on extension but it had no functional effect in flexion. In both these cases the anastomosis had been done with the flexor profundus at the wrist level. It was therefore the absence of the flexor superficialis that was solely responsible, for the hyperextension of the proximal interphalangeal joint, since the lumbrical had been excised.

INFECTION AFTER THE FIRST STAGE OF GRAFT

Two rods placed in the same hand had to be removed because of early suppuration. Three months later two new Silastic rods were re-implanted and replaced six weeks later

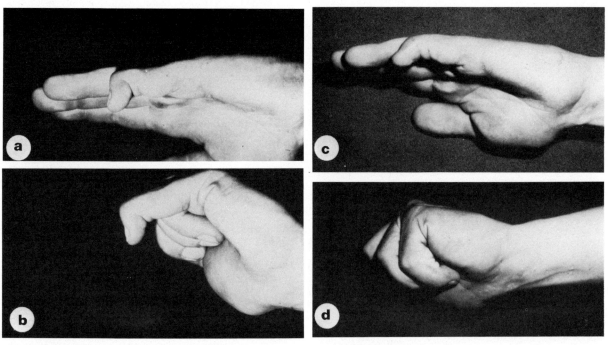

Figure 14.1
A 22-year-old mechanic had suffered a crushing injury on his left little finger in Zone II with section of both tendons. A suture of the flexor profundus, followed by tenolysis, was a failure. One year after the accident a two-stage graft was undertaken with reconstruction of the middle pulley and with a cross-finger skin flap. Subsequently graft adhesions and a 'swan-neck' deformity developed (a and b). A further tenolysis accompanied by arthrodesis of the distal interphalangeal joint and a Littler lateral extensor slip-plasty led to only moderate improvement (c and d).

by tendon grafts. Although passive motion was good, both cases were failures despite tenolysis. The tenolysis showed numerous adhesions along the whole length of the new sheath.

DISCUSSION

If preoperative and postoperative function of digits given a two-stage graft is compared it will be seen that there was an improvement in 18 digits, six were unchanged and two were made worse. In these two cases there was a functionally unacceptable stiffness in extension caused by total blockage of the tendons in their sheath.

The two-stage graft technique can be used in Boyes' groups 3, 4 and 5 with some hope of obtaining a partial recovery of function. However, some reservations in regard to the quality of the results are called for. It must not be expected that a scarred and partially dystrophic digit will regain after the second stage of the graft the range of passive motion that it had recovered after the first stage.

Two reasons can be adduced to explain the mediocrity of our results. The first lies in the selection of our cases. In this series our indications for a two-stage graft related for the most part to digits whose functional status had already been greatly jeopardized by scarring resulting from previous injury and surgical procedures.

The second reason lies in the concept of postoperative treatment and re-education. Indeed, our adherence to the conventional principle, accepted by most authors, that grafts should be immobilized for three weeks to enable revascularization to take place is probably the main reason for the large number of failures. It may be recalled that Hunter mobilizes his grafts very rapidly—five to seven days after the second stage of the operation. Our more recent clinical experiences, of which results have been more favourable, confirms this fact and suggest that early mobilization of tendon grafts in their new sheaths makes it possible to preserve the gliding surfaces induced by the implant and thus to avoid secondary adhesions. This of course, implies that the two ends of the graft must be soundly united surgically.

We included in our indications for two-stage grafts stiff fingers with radiologically and anatomically intact joints, thinking, quite rightly, that it is often enough to resect the flexor tendons that are adhering to the digital canal for good joint motion to be recovered after a few sessions of kinesotherapy. The first stage of the operation has a double purpose: reconstruction of the digital canal and restoration of joint motion.

It is altogether wrong to go on to carry out the tendon grafting itself without having restored complete or almost normal joint function through passive exercise, since after the second stage a certain proportion of this hard-won range of motion is always lost. As for the reconstruction of the pulleys we must draw attention to the need to preserve or reconstruct two or three pulleys for otherwise the graft will bowstring, causing a hook deformity of the digit with restriction of both flexion and extension.

At the present time we are using the two-stage grafting procedure wherever there is a layer of scar tissue in the immediate vicinity of the future graft or wherever the digital canal is obliterated by connective tissue and/or it is necessary to reconstruct a pulley system.

However, we refrain from undertaking any new operation on the flexor apparatus of a digit whose two pedicles have been sectioned and which shows considerable stiffness and scarring, since we know in advance that such a graft will be doomed to failure.

REFERENCES

BOYES, J.-H. & STARK, H. H. (1971) Flexor-tendon grafts in fingers and thumb. A study of factors influencing results in 1000. *J. Bone Jt Surg.*, **53-A**, 1332–1342.

CHONG, J. K., CRAMER, L. M. & CULF, N. K. (1972) A combined two-stage tenoplasty with silicone rods, for multiple flexor tendon injuries in 'No man's land'. *J. Trauma.*, **12**, 104–121.

FARKAS, L. G., McCAIN, W. G. *et al.* (1973) An experimental study of the changes following silastic rod preparation of a new tendon sheath and subsequent tendon grafting. *J. Bone Jt Surg.*, **55-A**, 1149–1158.

GAISFORD, J. C., HANNE, D. C. & RICHARDSON, G. S. (1966) Tendon grafting: A suggested technique. *Plast. reconstr. Surg.*, **38**, 302.

HELAL, B. (1973) The use of silicone rubber spacers in flexor tendon surgery. *The Hand*, **5**, 185–190.

HUNTER, J. M. (1971) Flexor tendon reconstruction in severely damaged hands. A two-stages procedure using a silicon dacron reinforced gliding prosthesis prior to tendon grafting. *J. Bone Jt Surg.*, **53-A**, 829–858.

LINDSAY, W. K., & THOMPSEN, H. G. (1960) Digital flexor tendons: an experimental study. Part I. The significance of each component of the flexor mechanism in tendon healing. *Brit. J. Plast. Surg.*, **12**, 289–316.

MICHON, J., & VILAIN, R. (1974) *Lésions traumatiques des tendons de la main.* Paris: Masson et Cie.

PEACOCK, E. E. (1965) Biological principles in the healing of long tendons. *Surg. clin. N. Amer.*, **45**, 461.

PEACOCK, E. E. (1964) Fundamental aspects of wound healing relating to the restoration of gliding function after tendon repair. *Surg., Gynec. Obstet.*, **119**, 241–250.

POTENZA, A. D. (1964) The healing of autogenous tendon grafts within the flexor digital sheath in dogs. *J. Bone Jt Surg.*, **46-A**, 1462–1484.

PULVERTAFT, R. G. (1956) Tendon grafts for flexor tendon injuries in the fingers and thumb. *J. Bone Jt Surg.*, **38-B**, 175–194.

TUBIANA, R. (1960) Greffes des tendons fléchisseurs des doigts et du pouce. Technique et résultats. *Rev. Chir. orthop.*, **46**, 191–214.

URBANIAK, J. R., BRIGHT, D., LOWELL, H. G. & GOLDNER, J. L. (1974) Vascularization and the gliding mechanism of free flexor tendon grafts inserted by the silicone rod method. *J. Bone Jt Surg.*, **56-A**, 473–482.

VERDAN, Cl. (1972) Half a century of flexor tendon surgery. *J. Bone Jt Surg.*, **54-A**, 472–491.

VERDAN, Cl. (1960) Primary repair of flexor tendons. *J. Bone Jt Surg.*, **42-A**, 617.

VERDAN, Cl. & CRAWFORD, G. (1971) Flexor tendon suture in the digital canal. *Transactions of the Vth international Congress of plastic and reconstructive surgery*, p. 485. Melbourne: Butterworth.

VERDAN, Cl. & MICHON, J. (1961) Le traitement des plaies des tendons fléchisseurs des doigts. *Rev. Chir. orthop.*, **47**, 285.

We shall discuss here the particular indications concerning the topographical surgical Zones V, VI and VII (Fig. 8.16, page 63) of the fingers, and the special case of the thumb.

ZONE VII: THE WRIST

At this level we are dealing with twelve tendons whose sliding amplitude is considerable:

1. flexor carpi radialis: 40 mm
2. flexor carpi ulnaris: 33 mm
3. flexor digitorum superficialis: 60 (little) to 88 mm (middle)
4. flexor digitorum profundus: 70 (little) to 85 mm (middle)
5. flexor pollicis longus: 52 mm.
6. palmaris longus is generally not repaired.

Repair of sectioned tendons in this region may seem easy due to the nearby musculo-tendinous junctions but these wounds can be very serious for the following reasons:

1. concomitant median and/or ulnar nerve injury
2. multiplicity of sectioned tendons
3. interruption of radial and/or ulnar arteries
4. difficulty in locating the retracted ends of the tendons; proximally in the muscular and haemorrhagic mass, distally under the flexor retinaculum when section has occurred with the fist closed and/or the wrist flexed.

An extensive exposure of the carpal canal is therefore often necessary. The cutaneous incision presented in Figure 8.2, page 58 is performed; 'T' incisions are to be avoided since tendinous scar junctions adhere to them easily and movement is blocked.

We proceed to careful identification of the tendon ends by their position, form of section surface and function by traction on the distal extremity. Marker threads are placed to avoid possible confusion.

Above all, care must be taken to avoid confusing tendons and nerves. During secondary repair operations the author has observed this on numerous occasions, to the point where he considers it almost the rule when the primary suture is performed without a pneumatic tourniquet, under incorrect anaesthesia by a surgeon not trained in hand surgery.

The pattern of functional loss is complicated at this level by paralysis of the intrinsic muscles innervated by the median and/or ulnar nerve.

TREATMENT

Primary suture: Primary suture is indicated in the majority of cases. The palmaris longus tendon is of no importance and can be ignored or resected. The tendons of flexor carpi radialis and flexor carpi ulnaris are important stabilizers of the carpus and must be firmly sutured using lace stitches (Bunnell) or lateral anchorage (Wilms-Kessler).

For the flexors of the fingers, since speed is important and the sheaths are not closely adjusted, Bunnell's 'double right angle' stitch can be performed quickly and efficiently. Its resistance to traction is relatively low, but suffices in this region since the immobilization position necessitates a flexed wrist. Several authors suture only the flexor digitorum profundus and flexor pollicis longus, sacrificing flexor digitorum superficialis to make room for profundus and the nerves. Though this does diminish the volume of the scar tissue mass, it results in the following difficulties:

1. diminished prehensile strength;
2. lack of independent movement of the fingers;
3. use of a flexor digitorum superficialis tendon for tendon transfer in case of non-regeneration of the nerves (paralysis of thumb opposition, claw hand) is no longer possible.

We try to repair all flexor tendons including flexor digitorum superficialis taking care to separate the groups of tendons by a flap of synovial sheath. If necessary the flexor digitorum superficialis of the little finger can be sacrificed.

Needless to say, when only the flexor digitorum superficialis tendons are sectioned, they are all repaired.

Care is taken not only to avoid suturing the ante-brachial fascia, but to remove constriction using a lateral longitudinal incision or even to partially excise it. The flexor retinaculum often must be partially or totally severed depending upon whether or not the suture level of the tendons comes into this region upon complete extension of the fingers and wrist.

Concerning concomitant nerve section, although we have earlier advocated primary simple face to face approximation followed six to eight weeks later by precise secondary suture, we now practice primary suture of nerves for both children and adults. This is due to the improvement of nerve suture technique under the microscope and use of very fine material, providing a new, higher level of precision.

Also, for concomitant radial and ulnar artery section we no longer ligate but repair by microsurgical anastomosis.

Secondary repair: In certain exceptional cases, when the wound is very contaminated, bruised, lacerated or the patient arrives too late after the accident, we are forced to clean and trim the wound and either leave it open or close and drain it. Later, between the ninth and twenty-first day the major elements can be repaired under antibiotic therapy. Sometimes it is even necessary to start by replacing skin losses using a skin-flap. Whenever possible at least flexor digitorum profundus and flexor pollicis longus should be repaired at the same time.

Late operations: On several occasions we have seen cases

where all is fused in a massive block of scar tissue with no nervous regeneration and where the fingers have become stiff. First, it is essential to repair the nerves to improve the trophic state of the hand. Then either a concomitant tenolysis to restore modest prehensile function (especially to the first 3 fingers) or tertiary tendon repair after a long period of mobilization physiotherapy may be performed.

ZONE VI: THE CARPAL CANAL

This region is characterized by a narrow passage formed by three bony walls and an anterior wall which is fibrous, rigid and inextensible. The nine flexor tendons are accompanied by the median nerve located anterolaterally. The flexor retinaculum is rarely sectioned by accidental traumatic injury since the lacerations object is stopped by the lateral bony edges. In any case it is necessary to completely section the flexor retinaculum to allow suture of the flexor digitorum profundus, flexor pollicis longus and the median nerve. Repair of the flexor digitorum superficialis is optional. The flexor retinaculum is not sutured, and a few Dexon stitches are placed in the superficial palmar aponeurosis.

But often we are dealing with a smaller wound, sometimes a mere puncture with only a few divided structures. Rather than open the carpal canal and proceed to primary repair, it seems wiser to simply excise the edges of the wound, clean it and immobilize the hand under antibiotic therapy (this exception is justified due to the endosynovial contamination) and two to three weeks later under perfectly aseptic conditions proceed to complete repair of all elements.

ZONE V: THE HOLLOW OF THE HAND

At this level the flexor tendons fan out in groups of two superimposed tendons. They are much more vulnerable here than in Zone VI and their section is frequently accompanied by that of the interdigital arteries and nerves. Recall that the index, middle and ring finger tendons have no sheath, and are simply enveloped in a paratendon. The proximal insertion of the lumbricals on the flexor digitorum profundus occurs in this region. The superficial arterial palmar arch is also often injured.

Isolated section of flexor digitorum superficialis can go unnoticed. It must be systematically investigated according to the method previously described. Partial sections can form small 'pedunculated tendinomas' that can catch under the first pulley and need be resected secondarily.

TREATMENT

Primary suture: Primary suture is generally indicated especially for flexor digitorum profundus. If flexor digitorum superficialis is seriously damaged and difficult to repair, it can be sacrificed with no serious repercussions. When both tendons are sectioned, the two sutures must be separated by the interposition of a paratendinous flap, and care taken to place the finger in an immobilization position that avoids superposition of the two planes of section.

Secondary repair: In late cases where healing has begun, frequently there exist degenerative modifications accompanied by retraction of the tendon ends, necessitating their resection. Suture is then impossible. Usually a tendon graft is indicated, using a superficialis when it has also been sectioned, to repair profundus. When the distal anastomosis of this graft just barely touches the entrance of the digital canal, a short end-to-end graft is acceptable. If on the contrary it passes into the digital canal, a long graft is needed extending to the tip of the finger (as for a wound in Zone II).

At this point we may again note that the real level of the tendon section can only be appreciated with the finger in complete extension; this is true for all the topographical zones.

On the other hand, we must remember the recent experimental work of Matthews and Ritchard (1977) on dogs, showing that partially severed and sutured tendons outside the sheath, and then reintroduced inside the intact digital canal, can heal without noticeable adhesion formation. It may be the same for total section in the human, and it may allow a change in policy, provided that the tendon anastomosis has been done accurately in the palm.

THE THUMB

For primary repair, the problem is the same in Zones I and III and in Zones I and II for the other fingers, except that here we are only dealing with one tendon, making repair much easier.

In Zone I: If the tendon ends are ragged, we can resect them and advance the proximal end by elongating it at the wrist by a stepwise incision and reinserting it on the bone of the distal phalanx. During incision care is taken to preserve the small sensitive branch of the median nerve destined to the thenar eminence; we have often observed painful neuromas at this level.

This lengthening of the tendon at the wrist allowing its peripheral extension is easier here than with the other fingers where the flexor digitorum profundus have lumbricals and various tendinous interconnections attached. It can be performed as a primary or as secondary repair, and advantageously replaces a graft. This lengthening can be up to 3 cm, and can therefore also be performed on wounds in the distal half of Zone III.

In the proximal half of Zone III, it is sometimes possible to perform primary suture, but this implies resection of the pulley which can lead to dislocation of the repaired tendon. It is best then to perform primarily or secondarily a tendon graft that can be short (digito-thenar) or long (digito-carpal) (cf. chapter by Boyes and Stark).

In Zone IV, the thenar muscles are partially or totally sectioned by the accidental wound. Direct tendon suture is normally possible, though technically difficult due to retraction of the superior tendon end. It can sometimes be brought down distally, by massage of the forearm musculature and bending the wrist, or it can be necessary to make another incision, using a leading thread, from as far up as the wrist.

The two collateral nerves are often also damaged and must be sutured at the same time. The most delicate region is the superior part of Zone IV, at the edge of Zone VI of the carpal canal, where the tendon changes direction. Direct suture is not possible here. A tendon graft is indicated extending from the wrist to the thenar eminence, bridging the carpal canal. It is useless to extend the graft as far as the tip of the thumb.

At all levels, recall that if the muscular body of flexor pollicis longus is nonfunctional (fibrous retraction, scar tissue blockage at the wrist, etc.) it is possible to use the flexor digitorum superficialis of the annular, transferring it to the digital canal of the thumb and inserting it on the distal phalanx.

SURGERY OF THE EXTENSOR TENDONS

R. Tubiana

These very common wounds pose problems of repair far greater than when the extensor tendons are injured on the dorsum of hand. In fact, at the finger level, we will have to deal not merely with extensor tendon injuries, but with injuries of an entire extensor apparatus shaped as a fibrous fascia, spread out all over the dorsal aspect of the finger, close to bones and joints, to which it adheres as soon as it is traumatized.

This fascia consists of the terminal fibres of long extensor tendons and of the intrinsic muscles, supplemented by passive fibrous structures, called retinacula.

These multiple tendon bundles compose, together with the flexor apparatus a most compound mechanism, whose balance must be preserved (Tubiana and Valentin, 1963) (Fig. 16.1).

We consider here only injuries of the fingers, omitting the thumb and adopting the local topography of Verdan (1966), with five zones for the fingers. Thus injuries are identified for the extensor apparatus at the level of each digital joint and in the two intermediary areas.

AT THE DISTAL INTERPHALANGEAL JOINT (DIP)

The terminal extensor tendon, formed by the two lateral bands united, is inserted on the dorsal aspect of the distal phalanx at its base, throughout nearly all its width. It is a thin fibrous membrane, tightly fastened to the joint capsule with which it partly merges. The tendon has an excursion of about 4–5 mm. We must remember that the extension of the distal phalanx results from both the common extensor and the intrinsic muscles, a part of this extension being a passive movement which only follows the extended middle phalanx by means of the oblique fibres of the retinacular bundle. These different structures explain the various amounts of deformity and the possibility to compensate partially for the lack of extension, according to the injuries. Every impairment of the ruptured extension mechanism produces a dropping of the distal phalanx, more marked the more distal the injury. The torn joint capsule is responsible for the worst deformities. An avulsion of the bone insertion of the tendon involves similar deformities (Fig. 16.2).

Any surgical repair in this area is particularly difficult to perform, on account not only of the joint itself being directly concerned, but also because of the thinness of the covering layers. The skin is extremely fine and frail, its blood supply is poor, especially since when the finger is hyperextended it loses colour immediately. The nail matrix so near makes a good approach difficult.

Complications are to be expected when the operation is not made with the utmost care.

It is advisable to put the proximal interphalangeal joint in flexion during part of the treatment, so as to release all tension from the interossei; it will be necessary to keep the distal joint still in hyperextension, for some weeks.

PRIMARY REPAIRS

In the presence of a wound, when this one is tidy, a primary suture will be performed.

The wound, usually transverse or oblique, is extended longitudinally and the flap so created may form an obtuse angle (Fig. 16.3). The skin should be manipulated with care, by sutures. We must remember that the nail matrix extends itself proximally about 5 mm beyond the visible part of the nail.

The tendon, near its insertion, is thin, so the suture itself must be fragile; it has to be relaxed by putting the distal phalanx in hyperextension. This position can be more easily held by putting in advance a Kirschner wire 10/100 before the suture, the distal interphalangeal joint being fixed in slight hyperextension (5°). Hyperextension must not be excessive, for the skin does not tolerate it for long. The wire is placed on the lateral side of the digit and crosses the joint obliquely. We do not put any more mid-longitudinal wire, since we had fibrous scars on the pulp, quite disturbing on pressure.

The tendon is usually repaired by means of a loop inserted into the lateral bands, the suture of both ends being improved with some 'U' points, using very thin nylon. Lorthioir recommends a double loop, laced through each band.

The digit is then dressed with a splint, keeping the proximal interphalangeal joint at a 40 degrees flexion, to release the extensor lateral tendons by the gliding of the dorsal fascia, which is drawn down by the central tendon insertion. The splint is removed on about the 25th day, to permit the motion of the proximal IP joint, the wire is also taken away, but the distal joint is kept immobilized during two further weeks by a short moulded splint. The same splint will then be applied every night for two more weeks.

When the conditions for a primary suture are not present, especially with a contused wound, an effort can be made to treat such injuries conservatively, the distal joint being kept in extension during six to seven weeks. Another operation, such as a tendon repair or arthrodesis will sometimes be necessary.

RUPTURES

Distal ruptures of the extensor apparatus follow after closed injuries. It is sometimes a violent injury, easy to detect as dur-

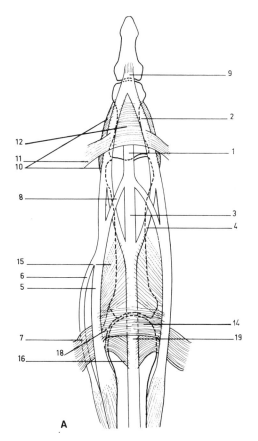

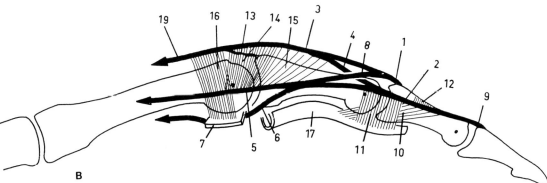

Figure 16.1
The extensor system of the fingers. (a) Dorsal view. (b) Sectional view (internal view) showing the endings of the extensor and specific muscles, as well as the retinacular ligaments. There is a certain symmetry between the fibrous formations at the level of the metacarpophalangeal articulations and the proximal interphalangeal articulations.
1. Median extensor tendon.
2. Lateral extensor tendon.
3. Median strip of the long extensor.
4. Lateral strip of the long extensor.
5. Tendon of the interosseous.
6. Tendon of the lumbrical.
7. Transverse intermetacarpal (or interglenoid) ligament.
8. Median strip of the interosseous.
9. Terminal extensor tendon.
10. Oblique retinacular ligament.
11. Transverse retinacular ligament.
12. Triangular ligament.
13. Insertion of the common extensor into the first phalanx.
14. Transverse fibres of the back of the interosseous muscles.
15. Oblique fibres of the back of the interosseous muscles.
16. Sagittal strips.
17. Fibrous sheaths of the flexor tendons.
18. Insertion of the interosseous muscle into the base of P1.
19. Tendon of the common extensor.

ing a football game; in other cases trauma is mild and we see ruptures happening in housewives turning up mattresses or folding sheets, it can even go unnoticed. The most frequent mechanism is a blunt flexion of the distal phalanx, previously held in extension. A blow on the head of the finger can involve a fracture by compression of the base of the distal phalanx with sudden flexion. Those injuries are seen on every finger, but rarely on the thumb. They show a permanent flexion of the distal phalanx, from 30 degrees to 40 degrees, according to cases, no matter what the position of the other joints may be. The patient can increase the flexion of the injured phalanx, but he cannot extend it beyond the starting position. Passive extension remains normal. The oedematous infiltration and fibrosis progressively reduce the joint range. This rather mild

symtomatology bothers the patient only a little and spontaneous healing is expected. The persisting deformity ultimately brings the patient to the surgeon.

X-rays examination can show a bony avulsion.

Ruptures are mostly treated conservatively by splintage (Fig. 16.4).

As after suture, the distal joint may be fixed in extension by a wire and immobilization completed by a splint maintaining the PIP in flexion. In case of spontaneous rupture, we protect the tendon healing by longer immobilization.

The Kirschner wire, has to be placed with the utmost precautions, and removed as soon as inflammation is detected.

We do not use, as Pratt proposed it, the same wire to fix both the DIP in extension and the PIP in flexion.

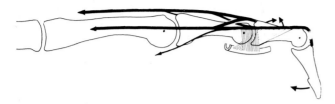

Figure 16.2
Mallet finger deformity.

Use of a wire, on account of its dangers leading to infection, might be criticized, but even a mere splint, apparently harmless may produce pressure sores. In lieu of wire, a plaster cast is best for immobilization. Bunnell pointed out that the patient is best holding the corrected position of his finger against his thumb. A narrow plaster splint is first set upon the dorsal surface of the finger, covered with jersey from its base; its end has to reach the nail. After it is dried, a palmar narrow splint is placed up to the pulp and left until dry. Both splints are then joined in a case.

A prognostic distinction should be made, between: spontaneous ruptures, secondary to light trauma and pathological ruptures from injuries such as a heavy blow on the end of the digit, often with bony avulsion. In these cases the repair seems to be easier.

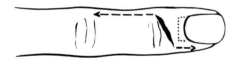

Figure 16.3
Wound of the extensor system at the distal interphalangeal level. It is necessary to make the wound larger at its extremities to avoid creating acute angles with a poor blood supply.

Our experience is too limited to allow me to say more than that in cases showing deformation up to 60 degrees, it would seem best to resort immediately to a surgical re-insertion of the tendon, using the technique pointed out by Esteve (1964): viz. a nylon thread, with a needle at both ends is fastened to the proximal extremity of tendon; both needles pass into the periosteum of the distal phalanx, out through the nail at the two corners of the lunula, stretched to draw up the tendon, and then knotted firmly, until a slight hyperextension of distal phalanx is attained.

Surgery is also indicated in the rare cases of major bony divulsion, with palmar subluxation of the distal phalanx. If the DIP is put in hyperextension, the displacement is even accentuated, so fixing the bony fragment, together with a transarticular wire allows for stable correction of the deformity.

We have never carried out a primary arthrodesis of the DIP joint and reserve it for late failures.

SECONDARY REPAIRS

We make no distinction from the indication of secondary treatment, whether for wounds or for ruptures, except in those cases when bad scars endanger a direct surgical approach.

It is difficult to fix a time limit for conservative treatment. We have been able to succeed with simple immobilization even six months after an accident, but it is likely, and statistics of Stark, Boyes and Wilson clearly confirm that the miscarriage percentage increases with the delay after the 10th day.

Besides, a long and uncertain orthopaedic treatment brings about considerable annoyance to a manual worker, so that we hesitate to prescribe it after the second month, having discussed with the patient other possibilities: either surgery or acceptance.

Acceptance is often recommended. One tends to take lightly the after-effects of a mallet-finger: the *functional impairment* is usually of little import, although catching the extremity of a deformed finger be not without inconvenience. Moreover, the pulp grasp with forefinger and middle finger against the thumb, is far more frequent than the terminal grasp in flexion of DIP. Therefore, stiffness in flexion of this joint can be an important functional loss, in certain jobs. Pain is not infrequent and may persist for a long time. Finally, the *aesthetic* problem is not to be underestimated for many subjects, especially women.

Leading people to believe that deformation will lessen with passing of time is actually to hope that the patient will adapt himself to his handicap. Such adaptation is possible to some degree, by means of a growing hyperextension at the PIP to compensate for the falling of the DIP.

One ought to admit that these conservative advices have arisen from lack of a confident treatment.

The *surgical treatment* is not without inconveniences, the results being not always satisfactory. We therefore only operate on troublesome deformations of over 40 degrees.

A number of proceedings have been recommended, but all leave a percentage of disappointments.

Instead of merely folding the callus, it is preferable in our opinion to practice a callus resection, and a suture.

Vilain obtained good results by shortening the tendon, approached in the sound area, above injury; the tendon is cut, then overlapped and sutured while Esteve (1964) remains faithful to tendon re-insertions.

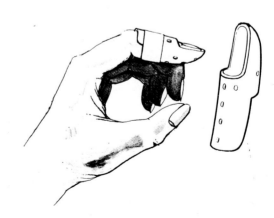

Figure 16.4
Stack's splint in polyethylene.

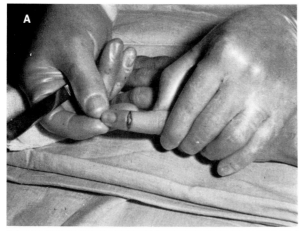

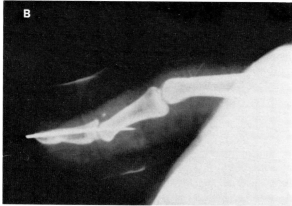

Figure 16.5
Brooks and Graner's operation for mallet deformity. (A) Elliptic (sic) excision of the skin and of the tendon callus. (B) Immobilization of the distal interphalanx by a pin.

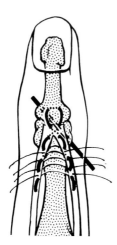

Figure 16.6
Grafting technique used by the author for old mallet deformities. The graft is fixed to the base of P3, the two extremities are crossed on the median line, then are slipped into the lateral extensor tendons. The tension is regulated by the transverse points more or less bringing together the lateral tendons.

We, of our part, when a late operation is decided, increase our probabilities of success by using a graft (Nichols). The graft has the advantage of strengthening the stretched scar callus, providing a strong grip on the proximal part of tendon and drawing it distally and reducing any tendency to retraction.

The skin flap has a longitudinal axis, and small vascular pedicles, at the distal end and directed to the nail matrix, are to be spared. A fine wire, obliquely implanted, maintains the joint slightly hyperextended. The extensor apparatus is tenolysed above the articulation, but care must be taken not to destroy, on both sides, the oblique fibres from the retinacular ligament.

A narrow tendinous band, 2 mm wide and 6–7 cm long is taken from a wrist flexor, attached by its middle at the base of DP, through fibrous tissue if it is firm enough, otherwise we would rather drill a small hole into the bone. Both ends of the graft are first crossed on the mid line, at the level of the DIP joint, then each end of graft is laced into the lateral bands; the PIP joint is bent and the graft tension carefully set with the help of some stitches joining both segments of the graft.

The finger is immobilized, PIP in flexion. Operation results are comparable to those described after suture.

Tenotomy of the central extensor tendon insertion was first proposed by Fowler, to correct the falling of the DP in late injuries—thus allowing a proximal retraction of the terminal bands and the fibrous scar. A buttonhole is not to be feared, for the triangular ligament preventing any subluxation of the lateral bands. A splint immobilizes PIP in slight flexion and DIP in extension during three weeks; then, the PIP and DIP are kept in extension up to two weeks.

Arthrodesis is reserved for cases where the joint becomes stiff in a bad position. When the PIP is mobile, the distal joint will be fused in slight flexion, this position having been discussed with the patient himself.

AT THE MIDDLE PHALANX

Injuries in this area are due to open wounds, and dropping of the distal phalanx is generally limited, since the distal joint capsule is intact and only rarely does the injury extend the whole width of finger.

The technique of primary suture is similar to that previously described. Deep adhesions are often found after fracture of the middle phalanx, demanding sometimes a secondary tenolysis.

AT THE PROXIMAL INTERPHALANGEAL-JOINT (PIP)

Most complexity is found in this area, both anatomically and physiologically.

The extensor apparatus comprises at this level, essentially one central and two lateral tendons.

The central slip of the common extensor receives the so-called spiral fibres from the interosseous muscles, forming together the *central extensor tendon*, crossing the dorsal side of PIP fused with the capsule, inserting itself on the base of the middle phalanx. The amplitude of movement attained here, is about 8 mm (Stack). This middle tendon has physiologically a most important role in extension of the three phalanges: it extends the middle phalanx where it inserts, except when the metacarpophalangeal is in hyperextension. It also has an indirect action on both other phalanges. It helps to extend the P.Phalanx pushing back its head when the PIP joint is flexed. It still extends the DP along the first half of its amplitude, owing to passive coordination through the retinacular ligament.

Both the lateral bands of the interosseous muscles receive fibres from the common extensor, thus forming *the lateral tendons*. Each of these fibrous structures glides along the postero-lateral side of the joint during flexion, but any side-displacement is checked by two fibrous structures: the *triangular* ligament and the *retinacular* ligament. The transverse fibres of the latter prevent the lateral extensor tendons from gliding toward the middle line during extension of PIP and in flexion, the tension of these transverse fibres draws the lateral extensor tendons on the sides of joint. This ventral displacement is then limited by the triangular ligament which joins lateral extensor to the central tendon on the back of the middle phalanx.

Any disturbance to that delicate mechanism produces finger deformities. The digits can actually be compared to a chain of bones and joints. In such a multiarticular system, an intercalated bone, such as the proximal phalanx, can only be kept in balance by a minimum of three muscles (Landsmeer). If the balance of this chain is broken, three varieties of deformation are to be found; each with a characteristic name:

The 'claw-hand' resulting from an hyperextension of the MP, and flexion of the PIP; it is the result of a paralysis of the interosseous muscles.

In the 'swan-neck', (Fig. 16.7a) the PIP joint is in hyperextension and DIP in flexion. This deformation may be due to many causes, including excessive traction on the extensor apparatus, inserted on the base of the middle phalanx. It is not a true injury of the extensor apparatus.

With the *'button-hole'* (Fig. 16.7b) deformity the initial injury involves the central extensor tendon, allowing a flexion deformity of PIP joint, together with DIP hyperextension.

'BUTTON-HOLE' DEFORMITIES

Any section, avulsion, rupture or progressive destruction of the central extensor tendon, is followed, whenever the triangular blade is also torn, by a volar luxation of the lateral tendons, producing a kind of 'button-hole', through which the head of the proximal phalanx prolapses.

The result thereof is a digital zig-zag deformity—first by action of the superficial flexor tendon; and then the distal phalanx passes into hyperextension, because it now receives all the extension forces since the middle tendon has become disinserted. Moreover, the lateral tendons being volar dislocated become stretched from the bulk of the PIP joint.

The retinacular ligament has a two-fold role in fixing that deformity—by its transverse fibre maintaining palmar luxation of the lateral bands and by retraction of its fibres

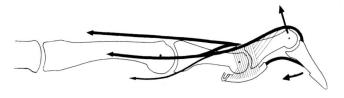

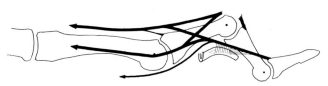

Figure 16.7
Deformities (a) swan neck (b) buttonhole.

fastening middle phalanx in flexion and distal phalanx in extension.

AETIOLOGY

Button-hole deformity is due to various causes: trauma (sections, avulsions or ruptures of the middle extensor tendon) or rhumatoid polyarthritis. In a series of 32 operated post-traumatic button-holes, we found 20 sections and 12 ruptures. A male predominance occurs in two-thirds of cases, both for section and for rupture.

The average age for sections is 39, for ruptures 27. That average is far below the age of subcutaneous ruptures of other tendons.

The causal trauma for ruptures accounting for a button-hole is important: among 12 ruptures, we found four IP luxations, five violent blows, and that suggests a traumatic rupture of previously normal tendon. In our series, the left hand is most often involved, the lateral fingers being more frequently injured.

TREATMENT

We ought to distinguish recent lesions, easy to reduce, from late lesions with retractions.

Recent injuries: *A wound* of the extensor tendon, on the back of the PIP joint does not usually produce an immediate button-hole deformity but one usually appears later, when the lateral tendons, after retractions are drawn forwards. The opening into the joint, has to be closed as soon as possible, to prevent infection. The soft tissue conditions decide the possibility of repairing tendon injuries. When local conditions are favourable, an immediate repair is undertaken, as anatomical as possible. A methodical exploration of injuries is obviously required.

The central tendon, if divided, will be re-implanted or sutured. Injuries to lateral tendons have also to be repaired. They are to be kept in their physiological position, partially reconstructing the triangular ligament with a few sutures, which approximate the distal portion of the lateral tendons to the central tendon margins.

A splint immobilizes the wrist in extension for three weeks, metacarpo-phalangeal joint in very slight flexion in order to release tension on the tendon suture.

Results of repairs of those wounds of the PIP joint, are usually satisfactory when the skin and extensor apparatus are cleanly cut. On the contrary, repairing of contused wounds, irregularly shaped, is often complicated by stiffness in extension, mostly due to adhesions, even if there was no joint involvement at the outset.

Re-education has little success when scars are dense. A tenolysis, undertaken not earlier than three months after the primary operation (Verdan, 1966) can be useful; yet it happens that superficial adhesions are such, that their section may leave a weakened tendinous apparatus, tending towards relapse of the initial button-hole injury. In these cases, our aim is to place the finger in a functional position, where a certain range of mobility, though limited, can be of use. A temporary wire fastens the PIP joint in such a position and movements of the DIP are rather encouraged.

When local conditions are bad, arthrodesis or amputation can be considered.

Recent ruptures are usually treated conservatively. A metal splint together with a cast maintain the wrist in extension, metacarpo-phalangeal joint slightly flexed at 10 degrees, PIP in extension and DIP at 45 degrees flexion for four weeks. Then, only PIP is kept immobilized in extension, with the help of a short splint, for another week.

Surgical repair seems to be indicated for such recent ruptures, in two circumstances:

1. In ruptures with bony avulsion, when control X-rays taken after PIP immobilization in extension show persistent displacement of the bony fragment which depending on its size, should either be directly fixed or, if it is too small, reimplanted by the tendinous end to the base of middle phalanx. The joint can be effectively maintained in extension by a fine Kirschner wire, obliquely placed. This is left for 10 days, then replaced by a splint.

2. In ruptures following a PIP joint dislocation, it can be of interest to operate, so as to make an exact assessment of injuries and to repair, beside the extensor apparatus, the articular capsule and cartilage, and the lateral ligament as well.

OLD LESIONS

Old button-hole deformities, either after non-treated wounds or to ruptures, pose similar problems, which can be considered together.

Late repairs of button-hole deformity are delicate and operations justified only when such deformities produce a functional disturbance. Attempts should be made only when the joints have sufficient suppleness. Physiotherapy is often necessary before operating, stressing mainly the active mobilization of the DIP whose flexion requires for a distal displacement of the extensor apparatus. Physiotherapy can involve serial corrective splints, to reduce flexion of the P2. It often happens that such precautions suffice to correct the deformity, making operation unnecessary.

Operation in selected cases, when a decision is made, will involve:

1. correction of the deformity
2. repair of the extensor apparatus.

We use a sinuous incision.

Correcting the deformation. Freeing the lateral bands and drawing up all the extensor apparatus is essential as the displaced ligaments adhere forward to the capsular layer. One must carefully dissect them to replace them back in their normal dorso-lateral position and thus the transverse fibres as well as most of the oblique fibres of the retinacular ligament are disinserted.

Sometimes, when the deformity is late and severe, the distal joint cannot be flexed, by merely liberating the lateral tendons. *Those are precisely the cases where their tenotomy has to be considered.*

Repair of the extensor apparatus. As normal as possible anatomical conditions have to be restored, therefore the most urgent step consists in repairing the middle tendon, which must be stretched and reimplanted on the base of the middle phalanx. With this principle in mind, several repair procedures were described.

1. *Shortening of callus.* Mere plication has always disappointed us.

2. *Reconstruction of the middle tendon.* If it has not degenerated, the central tendon can be reconstructed and

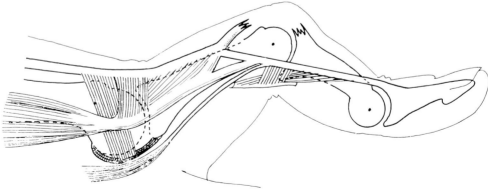

Figure 16.8
An old buttonhole deformity. The loss of insertion of the median flexor tendon into the base of the second phalanx allows the proximal sliding of all the extensor system. The lateral displacement of the lateral extensor tendons is fixed by the retraction of the transverse and oblique retinacular ligaments, resisting little by little the flexion of the distal phalanx.

reimplanted either on the distal stump or directly into the bone, after the proximal end has been freed. The fibrous callus is resected, care being taken to retain any distal tendon insertion on the base of middle phalanx.

Many choices can be considered: It may happen that the proximal end allows without excessive strain the extensor apparatus to be drawn forwards and either reimplanted on the middle phalanx base or sutured with the distal tendon end. In other cases, when the defect is too large, some local fibrous tissue, can be used, else a lateral tendon or a tendinous graft is inserted.

Local fibrous tissue. A small flap from the dorsal aponeurosis, may be capable, once folded, of filling the gap between both tendon ends. Moreover, the lateral bands must be drawn toward each other in their distal part, to reconstruct the triangular ligament. The results can be satisfactory, but seldom perfect!

Using the lateral tendons. These can be utilized in a variety of ways:

Pushing upwards the lateral bands all along their rim is not physiological and impairs flexion.

Planas uses one of the tendons, severed at its proximal end, leading it over to the midline, yet criticizes his own procedure, and he admitted being unable to get a good flexion of the distal joint. Flexion is only possible when the lateral tendons remain free to glide over the lateral aspects of the proximal joint letting the terminal tendon run about 4 mm, the medial one running on its part 8 mm. For that reason Matev lengthens one lateral band running to the distal joint and fixes the other on the base of middle phalanx (Fig. 16.9).

Littler, as we will see it, uses both lateral tendons, after their tenotomy, overturning them in order to remake a middle tendon.

Tendon grafts. These can also be used, using as motor either the extensor longus, the interossei or even the flexor digitorum superficialis. The middle tendon can be reconstructed by a single graft or by lacing a fine tendinous strip, inserted through the tendon (Nichols) (Fig. 16.10A). This lacing can be to the distal stump or to the bone when it is implanted at the site of insertion of the original tendon, in the middle part of the base of middle phalanx. When a tunnel is made in the bone, one must make sure that it is not too anterior nor too long transversely.

Fowler uses a thin graft the middle of which he attaches to the base of the middle phalanx; he then crosses the two ends over the dorsal aspect of the PIP and sutures them laterally to the interossei tendons at the root of the finger, (Fig. 16.10B) or, if these muscles are not utilizable, to the two terminal bands of the flexor superficialis in the palm.

We have used a Y-shaped graft, and then three-pronged grafts; the proximal end is laced into the dorsal aponeurosis, bringing it distally; it is then fixed to the base of the middle phalanx and split longitudinally before running over the joint, the two halves being fixed at their end to the lateral tendons, thus preventing their volar displacement (Fig. 16.11).

3. *Tenotomy.* This procedure has been suggested by Fowler for old, deep, fixed lesions. By dividing the distal insertion of

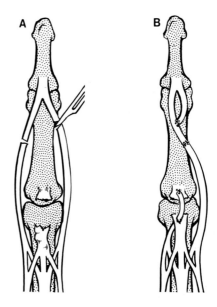

Figure 16.9
1. Matev's procedure using the lateral extensor tendons. (A) the lateral extensor tendons are sectioned at different levels. (B) one of the lateral tendons of which the section is most close, is passed into the proximal end of the median extensor tendon across which it slides, then is fixed to the base of the second phalanx. The other lateral tendon for the second phalanx is lengthened using the distal end of the preceding tendon.

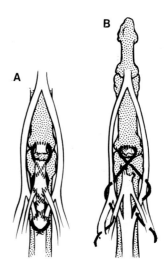

Figure 16.10
Repair of the buttonhole deformity using tendon grafts. On the left the procedure of Nichols using the common extensor as a motor. On the right the procedure of Fowler using the interosseous muscles.

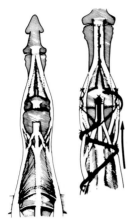

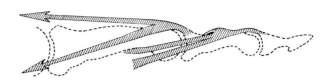

Figure 16.13
Littler's procedure for the correction of buttonhole deformities. The insertion of the lateral tendons into the base of P2, in association with tenotomy, permits a redistribution of the extensor forces at the level of the two distal phalanges.

Figure 16.11
The trident graft (R. Tubiana). The graft slipped into the whole of the extensor system at the proximal part of the finger is fixed to the base of the second phalanx. The graft, before crossing the articular space of the proximal interphalanx, sends out small strips which are fixed to the lateral extensor tendons.

the terminal extensor tendon on the distal phalanx the hyperextension dislocation of the lateral tendons is reduced. If, however, the tendon is divided more proximally, so as to spare the distal insertions of the retinacular ligament, extension of the distal phalanx can be partially preserved (Dolphin) (Fig. 16.12).

4. *Tenotomy combined with reconstruction of the middle tendon.* Tenotomy of the lateral tendons, so as to flex the DIP can be combined with one of the procedures of reconstruction of the middle tendon. In these cases, according to Littler (Fig. 16. 13 and 16.14), it will be of interest to resort to *selective tenotomy*. He cuts the two lateral tendons at the level of the middle phalanx and spares the distal oblique fibres of the retinacular ligaments which run to the terminal tendon, as well as the more peripheral portion of the lateral radial tendon in continuity with the tendon of the lumbrical. The lateral tendons, once they have been cut, are folded over on themselves and fixed to the base of the middle phalanx so as to replace the middle tendon. In this way, two extensor systems are constructed, one

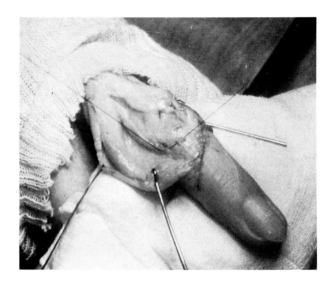

Figure 16.14
Littler's procedure. The lateral tendons sectioned at the level of the diaphysis of P2 are cut back on the median line and fixed to the base of P2 to reconstruct a lesser extensor tendon. The lumbrical tendon and the oblique fibres of the retinacular ligaments make up an extension system for the last phalanx. A pin maintains the IPP in extension.

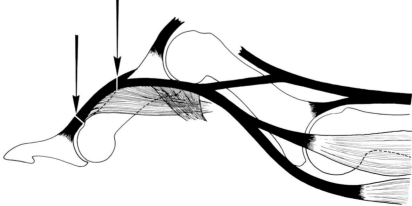

Figure 16.12
Treatment of buttonhole deformities by tenotomy. The proximal tenotomy (Dolphin) allows conservation of the oblique retinacular ligament insertions.

for each IP joint; all the active extension takes place at the PIP joint, while the oblique retinacular ligaments exert an 'active tenodesis' effect which is reinforced by the lumbrical so as to prevent dropping of the distal phalanx.

5. *Arthrodesis of the Proximal Interphalangeal Joint.* This is proposed for either painful stiffness of the joint, deformities of the joint surfaces or to correct severe fixed flexion deformities. The indications for this procedure must be weighed carefully, as fixation of the PIP joint must be functionally less crippling than the 'boutonnière' primary lesion.

6. *Articular Implants.* They represent now another alternative to arthrodesis, in old cases with fixed deformities. Arthroplasty with the help of a small silicon implant (Swanson) can be taken into consideration but only with intact flexor tendons.

The extensor apparatus is longitudinally incised, to insert the implant; with possible plication in order to keep it taut (see chapter on articular implants).

DISCUSSION

It would appear that the main object must be the restoration of the normal balance between the various elements of the extensor apparatus. In particular this involves:

1. Reinserting an active extensor tendon on the middle phalanx; and

2. Replacing lateral extensor tendons in their physiological position and relaxing the oblique fibres, thickened and bent, of the retinacular ligament.

In every case, the tension of the central tendon must be accurately balanced with that of the lateral because there is a real risk of transforming the 'boutonnière' into 'swan neck' deformity.

Several procedures, need to be combined. Reinsertions or sutures of the middle tendon have produced fairly good results, but they are feasible only when there is minimal retraction of the proximal part of the severed tendon. Tenoplasty of lateral tendons ought to be considered only when the latter are in good condition, its indication remains therefore quite limited.

Grafting is useful to repair defect in the extensor apparatus, after having freed retractions, when the loss cannot be filled by using adjacent scar tissues. Lacing the graft into the extensor apparatus contributes to its good tension.

Grafting can give excellent results. The long extensor can be used as a motor when its tendon is available at the level of the proximal phalanx and if adhesions at that level are not severe. Otherwise, it is preferable to use Fowler's procedure, on the interosseous muscles.

Tenotomy is considered in some cases with late lesions to correct hyperextension of the distal phalanx, combined with moderate deformity of the middle joint. But one has to bear in mind that the deformity in flexion of the PIP joint is compensated functionally by the hyperextension of the distal joint. Selective tenotomy combined with other procedures of restoration of the middle tendon, is not sufficient to achieve flexion of the second phalanx.

Arthroplasty and arthrodesis are reserved for cases showing severe and irreducible deformity of the PIP joint. Arthroplasty

with implants is more attractive, but it requires a good flexor tendon and a retrievable extensor apparatus still. It would be wiser to be content with arthrodesis, if the patient performs heavy manual labour.

AT THE LEVEL OF THE PROXIMAL PHALANX

The extensor apparatus is stretched out on all the dorsal aspect of the phalanx.

Lesions at that level are mainly traumatic: division, total or often partial occur, as well as adhesions after fracture of the phalanx.

Wounds require primary suture. Secondary tenolysis is frequently required.

AT THE LEVEL OF THE METACARPO-PHALANGEAL JOINT (MP)

Each long extensor tendon (proper tendon of index finger and of fifth digit merge with the common extensores at this level) crosses the dorsal aspect of the MP joint at this level. They are maintained along the axis of each digit, first by irregular and lax insertions at the base of the proximal phalanx and then chiefly by the sagittal bands crossing the lateral aspects of the joint, fixing themselves to the deep transverse metacarpal ligament. They actually represent the true proximal insertions of that tendon thus kept over the dorsal aspect of the joint.

The excursion of extensores longi digitorum is about 15 mm.

Extension of the proximal phalanx depends on two motor systems:

1. A direct motor: the common extensor insertion on the base of the proximal phalanx. However this is slackened by flexion of the IP joints involving a distal gliding of the dorsal aponeurosis whose action is effective only when the PIP is extended.

2. An indirect motor: the pressure exerted on the head of proximal phalanx through the base of the middle phalanx which pushes it dorsally, acting so more and more as the PIP is more flexed.

When the MP joint is in hyperextension, all effort of the extensor longus is absorbed by its proximal insertions on the first phalanx and by the sagittal bands. Such hyperextension must be prevented whenever the extensor longus has to fully act on the distal phalanges as in the correcting of claw deformity.

Two types of lesions may be encountered at the level of the MP joint: the tendon may be severed or it may be displaced laterally.

Section of the extensor tendon results in loss of extension at the proximal phalanx. Extension of the distal phalanges is performed by the interossei and lumbrical, when these muscles are intact. Retraction of the tendinous extremities is limited by the sagittal bands and by the junctura tendinum.

After tendon injury one usually finds an open joint capsule and sometimes a tear in the sagittal bands and the dorsal axis of the joint. These three structures must be carefully sutured and immobilized for four weeks, the wrist and finger in extension and the MP joint in 10 degrees of flexion, to prevent joint stiffness. Secondary suture at that level is usually possible.

Lateral displacement of the extensor tendon. The long extensor tendon is maintained on the dorsal aspect of the MP joint by the interosseous aponeurosis and its fragile proximal insertions, the sagittal bands, loose adhesions to the capsule and inconstant insertion on the base of the first phalanx.

When these structures are torn by trauma or stretched by rheumatoid arthritis, the tendon, when submitted to passive tension, as in flexion, will tend to slide over to the ulnar side of the joint. As the lesions become more severe, the tendons are displaced into the intermetacarpal valley and contribute to maintaining the flexion deformity and ulnar deviation of the MP joint.

In addition, freed from its proximal attachment, the extensor tendon will exert an even stronger action on the middle phalanx, forcing it into hyperextension.

Such tendon displacement must be corrected, the difficulty being to maintain the tendon in its axis without impeding its gliding movement.

In rheumatoid arthritis, a synovectomy is performed and an overlapping suture is placed on the lateral border of the distended sheath in order to recentre the tendon.

In cases presenting an old tear of the sheath, correction is achieved by a plasty using a junctura tendinum (Wheeldon) or a strip of tendon (Michon), which is fixed to the external edge of the tear.

The sagittal bands can also be reconstructed to a more anatomical pattern, though more difficult surgically, directly into the intermetacarpal transverse ligament, with the help of a small band taken from the tendon, or by means of a graft attached on the sheath, on both sides of the tendon (Curtis).

The length of such mooring must exactly balance flexion and extension movements of the whole finger.

REFERENCES

ALBERTONI, W. *La technique de D. Brooks et O. Graner pour la correction des Mallet fingers.* Thesis, Sao Paulo.

BOYES, J. (1964) *Bunnell's surgery of the hand.* 4th edn. Philadelphia: J.-B. Lippincott.

BUNNELL, S. (1956) *Surgery of the hand* 3rd edn. London: Pitman Medical Publishing.

BUTLER, B., Jr. 'Another' Boutonniere procedure. *American Society for Surgery of the Hand letters.*

DOLPHIN, J.-A. (1965) The extensor tenotomy for chronic boutonniere deformity of the finger. *J. Bone Jt Surg.*, **47-A,** ECE-ECG.

ENTIN, M.-A. (1960) Repair of extensor mechanism of the hand. *Surg. Clin. N. Amer.,* **40,** 275.

ESTÈVE, P. (1964) Traitement de la rupture distale des tendons extenseurs. *Entretiens de Bichat, Chirurgie,* Paris: Expansion Scientifique Française.

FOWLER, S.-B. (1949) Extensor apparatus of the digits. *J. Bone Jt Surg.,* **31-B,** 477.

LANDSMEER, J.-M.-F. (1949) Anatomy of the dorsal aponeurosis of the human finger, and its functional significance. *Anat. Rec.,* **104,** 35–45.

LITTLER, J.-W., & EATON, R.-G. (1967) Redistribution of forces in correction of boutonniere deformity. *J. Bone Jt Surg.,* **49-A,** 1267–1274.

LORTHIOIR, G., EVRARD, H., & VANDERELST, E. (1958) Le traitement des traumatismes récents de la main. *Acta orthop. belg.,* **24,** Suppl., I, p. 157.

MAISELS, D.-O. (1965) The middle slip or boutonniere deformity in burned hands. *Brit. J. plast. Surg.,* **18,** 117.

MATEV, I. (1964) Treatment of long-standing boutonniere deformity of the fingers. *Brit. J. plast. Surg.,* **17,** 281.

MICHON, J., & VICHARD, P. (1961) Luxations latérales des tendons extenseurs en regard de l'articulation métacarpo-phalangienne. *Rev. Méd. Nancy,* **86,** 595–601.

NICHOLS, H.-M. *Manual of hand Injuries* 2nd. edn. Chicago, Year Book Publishers.

PLANAS, J. (1962) Buttonhole deformity of the fingers. *The Second Hand Club,* Réunion de Paris.

PRATT, R.-R. (1952) Internal splint for closed and open treatment of injuries of the extensor tendon at the distal joint of the finger. *J. Bone Jt Surg.,* **34-A,** 785–788.

PULVERTAFT, R.-G. (1962) Discussion. *The Second Hand Club. Réunion de Paris.*

SALVI, V. (1969) Technique for the buttonhole deformity. *The Hand,* **1,** 96.

SOUTER, W.-A. (1967) The boutonniere deformity. *J. Bone Jt Surg.,* **49-B,** 4, 710–721.

STACK, G. (1962) Muscle function in the fingers. *J. Bone Jt Surg.,* **44-B,** 899–909.

STACK, G. (1971) Buttonhole deformity. *The Hand,* **3,** 152.

STARK, H., BOYES, J. & WILSON, J. (1962) Mallet finger. *J. Bone Jt Surg.,* **44-A,** 1061.

STEWART, I.-M. (1962) Boutonniere finger. *Clin. Orthop.,* **23,** 220.

TUBIANA, R. (1968) Surgical repair of the extensor apparatus of the fingers. *Surg. Clin. N. Amer.,* **48,** 1015-1031.

TUBIANA, R. & VALENTIN P. (1969) L'extension des doigts. *Rev. Chir. orthop.,* **53,** 2, 111–124.

VERDAN, Cl. (1966) Primary and secondary repair of flexor and extensor tendon injuries. In: *Hand Surgery.* ed. Flynn, J. E., Baltimore: Williams and Wilkins Co.

VILAIN, R. (1962) Repair of the extensor of the finger at its distal extremity. *The Second Hand Club, Réunion de Paris.*

17. Extensor Tendon Lesions on the Dorsum of the Hand and Wrist

J. Cantero A. Chamay

The extensor apparatus on the dorsum of the hand and wrist is composed of:
1. the extensor digitorum communis for the four fingers,
2. the extensores indicis proprius and digiti quinti proprius,
3. the extensores pollicis longus and brevis,
4. the abductor pollicis longus,
5. the extensores carpi radialis longus and brevis,
6. the extensor carpi ulnaris.

The tendons of the extensor communis are connected to one another by transverse and oblique bands called Juncturae tendinum thereby permitting, in case of laceration of one of the tendons and depending on the level of the injury, a certain amount of function supplied by the neighbouring tendon. But the extensor system of the thumb is entirely individual.

On the dorsum of the metacarpal phalangeal joint (Verdan's Zone V, Fig. 18.2, page 135) the tendons are flattened to form three bands. They each receive lateral expansions from the palmar and dorsal interosseous muscles to intermingle with its own fibres to form the dorsal 'hood'.

A laceration of the extensor tendon on the dorsum of the hand or at the metacarpal head level leads to a drop of the proximal phalanx only. The extension of the middle and distal phalanges is preserved due to the integrity of the intrinsic system. Not infrequently, in cases of recent extensor tendon lesions, the undamaged lateral expansion may extend the proximal phalanx. This phenomenon is similar to the one observed in certain patellar fractures in which the extension of the knee is possible when the lateral and medial retinaculi of the patella are undamaged. In injuries at the aforementioned levels the extensor tendon does not retract very far. At the wrist level (Verdan's Zone VII the extensor tendons are ensheathed in six compartments beneath the extensor retinaculum. These sheaths are separated by vertical fibrous septa which unite the extensor retinaculum with the radius. The sheath of the abductor pollicis longus and extensor pollicis brevis is at the extreme radial side. Aligned on the same plane are the sheaths for the extensores carpi radiales, longus and brevis, the extensor pollicis longus, the extensor digitorum communis with the extensor indicis proprius, the extensor digiti quinti proprius and finally, the extensor carpi ulnaris.

EXTENSOR TENDON DIVISION AT THE METACARPOPHALANGEAL JOINT LEVEL
(Zone V)

The diagnosis of a lesion of an extensor tendon at this level does not present any problem when seen early. However, in late cases, the diagnosis may not be so easy because a fibrous bridge is generally formed uniting the two extremities. Nevertheless, a transverse depression may be felt when palpating the tendon. The best way to test the function of the extensor tendon is to place the hand of the patient on a flat surface as a pianist would to play the piano. Then the patient is asked to lift each finger at a time as if he were to play a gamut. This particular movement can only be made by the extensor tendons since the intrinsic muscles could not possibly compensate.

At the metacarpophalangeal joint level, the extensor apparatus is intimately united to the joint capsule. Very frequently the latter is severed at the same time as the tendon, leaving a large gap. In 'tidy' injuries, repair is done in one whole layer, using Polydeck 4–0 (braided polyester thread). The stitch is done by passing the thread through the tendon in a horizontal 'U' manner, being careful not to penetrate the synovial layer. The lateral expansion is then sutured by a few simple stitches with thinner thread (Polydeck 5–0).

However, in cases of 'untidy' injuries (Fig. 17.1), which are ragged, crushed or torn at the margins and are more widely damaged in depth severing the bone structure of the joint, it is preferable to suture each different plane separately; that is: capsule, tendon and paratenon. Doing so, the massive scarring that might hinder later function is avoided. Steel wires should not be used since they can easily break and the fragments may become annoying, rubbing against a bony surface in each to and fro movement. After tendon repair, the hand is immobilized for four weeks in a standard plaster cast in the following position: the wrist dorsally flexed, the finger rests on an aluminium splint which is fixed buried within the plaster cast. The MP joint should be flexed at about 60 degrees and the PIP joint extended. The DIP joint may be left free permitting a certain amount of movement and thus maintaining the function of intrinsic muscles. Recently we have replaced this type of immobilization by a double plaster splint (volar and dorsal) wrapped by an elastic bandage maintaining the same position as described before. In some cases of untidy injuries when it is not possible to suture the tendon because of an important gap or because the tendon is ragged, crushed or torn, a graft then must be done. Ducourtioux tacks a thin tendon graft (palmaris longus) through the capsular-tendon layer at its distal end obtaining a sort of U-form stitch. The two ends of the graft are crossed in 'X' on the dorsum of the hand and are sutured to the proximal end of the extensor tendon, thus obtaining a solid bridge. This technique is interesting because the repair can be made without any suture material being used in anastomosing of the distal end.

If at the site of the injury, the missing or nonviable skin or the shape of the tendon does not permit the tenorrhaphy, the

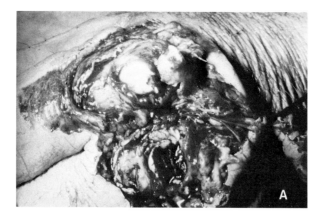

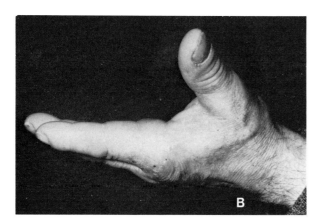

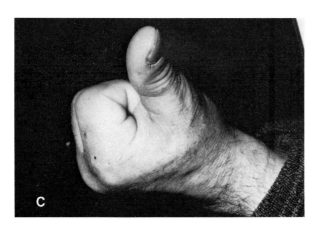

Figure 17.1
(A) 'Untidy' wound on the dorsum of the hand with extensor tendon lacerations of the index and middle finger *exposing* the MP joint. (B) and (C) Results five months after having sutured each different plane separately.

best procedure to cover the defect would be an advancement flap or a bipedicled transposition flap, leaving the tenorrhaphy for later. This is also true for late cases where areas of massive fibrous adherences predominate.

In cases of secondary repair, the skin incision should be made around the scar passing through the interjoint space making a sort of half-circled flap. After liberating the adhesions between the skin and the tendons, the fibrous bridge is then resected transversely. On extending the proximal phalanx, the two ends can be approached and the repair can be done either by a simple 'U' stitch or by grafting.

EXTENSOR TENDON DISLOCATIONS

The extensor is held in the centre of the metacarpophalangeal joint by the dorsal expansions of the interosseous muscles and by two sagittal bands which insert on the deep transversal intermetacarpal ligament.

In cases when one of the lateral expansions is severed, or when there is a subcutaneous rupture or elongation of one of the lateral expansions with synovitis, the tendons may be displaced towards the ulnar side of the joint leading to the ulnar drift deformity, typical of rheumatoid disease. These tendons, once dislocated towards the intermetacarpal space, cannot extend completely the MP joints. The surgical treatment should be the direct suture of the lateral expansion whenever possible. Otherwise, a plastic repair can be made using a thin slice of the same tendon or of a junctura tendinum. If several tendons are dislocated, a graft is passed transversely through each tendon and it is sutured at each passage. Then the radial end of the graft is sutured laterally to the tendon of the first dorsal interosseous muscle in order to counterbalance the system. Moreover, the extensor indicis proprius can be transferred to the tendon of the first dorsal interosseous to contribute in a dynamic manner to oppose the ulnar drift of the fingers.

TENDON DIVISION ON THE DORSUM OF THE HAND (Zone VI)

The clinical signs of tendon injury within this zone may be similar to that of Zone V. However, several differences may be found mainly due to the presence of intertendinous connections which more or less modify the degree of tendon retraction giving different functional values. Moreover, the retraction of the proximal end may be greater if the tendon is divided proximally to the connexus intertendineus. Consequently, the functional limitation may vary.

When one of the communis tendons of the index finger or of the little finger is divided, there is hardly any functional deficit noticeable. Yet, a lack of independence of extension may be demonstrated if the tendon severed is the proprius.

In late cases, the distal end of the severed tendon may adhere to the scar tissue producing a tenodesis effect which might be difficult to differentiate from cases of simple adherences without tendon injury. This is also true in injuries to Zones VII and VIII.

TREATMENT

With the exception of the extensor pollicis longus, the treatment in this zone does not raise any particular problem. Primary suture is indicated each time that the lesion presents satisfactory conditions. In searching for the proximal end of the severed tendon it might be necessary to make a small transverse incision proximal to the lesion. However, by enlarging the wound at its extremities and massaging the muscle of the tendon distally, the proximal end will often appear at the site of the wound. It is desirable to block the tendon within its compartment at the wrist by a pin passed through the skin, picking up the tendon transversely, until the suture has been achieved. The suture should be covered by surrounding paratenon in order to avoid adherences between the cicatrice of the tendon and that of the skin.

Secondary suture is indicated in cases of unsuccessful results of primary suture, untidy wounds and in certain degenerative diseases with partial or total ruptures of one or several tendons. The hand should be immobilized for four weeks with the wrist dorsally flexed, the MP joints flexed and the PIP joints extended avoiding hyperextension of MP joints.

TENOLYSIS

In cases where adherences lead to dimpling of the skin and to limitation of function, tenolysis is then indicated. Complete excision of the scar might be necessary if the latter is too wide and ill-conditioned. However, as a general rule, it is best to approach the tendon by an incision at a certain distance from the site of the lesion in order to avoid recurrence of adherences directly to the scar of the skin.

On the ulnar half of the hand, the best site for incision is at the junction between the dorsal skin and the hypothenar mass. In the centre of the dorsum of the hand, a curved incision in the longitudinal axis forming small flaps should be chosen. One must take care not to lacerate the sensory branches of the ulnar and radial nerves.

EXTENSOR TENDON GRAFT

In the management of a large tendon defect, one of the following procedures may be chosen: anastomosis of the distal end with a neighbouring tendon, transfer of one of the extensors of the index or of the little finger, or tendon graft. The latter is only possible if the proximal end is easy to find and if the muscle is in satisfactory condition. The extensor tendon graft is the best procedure since it can be done without involving the rest of the hand. It is essential in cases of multiple tendon tissue losses and it can be combined with muscle tendon transfer depending on the circumstances.

One must not forget the possibility of using the flexor superficialis of the ring finger which can be passed through the interosseous membrane of the forearm to the dorsum of the hand to be used as an extensor tendon. This of course is possible due to the great independent function of each flexor superficialis muscle.

In cases of associated skin loss, the gap should firstly be covered by a flap. The grafting of the tendons is done secondarily and if possible by tunnelling through at a certain distance from the scars surrounding the flap. The anastomosis with the proximal end should be placed proximally to the extensor retinaculum.

EXTENSOR TENDON DIVISION AT THE DORSUM OF THE WRIST (Zone VII)

A systematic exploration of the function of each finger is necessary. The drop of the two middle fingers suggests a division of the four tendons of the extensor communis since the extensor indicis proprius and extensor digiti quinti proprius suffice to assure the extension of these two fingers respectively.

To explore the action of the extensores carpi radialis longus and brevis as well as the extensor carpi ulnaris, the patient should try to extend dorsally the wrist with a closed fist.

TREATMENT

Tendon repair at this level is rather difficult due to the fact that the tendons are ensheathed tightly in fibrous compartments beneath the extensor retinaculum (Fig. 17.2). Their excursion is of about 5.5 cm thus presenting a gliding problem similar to that of the flexor tendons.

If any limitation of function should occur, it will depend on the level of repair in relation to the extensor retinaculum. If the repair is distal to the retinaculum, extension may be limited, whereas if it is proximal to the retinaculum, flexion is limited.

Often, after repair, extension of the fingers is possible only if the wrist is in an attitude neutral or of partial flexion, whereas, in a hyperextended position, it is impossible. Inversely, complete flexion of the wrist is only possible when the fingers are extended; it is impossible when the fist is closed.

This partial block often justifies the tenolysis with transfer of the retinaculum under the extensor tendons as is often done in cases of rheumatoid arthritis. The interposition of paratenon or of a silastic sheet can also be done. Occasionally, the problem can be resolved by a tendon graft, anastomosing it far from the retinaculum. When all of the tendons are not severed, a transfer may be possible.

THE EXTENSOR CARPI TENDONS

There are usually two types of injuries at this level:

1. in the ulnar half of the wrist the severance of the extensor carpi ulnaris is often associated with that of the extensor digiti quinti;

2. in the radial half, the severance of the extensores carpi radiales brevis and longus is generally combined with the extensors of the index finger and the extensor pollicis longus.

The extensores carpi radiales are located in the deeper plane and their severance is often overlooked. They must be sutured primarily since they undergo fibrous retraction and adhere proximally rendering more difficult the secondary repair. It is sometimes necessary for the secondary repair to lengthen the tendons either by 'Z'-tenotomy or by tendon graft using one

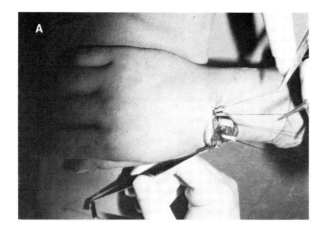

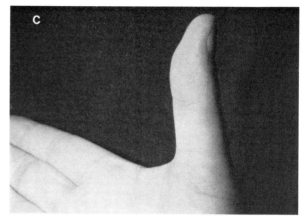

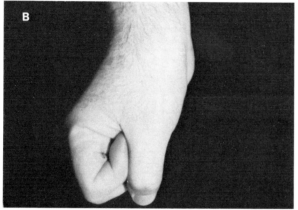

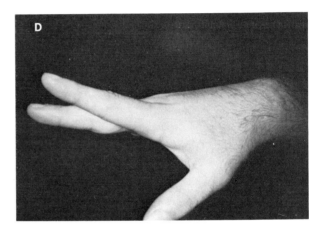

Figure 17.2
(A) Wound on the dorsum of the wrist with severance of the extensor pollicis longus, the extensor indicis proprius and communis, and

extensor carpi radialis brevis. Suture was done by Bunnell's shoelace stitch. (B) (C) and (D) Results two months after repair.

of the two tendons as a graft and suturing together the two proximal ends.

TENDON TRANSFER

The result of tendon transfer is not good unless the gliding amplitude of the tendon being repaired is the same as that of the tendon to be transferred. This is the reason why one obtains poor results when one of the extensor carpi tendons (amplitude of 37 mm) is transferred to replace the extensor of the index finger (amplitude of 55 mm) or the extensor pollicis longus (amplitude of 58 mm). In such cases a graft is the best procedure.

DIVISION OF THE EXTENSOR TENDONS OF THE THUMB

Tendon injury at the *metacarpophalangeal level of the* thumb differs from that of other fingers. The extensor mechanism of the thumb is more complicated since it comprises not only the extensor pollicis brevis and longus but also the dorsal expansions of the abductor pollicis brevis and of the adductor pollicis. These latter tendons can compensate to a certain degree, the extension of the distal phalanx when the extensor pollicis longus has been severed. Injuries in this area often only partially divide this wide tendinous band. Generally, the

retraction of the tendon is small and the repair is not difficult. Primary as well as secondary repairs often give good results. It is important that each tendon be sutured individually by a separate 'U'-stitch. The thumb should be immobilized by a plaster cast in the 'hitch-hiker' position during five weeks (Fig. 17.3). The isolated division of the *extensor pollicis brevis* may escape notice if the extensor pollicis longus is undamaged. However, a progressive drop of the proximal phalanx may be noticed months later. This is due mainly to a lateral ulnar displacement of the extensor pollicis longus causing a hyperextension of the IP joint and flexion of the MP joint. This deformity recalls the 'boutonnière' deformity seen in the long fingers.

The *abductor pollicis longus*, a stronger muscle, presents a more serious problem when severed because it glides through a close-fitting compartment. This fibrous compartment must be opened widely in order to suture the tendon. At the same time, one avoids a later block of the tendon that reminds one of the stenosing tenosynovitis of de Quervain. Aberrant tendons are not infrequently found in this compartment.

Injuries of the *extensor pollicis longus* merits special attention since it is particularly necessary for the function of the thumb. Its course is characterized by angulation around Lister's tubercule. It is ensheathed independently from the other extensor

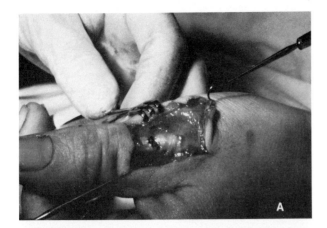

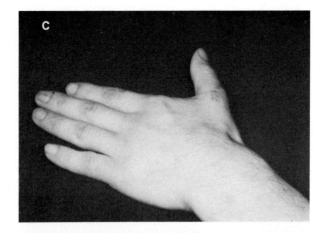

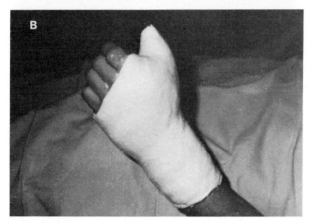

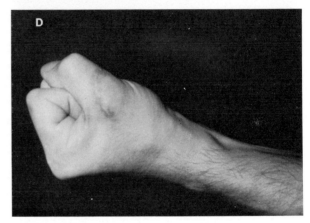

Figure 17.3
Wound on the dorsum of the MP joint of the thumb with severance of its two extensor tendons: (A) after the suture; (B) immobilization in a plaster cast in the hitch-hiker position; (C) and (D) results two months after surgery.

tendons. It crosses the course of the extensores carpi radialis brevis and longus. There may exist a communication between their sheaths at this point. When the tendon is severed, its proximal end retracts considerably and often as far as the extensor retinaculum. In order to search for the tendon, it is preferable to make a transverse incision rather than a longitudinal incision beginning at the wound. The suture is done by a shoelace stitch (Bunnell's) using Polydek 4–0. The thumb is immobilized for five weeks by a plaster cast in the hitch-hiker position. If the tendinous gap is more than 1 cm, then we prefer a tendon graft. If primary suture is not done immediately, it is generally impossible to do a secondary end-to-end suture. This is also true in cases of subcutaneous ruptures of the tendon. In these cases, we either graft, using the palmaris longus tendon or other tendons, or we proceed to the transfer of the extensor indicis proprius or communis. The graft is more physiological since it permits recovery of the function of the retracted muscle thus preserving the force of the extensors of

the index finger. However, it is a delicate and long procedure; the proximal anastomosis should be done at the muscle-tendinous junction whereas the distal should be performed at about the middle of the metacarpal. The hand should be immobilized for five weeks. The tendon transfer of the extensor indicis is an easier and faster technique. The length adjustment of the transposed tendon is simple if one uses the interlacing technique for the anastomosis. One must take into consideration the fact that the index finger loses half of its force of extension as well as a certain degree of independence of movement. We consider that the transfer is only indicated in cases of extensor pollicis longus muscle atrophy. In certain complicated injuries, the extensor digiti quinti proprius may be used (Verdan, 1972). Its transfer to the extensor pollicis longus tendon is in general satisfactory. Regarding the transfer of the extensor pollicis brevis to the longus, we do not recommend this, since its gliding amplitude and approaching angles are different from those of the extensor pollicis longus.

REFERENCES

DUCOURTIOUX, J.-L. (1969) Une technique de réparation utilisant des greffes de tendon extenseur sur le dos de la main. *Ann. Chir. plast.,* **14,** 267–268.

THOMPSEN, M. *et al.* (1969) Tendon transfers for defective long extensors of the wrist and finger. *Scand. J. Plast. Surg.* **3,** 71–78.

TUBIANA, R. (1968) Surgical repair of the extensor apparatus of the fingers. *Surg. Clin. N. Amer.,* **48,** 1050.

VERDAN, Cl. (1968) Primary and secondary repair of flexor and extensor tendon injuries. In *Hand Surgery,* ed. Flynn, J. E. Baltimore: Williams and Wilkins.

VERDAN, Cl. (1972) *Die Operationen an der Hand.* Band X, Teil XII. ed. Wachsmuth, W. and Wilhelm, A. Berlin: Springer Verlag.

VARIOUS ASPECTS OF TENDON SURGERY

18. Tenolysis

C. Verdan

The aim of tenolysis is the release of adhesions or other obstacles that impede normal gliding of the tendon. It presupposes continuity of the tendon.

The delicate release of peritendinous adhesions can be performed on flexor and extensor tendons in all the topographical surgical zones (Fig. 18.1 and 18.2). But it is not an easy operation; release over a short distance such as near a scar junction is generally insufficient, since the adhesions can extend further than the primary suture or graft area, even as far as the musculotendinous junction. The technical difficulties encountered can be as great or greater than those of a tendon graft. The duration of such an operation can be an hour and a half, or more.

The incisions and mode of access are the same as those used for grafts (see Figs. 8.2, 8.3 and 8.4). We consider that the zig-zag incision on the palmar surface of the finger as described by Bruner (Fig. 18.3, index) can cause difficulties in the immediate functional rehabilitation. We prefer a classic mid-lateral incision, leaving the entire palmar surface intact (Fig. 18.3). We also take care that the original scar be avoided or included in the prepared flap such that early mobilization and daily exercises are not hindered.

Adherent tendons may result from:
1. primary or secondary suture;
2. tendon graft;
3. tendon transfer;
4. fracture located near a tendon;
5. infections;
6. untidy wound in the area;
7. foreign body;
8. post operative adhesions (for ganglions, tumors, etc.);
9. 'quadriga' syndrome after amputation.

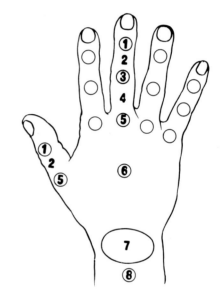

Figure 18.2
Surgical topographical areas: eight extensor tendon zones.

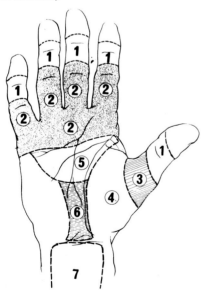

Figure 18.1
Surgical topographical areas: seven flexor tendon zones.

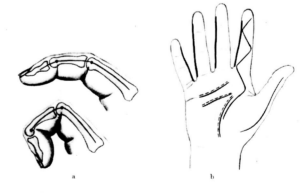

Figure 18.3
(a) Classical mid-lateral digital incision
(b) Combined various incisions.

CONDITIONS FOR SUCCESSFUL TENOLYSES

When the tendon is stripped over a certain distance, it is necessarily devascularized. Necrosis is avoided by the formation of connective granulation tissue very richly vascularized, which develops in the first days after the operation. New adhesions inevitably result, and if the tendon is immobilized, they will form a diffuse circular cushion leading to a new blockage.

Treatment must be aimed at transforming these 'vessel-carrying' adherences into nutritive mesotenons or at least a paratendon that will allow adequate sliding.

The fundamental conditions for successful tenolysis are:

1. that the interrupted vascularization be re-established without interfering with the gliding;

2. that the vascularization and trophicity of the finger be good overall, implying a satisfactory innervation;

3. that the operation be followed by a period of active re-education such that the sliding amplitude obtained surgically be maintained, allowing the tissue adaptation necessary to anatomical and functional normality.

These conditions imply total cooperation on the patient's part, whose will to recuperate is essential to success.

Six local factors condition this success:

1. the corresponding muscle must be functionally intact;

2. mobility of the joints involved must be good;

3. active and passive movements of the antagonist muscles must be free;

4. the freed tendon must be sufficiently resistant to rupture;

5. the surface of the liberated tendon must be smooth and its calibre regular;

6. the tendon bed must be free of bony spicules, surrounding fibrosis, bone stripped of its periosteum, etc.

TENOLYSIS OF EXTENSOR TENDONS

Because of the functional partitioning of the extensor system, it is often possible to perform a tenolysis over a limited distance. On the dorsal surface of the PIP joint and proximal phalanx, it is useful to find the sliding plane in healthy territory by separating the middle band from a lateral one by a longitudinal incision. The dissector will then have less difficulty in adherent zones and can diminish the risk of tendon damage. Often the small dorsal synovial sac of the PIP joint must also be liberated, and sometimes it is necessary to combine a tenolysis with excision of the dorsal part of the collateral ligaments.

Only when complete passive flexion of an articulation is attained can one be satisfied.

On the back of the hand and wrist the absence or limitation of sliding of the extensor system causes a tenodesis effect. This is manifested by the fact that the fingers alone or the wrist alone can be flexed passively, but not simultaneously. This means that the sliding amplitude of the tendons is not sufficient to allow both movements together; this is why it is so important at the end of the operation to verify that complete flexion of the fingers and wrist can be performed together.

TENOLYSIS OF FLEXOR TENDONS

Tenolysis of flexor tendons may be necessary at any level; most often at the *digital canal* and at the *wrist*.

In the *digital canal*, one must penetrate the sheath at different levels and therefore excise successive segments leaving strategically placed pulleys intact. However, Duparc and Alnot (1974) proposed incision of the sheath along the whole necessary length at its insertion raising it like a flap with a lateral hinge. This mode of access permits easy liberation of adhesions and traumatizes the tendon less. The sheath is resutured with separated stitches numerous enough to insure the strength necessary for early mobilization.

Whatever the method, it is important to be sure (using another incision in the palm or more often wrist) that selective traction on the tendon produces complete flexion (Fig. 18.4). The fingertip must touch the palm. It is important to keep a pulley as long and solid as possible in the region of the metacarpophalangeal articulation and the proximal phalanx. Resection of the entire sheath from this point distally can be sometimes necessary. It does not result necessarily in dislocation of the flexor digitorum profundus as it is held in the eyelet formed by superficialis.

Until six or seven years ago we excised the superficialis to give more room for the profundus; now we try to preserve both tendons. The reason for this is that the mesotenon of the flexor profundus at the level of the first phalanx is a vinculum arising in the region of the PIP joint and then passing *through* the superficialis to reach the profundus. Removing the superficialis tendon destroys this vascularization. Whenever possible we try to expose the vincula and leave them intact when mobilizing the tendon.

ANAESTHESIA

Instead of the usual regional or general anaesthesia, it may be helpful to apply a local anaesthesia, combined with Diazepam thus permitting voluntary muscle function. In this manner by alternatively opening and closing the tourniquet every 25 minutes to avoid muscle paralysis the patient may be asked to actively mobilize his own finger.

The operator can thus check the progression of his work: the amount of mobility obtained by the dissection of the tendon. This is especially valuable for the flexors (Hunter).

INTERPOSITION OF A SLICE OF PARATENDON OR PLASTIC MATERIAL

When dissection necessitates stripping bone surfaces or when it is not possible to excise all the surrounding scar tissue, new adhesions are likely to develop. Three possible courses of action exist:

1. excision of the tendon and sheath excepting one or two pulleys and reconstruction of a new sheath around a Silastic (R) or Hunter rod; a tendon graft is performed three months later;

2. a slice of tricipital paratendon envelops the liberated tendon; this method is mostly valid for extensors;

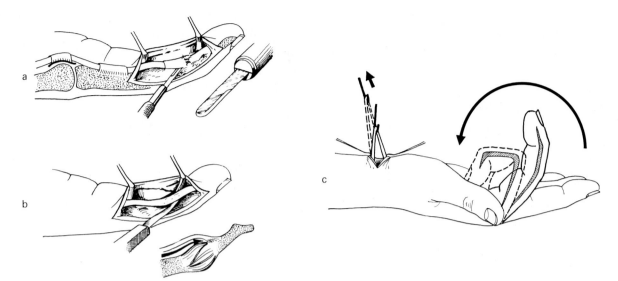

Figure 18.4
Tenolysis for jamming after suture of the deep flexor tendon in Zone I (Verdan, 1972)

3. interposition of a sheet of plastic (polyethylene or even better Silastic (R)). The risk here is that the sheet cannot be held in place and can fold over on itself during rehabilitation exercises, becoming a foreign body that hinders more then helps. Around an articulation such a set-up is contraindicated, but over short, more or less straight distances (e.g. over a diaphysial fracture callus) it can be useful for flexors and extensors.

USE OF CORTICOIDS

We have made limited use of corticoids when Carstam's (1953) experimental work seemed to favour them; but we are unconvinced of their utility either in general or local application. They may even increase the risk of rupture. We do not use salicylates, butazolidine or alphachymotrypsin as postoperative anti-oedema therapy, since their clinical utility seemed quite variable.

POSTOPERATIVE CARE

We mobilize the fingers as soon as we think haemostasis is satisfactory, i.e. after 48 hours of compressive bandage with the hand elevated. However, limited active movements can be encouraged immediately after surgery.

It is best to have the initial bandage in a flexed position such that its removal allows the surgeon to passively mobilize the finger to extension, which breaks the first adhesions caused by clotting of the blood. Following bandages should not limit movement amplitude; at this point we use a spray bandage (aerofilm, etc.).

OPERATIONS ASSOCIATED WITH TENOLYSIS

Examples of such operations are:
1. 'Z'-plasty in case of scar contractures;
2. excision of a scar or retractile subcutaneous fibrous tissue;
3. extraction of foreign bodies;
4. removal of osteosynthetic material;
5. neurolysis.

CONTRAINDICATIONS TO TENOLYSIS

Since success of the operation depends on active mobilization, any operation that prevents this is contra-indicated. This includes the following.
1. lengthening or shortening of a tendon;
2. free skin grafts;
3. corrective osteotomy; it is sometimes possible to obtain an osteosynthesis stable enough to permit immediate mobilization.

Sometimes tenolysis must be combined with resection of the lumbrical in the presence of 'lumbrical plus' syndrome (A. Parkes, 1970).

The frequent association of flexor tendon and collateral nerve damage raises the problem of concomitant neurorhaphy and tenolysis. These operations seem incompatible; often however we have seen that tenolysis does not exclude a nerve suture. We perform nerve grafts if tension is to be exerted on the suture line; this tension can also be controlled by limiting the finger extension in a special splint. The dorsal position permits full flexion but limits extension during the necessary three weeks (Fig. 18.5).

TENOLYSIS IN CHILDREN

A two- or three-year-old child cannot cooperate in the necessary active rehabilitation of this therapeutic method, but a four-year-old can replace adult exercises by games supervised by his mother. The games should be combined with passive mobilization in the presence of a physiotherapist (Fig. 18.6).

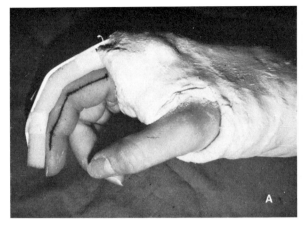

Figure 18.5
Splint allowing complete flexion of the finger:
(A) while limiting extension,

(B) permitting flexion when suture of a collateral nerve is performed with tenolysis.

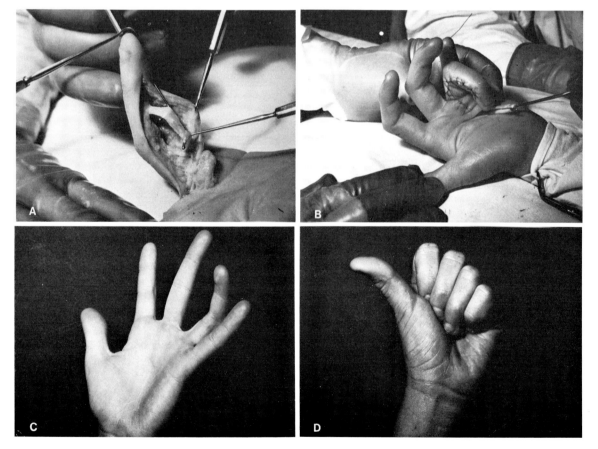

Figure 18.6
Child, age 12: Section of both flexors of left ring finger in Zone II. Primary suture of profundus and resection of superficialis in an emergency intervention. Complete blockage.
(A) Extensive tenolysis of profundus eight months later;

(B) Check of tendon liberation by traction in the palm;

(C) and (D) Result at check-up six months later: limitation of extension liable to diminish in a dynamic splint.

RETRO-SYNOVIAL PANNUS OF FLEXOR TENDONS AT THE PROXIMAL PHALANX

Several times during tenolysis to restore extension of the PIP joint, fixed after suture of a flexor tendon in Zone II, we have found that this fixation was not due to the tendons themselves but to a thick fibrous layer located behind the tendon. This covers the distal two thirds of the first phalanx and extends to the volar plate of the PIP joint. Only after its complete resection to the bone, implying also partial resection of the volar plate to which it is fused, can complete extension of the joint be obtained. Often this position must be held by an oblique Kirschner wire passing through the joint, as the musculo-tendinous traction could rapidly cause a relapse. After 10 days the wire is removed and a dynamic splint worn intermittently. Though we have no proof, we believe that this fibrous pannus develops when primary repair necessitated resection of the basal pulley over a long distance. The accidental wound that sectioned the flexors may also have penetrated the posterior wall of the synovial sheath through to the bone, producing connective tissue proliferation that can extend in both directions over the anterior surface of the PIP joint.

RESULTS

In 1971 we made a study with Crawford and Martini-Benkeddache of 92 patients (64 men and 28 women) aged four to 68 years, with 51 per cent between the ages of 21 and 40. One hundred and seventy-seven tendons were tenolysed on a total of 124 fingers. We remarked that a secondary tenolysis in zones I and II was especially useful in perfecting the result of primary treatment (Fig. 18.7 to 18.10). Zones VI and VII of the wrist and carpal tunnel also benefit from secondary tenolysis. For the detailed results refer to the 1971 publication. A summary follows:

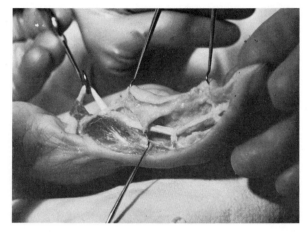

Figure 18.8
Factory worker, aged 28: open wound of extensors and open fracture of the proximal phalanx of the index finger. After consolidation of the fracture, block of both flexor tendons. Ten months later: tenolysis of profundus and resection of superficialis.

We adopted a grading system based on 5 numbers:

5 = excellent = normal flexion and extension;
4 = good = moderate improvement of flexion and/or extension, ability to flex the finger to 2.5 cm from the distal palmar crease;
3 = fair = some improvement but persistence of a notable deficit of flexion and extension, ability to flex the finger from 2.5 to 5 cm from the distal palmar crease;
2 = mediocre = no improvement;
1 = poor = worsening, amputations, etc.

Considering all tenolyses of flexors and extensors we objectively obtained 50 per cent excellent and good results $(5+4)$; the patient's subjective view was 65 per cent. If we include category 3 which does show some modest improvement, we attain 78 per cent favourable results.

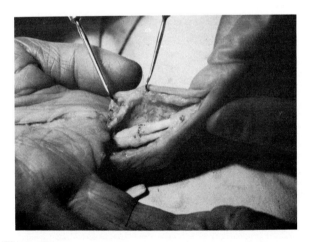

Figure 18.7
Nurse, aged 48: tenolysis four months after primary suture in Zone II of a flexor digitorum profundus and of a partially sectioned superficialis.

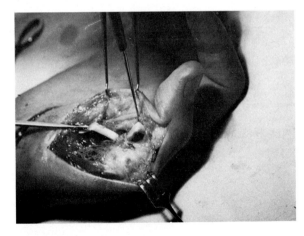

Figure 18.9
Child, aged 15: Partial section of flexor pollicis longus by a commissural dorso-medial axe blow sectioning the bone in Zone III; complete block after consolidation. Tenolysis six weeks later and verification of tendon sliding under the only preserved ring of the sheath.

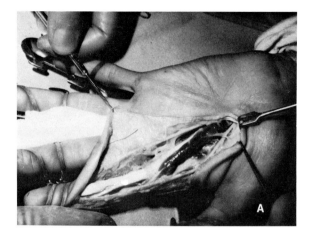

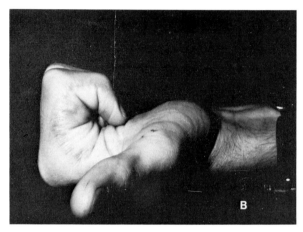

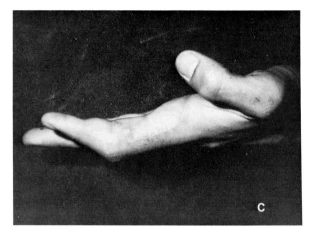

Figure 18.10
Teacher, aged 35: Suture of the two flexors of the left index in Zone II followed by complete block;
(A) Tenolysis 3 months later with liberation of the lumbrical (Simonetta);
(B) and (C): Functional result two months later.

Tenolysis applied to *extensors* sutured under emergency conditions showed that out of 29 blocks, 17 could be classed in groups 5 and 4. Only four cases gave no improvement, and they were all in juxta-articular Zones I–III–V (Verdan) (Fig. 18.2).

Tenolysis of *flexors* showed that out of 19 cases:

1. Eleven tenolyses in Zone I with 7 improvements (64 per cent).

2. Eight tenolyses in Zone II with 7 improvements (87 per cent).

In the two zones the 14 improved cases (4 excellent, 8 good, 2 fair) represent 74 per cent of the overall improved cases.

Considering the other flexor zones we obtained 81 per cent improvement.

There was overall improvement in 78 per cent of all flexor and extensor tenolyses performed.

A recent study (Egloff–Verdan, 1978) has been conducted to investigate the factors which worsen the result of tenolysis. A 100 tenolyses have been studied. It was statistically determined that the following situations were detrimental:

1. Patient over 40.
2. Concomitant surgery on the same digit, particularly
   (a) secondary nerve suture or graft of collateral nerve;
   (b) corrective osteotomy;
   (c) capsulotomy, (neurolysis of the collateral nerve, flexor sublimis resection, tenodesis or arthrodesis of the distal interphalangeal joint did not modify the results of tenolysis).
3. Tenolysis performed 1 year or more after the initial surgery or trauma.
4. Tenolysis performed after infectious or inflammatory conditions.
5. Tenolysis requiring a prolonged operative time.

The study, however, proved the value of tenolysis, as in 73 cases (73 per cent) the amplitude of active motion was improved by a mean of 24,5 degrees. Results were better after flexor tenolysis (28,35°) than after extensor tenolysis (15,60°). These results indicate the utility of this operation and that it must in selected cases become an accepted therapeutic measure.

REFERENCES

CARSTAM, N. (1953) Effect of cortisone on the formation of tendon adhesions and on tendon healing. *Acta chir. scand.* Suppl. 182, Stockholm.
DUPARC, J. & ALNOT V. (1970) Personal communication.
PARKES, A. (1970) The lumbrical plus finger. *Hand*, **2**, 164.
VERDAN, Cl., CRAWFORD, G. & MARTINI Y. (1971) Tenolysis in traumatic hand-surgery. *Educational Foundation of the American Society of Plastic and Reconstructive Surgeons*, vol. 3, Symposium on the Hand. Saint-Louis. C. V. Mosby.
VERDAN, Cl. & MICHON J. (1961) Le traitement des plaies des tendons fléchisseurs des doigts. *Rev. Chir. orthop.*, **47**, 285.
VERDAN, Cl. (1972) Die Eingriffe an Muskeln, Sehnen und Sehnenscheiden. In *Chirurgische Operationslehre*. Band X, ed. Wachsmuth, W. & Wilhelm, A. Teil III. Heidelberg: Springer Verlag.

C. Verdan

In the presence of a permanent disability following injury of peripheral nerves, with total or partial integrity of the joints and skeleton, one can be confronted with either an irreparable lesion at the first, or a failure in a previous attempt made to repair the nerves. It is sometimes difficult to decide within a given period of time, if this repair will really be a definitive failure.

Whatever the cause of the functional loss may be, many injuries leave a number of nervous lesions for which the question will be raised of palliative surgery. Also what is the role of the surgeon in a late partial palsy of motor muscles?

Operations on the motor apparatus, after nerve surgery has failed, will essentially concern muscle and tendon transplantations; these can secondarily be combined with procedures involving joints, so as to stabilize them by means of capsulorhaphy and still better of arthrodesis.

This chapter will only consider well established operations on motor, not sensory, apparatus.

We are indebted to the ingenuity of Carl Nicoladoni (1847–1902) (and later of Fritz Lange, Vulpius, Georg Perthes, Robert Jones, Harold Stiles, Sterling Bunnell and many others) for the idea of changing the direction of living muscles and thus modifying their mechanical action on joints. Owing to the fact that usually the vasculo-nervous pedicle penetrates a muscle in its proximal and middle part, the distal portion of muscle and tendon can easily be disinserted, then freed for some length in order to shift its direction and finally be reimplanted elsewhere, with minimal damage to its nutrition and contractility. However, there will be often a diminution of strength of about one-third.

One should take into consideration the mechanical results following loss of a given muscle and its insertion on the new site. The muscular power, the length of the lever arm acted upon, the angle of approach and chiefly the gliding range are the many factors to be considered in the surgeon's choice. Errors of choice, of implantation, and of direction are unfortunately responsible for a number of failures.

MUSCULAR SYNERGY

Former authors have overemphasized the role played by muscular synergy.

Muscles are called synergic wherever they act in concert with each other to enhance their effect. Thus they can contract together without having an antagonistic effect e.g. the extensors carpi with the flexors digitorum or otherwise the extensors digitorum with the flexors carpi. We must logically admit that two synergic muscles accustomed to contract both

at the same time would easily replace one another. Besides, the nervous centres controlling them will adapt themselves with less effort.

According to Boyes, the role of synergy at the level of the hand is far from outstanding, since here all usual motion is mainly voluntary and in direct relation with the brain. On the contrary the pelvic limbs move far more automatically, especially walking, and are more under the influence of the spinal cord.

Scherb of Zurich emphasized the necessity of using synergic muscles for transfers in the legs. In the upper limb there is a much wider choice for a new motor; nevertheless the difficulty of rehabilitation will often depend on the choice of muscle made.

BASIC CONDITIONS FOR TENDON TRANSFER

1. It is obvious that bones and joints in the concerned area must have been restored to their anatomical and functional integrity.

2. It would be absurd to require from a tendon transfer a new performance and expect by the same procedure a recovering of an old stiffness or deformity. The following cannot be overstressed: the importance of physiotherapy previous to the operation, and the early use for splints to correct deviations due to palsy (radial, opposition of thumb, intrinsic muscles, etc.). When deformities have been neglected, they will be so much more difficult to correct later.

3. Subcutaneous tissue and musculature ought to show a good state of suppleness and nutrition. Whenever confronted with scars or fibrosis, one will have to first replace these by a good tissue, by some plastic procedure, before undertaking any transplantation.

4. The transferred tendon should have an appropriate length and it is preferable, when possible, not to have to prolong it by a graft.

5. The motor muscle should have an adequate strength for the required function. It ought to be neither too strong nor too weak. The gliding amplitude of the chosen tendon must be convenient. It is sometimes possible to improve e.g. with the brachioradialis, which is frequently overlooked because of its short gliding range. Yet the amplitude can be greatly increased if that muscle is freed well proximally and it is a useful transfer for palsy of the flexor pollicis longus.

6. The mobility of the wrist plays an important part in some procedures, to compensate a too short gliding range and supply a sort of active tenodesis.

7. The effectiveness of the transfer will largely depend upon

the direction of the transplant: it must follow as straight a course as possible. The interosseous membrane, for instance, should be widely excised, in order to replace a lacking extensor digitorum longus by a flexor superficialis transferred to the dorsal compartment.

8. In a number of special situations, new pulleys must be created so that the direction of approach of the tendons can be changed and yet its dislocation prevented, for that would mean an impairment and even an ineffectiveness of its force of traction. This shift of direction is a classic step during palliative surgery for thumb-opposition palsy, where a pulley is essential: but special attention must be given to keep the angle within 45 degrees. The same angulation is found in creating a new adductor pollicis, by means of one of the extensors carpi radialis, to which a tendinous graft will be added as it is passed through the third interosseous space. All these deflections in the course of the tendon account for a considerable amount of friction, of adhesions and reduced gliding and therefore they all entail a functional impairment.

9. It is not wise to take a preoperatively useful muscle and convert it into an uncertain transplant. Every muscle representing an element of joint stabilization has always to be respected. Therefore the flexor carpi radialis, stabilizing factor of the wrist, cannot be utilized unless the wrist is fixed with an arthrodesis. Remember also that flexor carpi ulnaris is the strongest flexor of the wrist.

10. We must always keep in mind that our operations aim at correcting functional imbalance. We cannot add new forces, only re-distribute the remaining ones. Any palliative operation should therefore be conceived with simplicity, accepting in anticipation a limited functional achievement.

11. The point of insertion is important:

Nicoladoni would implant the tendons of the functioning muscles on the tendons of the palsied ones. It was wrong to forsake that technique, fearing a progressive elongation of the receptor tendon and then weakening of the muscular contractility. Bielsalski substituted a subperiosteal insertion, directly on the bone. Putti improved this procedure by introducing the tendon in a bony ditch, so as to fold its end and suture it back on the tendon itself. Yet too often the transferred tendon is too short for this. Periosteal reinsertion is still often recommended. It is a false term, since the periosteum allows no real insertion of a contracting muscle, except with children. It is by far preferable to create a hole into the bone, where the tendon will be fastened by means of a pull-out steel suture, technique of Bunnell.

Today implantation into the tendon itself has regained much favour for it allows action exactly at the site where the palsied muscle is inserted and moreover the surrounding mechanism can occasionally benefit from the new gliding apparatus.

12. A fair gliding range is essential. Three possible ways exist, for the passage of the tendon:

    (a) a subcutaneous route, with or without an artificial pulley;
    (b) an intrasynovial route;
    (c) an interosseous route.

The subcutaneous route, while it looks favourable most of the time, is unsuitable when the contracting muscle moves too far from the axis of the joint and gives the tendon a prolapsed tangential direction which impairs its activity.

Whenever anatomical conditions make it possible, the synovial passage produces more physiological results, because the tendon will have a proper pulley to control it. This pulley must yet be short, to avoid adhesions which must be loosened by exercise.

The interosseous route, between both bones of the forearm or the metacarpal bones permits direct and effective transfers. Max Lange described two main types of transfer:

    (a) The ascending tendinous transfer, consisting in joining the tendon of a palsied muscle to the tendon of a proximal healthy motor muscle. The strength of the latter will be transmitted not only to the site of its insertion, but further along to the palsied muscle, proximal to its tendon. One can either simply anastomose both tendinous segments or divide the tendon from its palsied muscle and suture it to the tendon of the motor muscle. This method seems to have an advantage, namely to let the healthy muscle maintain a normal insertion. But this muscular body will then have a twofold assignment and neither can be really effective. '*Qui trop embrasse, mal ètreint.*' The foregoing procedure will be valuable just for cases where the function of the palsied muscle was parallel with that of the new motor. Topographic situations allowing such a type of junction are few. We could cite mainly sutures of the tendons of profundus flexors of the two last fingers (ulnar nerve) with those of the middle and index finger, in the median nerve palsy at arm level.

    (b) The descending tendinous transfer consists in dis-inserting the distal insertion of the motor muscle tendon and transferring it on to the new site of insertion. The latter might well be the tendon of the palsied muscle itself or a new bony insertion.

THE ROLE OF ARTHRODESIS

Arthrodesis is justified especially in two situations:

1. When active muscles are either too few or too weak to supply the desired motion and a sufficient force. It will then be possible, by immobilizing the joint, to free a number of tendons previously destined to actively move the joint and utilize them for other purposes. As a principle, the weaker the muscular force, the greater is the opportunity of an arthrodesis. In the upper limb, the most important joint will be the wrist: its arthrodesis allows, theoretically, a number of muscles to become disposable, namely the extensors and flexors carpi.

2. When severe joint deformities are present and it is impossible to have them corrected by conservative means, i.e. physiotherapy, splints, traction, successive plaster cast with frequent changing, etc. Eventually, blocking the excursion of some joint movement with a bony graft, *arthroereisis*, can render considerable service, chiefly at the elbow in plexus palsies.

DURATION AND MEANS OF IMMOBILIZATION

As a rule, an immobilizing plaster is indispensible after every musculo-tendinous transfer, with ample padding, especially along the transplanted muscles and tendons. It can even be necessary to remove a section of plaster along the excursion of the new motor system, to avoid the slightest ischemia and compression at this level.

Immobilization after a tendon transfer upon another tendon, need not be different from that of a tendon suture, namely three to four weeks. It is wrong, whatever handbooks might suggest, to advise early mobilization because this can result in elongations and even ruptures.

The implantations on bone, with the 'pull-out wire' Bunnell's technique, require an immobilization time of six weeks.

FUNCTIONAL REHABILITATION

The success of tendon transfer surgery depends largely upon physical therapy. These cases are to be entrusted only to well-trained physiotherapists. Max Lange suggests commencing with minimal muscular exercises, even during the second week, either without removing the cast, or the plaster cast being merely opened like a shell. Those light early exercises of active contraction by the muscle prevent its atrophy and facilitate early and late gliding of the new tendon. Most care will be given to avoiding movement on the part of the antagonists of the transferred muscle. The therapist will find it useful to ask the patient first to contract the corresponding muscle on his healthy side, then on both sides and finally just the transplanted muscle. This new function may require a difficult apprenticeship from the patient, especially when surgery has transferred non-synergic muscles. A long time may be necessary before he will be able to produce a well coordinated movement.

A muscle previously impaired and only partially innervated cannot usually be used as a motor. Its force will generally remain below the functional level for this kind of reconstructive surgery.

All proceedings of anastomosis, approximation, implantation for each single case are to be found in specialized manuals.

REFERENCES

BATEMAN J.-E. (1962) *Trauma to Nerves in Limbs.* Philadelphia: W. B. Saunders Co.

BIESALSKI, K. & MAYER, L. (1916) *Die physiologische Sehnenverpflanzung.* Berlin: Springer.

BOYES, J.-H. (1960) Tendon transfers for radial palsy. *Bull. Hosp. Joint Dis.,* **21,** 97.

BRAND, P.-W. (1952) The reconstruction of the hand in leprosy. *Ann. roy. Coll. Surg. Engl.,* **11,** 350.

BRAND, P.-W. (1958) Paralytic claw-hand. With special reference to paralysis in leprosy and treatment by the sublimis transfer of Stiles and Bunnell. *J. Bone Jt Surg.,* **40-B,** 618.

BRAND, P.-W. (1961) Tendon grafting *J. Bone Jt Surg.,* **43-B,** 444.

BUNNELL, St. (1964) *Surgery of the Hand.* 4th edn. Revised by Boyes, J.-H. Philadelphia: J.-B. Lippincott, 1964.

BURKLE DE LA CAMP, H. & ROSTOCK P. (1956) *Handbuch der gesamten Unfallheilkunde.* I. u. 3. Band. Stuttgart: F. Enke.

CAMPBELL'S. (1963) *Operative Orthopaedics.* Saint-Louis: C.-V. Mosby C.

CLARKE, J.-M.-P. (1946) Reconstruction of biceps brachii by pectoral muscle transplantation. *Brit. J. Surg.,* **34,** 180.

CONVERSE, J.-M. (1964) *Reconstructive Plastic Surgery.* Vol. IV. Philadelphia: W.-B. Saunders.

DUCHENNE, G.-B. (1861) *De l'électrisation localisée et de son application à la pathologie et à la thérapeutique.* 2nd edn. Paris: J.-B. Baillière.

EDGERTON, M.-T. & BRAND, P.-W. (1965) Restoration of abduction and adduction to the unstable thumb in median and ulnar paralysis. *Plast. reconst. Surg.,* **36,** 150.

FOERSTER, O. (1930) Beiträge zum Wert fixierender Operationen bei Nervenkrankheiten. *Acta chir. scand.,* **67,** 251.

FOWLER, S.-B. (1949) Extensor apparatus of the digits. *J. Bone Jt Surg.,* **31-B,** 477.

FOWLER, S.-B. (1959) The management of tendon injuries. *J. Bone Jt Surg.,* **41-A,** 579.

JONES, R. (1908) On arthrodesis and tendon transplantation. *Brit. med. J.,* **1,** 728.

JONES, R. (1921) Tendon transplant in cases of musculospinal injuries not amenable to suture. *Am. J. Surg.,* **35,** 333.

LANGE, M. (1962) *Orthopädisch-chirurgische Operationslehre.* 2. Auflage. München: J.-F. Bergmann.

LITTLER, J.-W. & COOLEY. (1963) Opposition of the thumb and its restoration by abductor digiti quinti transfer. *J. Bone Jt Surg.,* **45-A,** 1389.

MERLE D'AUBIGNÉ, R. (1966) Technique et résultats de la réparation des plaies des nerfs médian et cubital. *Rev. chir. orthop.,* **52,** 578.

MERLE D'AUBIGNÉ, R. & DEBURGE, A. (1967) Traitement des paralysies du plexus brachial. *Rev. chir. orthop.,* **53,** 199.

MURPHY, J.-B. (1915) Infantile palsy of flexors of hand and fingers-tenoplasty. *Surg. Clin.,* **4,** 693.

NICOLADONI, C. Cited by SCHOLDER J.-C.

NIGST, H. (1955) *Die Chirurgie der peripheren Nerven.* Stuttgart: George Thieme.

PARÉ, A. (1664) *Œuvres du Conseiller et premier Chirugien du Roy. Des plaies des nerfs et parties nerveuses.* Lyon J. Grégoire 257.

PARKES, A. (1951) The treatment of established Volkmann's contracture by tendon transplantation. *J. Bone Jt Surg.,* **33-B,** 359.

PERIPHERAL NERVE INJURIES. (1954) *By the nerve injuries committee of the medical research council.* London: H.-J. Seddon.

PUTTI. Cited by SCHOLDER.

RANK, B.-K. WAKEFIELD, A.-R. & HUESTON, J.-T. (1968) *Surgery of Repair as Applied to Hand Injuries.* 3rd edn. Edinburgh: E. and S. Livingstone.

RIORDAN, D.-C. (1953) Tendon transplantations in median-nerve and ulnar-nerve paralysis. *J. Bone. Jt Surg.,* **3Ē-A,** 312.

RIORDAN, D.-C. (1959) Surgery of the paralytic hand. *Am. Academy of orthop. Surg.,* **XVI,** 79.

RIORDAN, D.-C. (1960) The hand in leprosy. A seven-year clinical study. *J. Bone Jt Surg.,* **42-A,** 661.

SCHERB, R. (1927) Uber die Gesetzmässigkeit der funktionellen Umstellung von Muskeln nach Transplantation ihrer Sehnen. *Z. orthop. Chir.,* **48,** 582.

SCHERB, R. (1934) Biologisches und Technisches zur Sehnen-transplantation. *Z. orthop. Chir.,* **61,** 303.

SCHERB, R. (1943) Uber den Ersatz poliomyelitisch gelähmter Daumenmuskeln durch Sehnentransplantation und über das Fehlen antagonistischer Bindungen an der oberen Extremität. *Schweiz. med. Wschr.,* **75,** 744.

SCHOLDER, J. C. (1948) Les séquelles musculaires de la poliomyélite et leur traitement orthopédique. *Rev. méd. Suisse Romande*, **68,** 2.

SEDDON, H.-J. (1956) Volkmann's contracture: treatment by excision of the infarct. *J. Bone Jt Surg.*, **38-B,** 152.

SEDDON, H.-J. (1960) L'ischémie de Volkmann une nouvelle étude de son traitement. *Rev. Orthop.*, **46,** 149.

SEDDON, H.-J. (1968) Progrès de la réparation les lésions nerveuses périphériques. *Triangle*, **8,** 252.

STAMPFLI, F. (1953) Uber Nervenverletzungen. *Z. Unfallmed. u. Berufskrh*, **46,** 228.

STEINDLER, A. (1918) Orthopedic operations of the hand. *JAMA*, **71,** 1288.

STEINDLER, A. (1939) Tendon transplantation in the upper extremity. *Amer. J. Surg.*, **44,** 260.

STEINDLER, A. (1954) Reconstruction of the poliomyelitic upper extremity. *Bull. Hosp. Joint Dis.*, IE, 21.

STILES, H.-M. & FORESTER-BROWN, M.-F. (1922) *Treatment of Injuries of Peripheral Spinal Nerves*. New York: Oxford Univ. Press.

TUBIANA, R. (1975) Ersatzoperationen bei irreparablen Nervenlähmungen. 13th annual assembly of the Austrian Society of Plastic Surgery, Vienna, 18 Nov.

VERDAN, Cl. (1969) Opérations palliatives dans les lésions nerveuses motrices irréversibles du membre supérieur *Zeitschrift für Unfallmedizin und Berufskrankheiten* **2,** 69.

WHITE, W.-L. (1960) Restoration of function and balance of the wrist and hand by tendon transfer. *Surg. Clin. N. Amer.*, **40,** 2, 427.

WITT, A.-N. (1953) *Sehnenverletzungen und Sehnen-/Muskel-Transplantationen*. Munich: J.-F. Bergmann.

WITT, A.-N. (1962) Die Wiederherstellungsoperationen bei irreversiblen Nervenlähmungen der oberen Extremität. *Langenbecks Arch. u. Dtsch. Zschr. Chirur.*, Bd. 301 u. 302.

ZANCOLLI, E.-A. (1957) Claw-hand caused by paralysis of the intrinsic muscles. *J. Bone and Jt Surg.*, **39-A,** 5, 1076.

ZRUBECKY, G. (1965) *Derzeitige Grenzen bei der planmässigen Versorgung schwerer Handverletzungen*. Hefte z. Unfallheilkunde, Heidelberg: Springer Verlag.

20. Tendon Involvement in Rheumatoid Arthritis

N. Gschwend

Rheumatoid arthritis is a systemic disorder of the mesenchyma, which leads to more or less typical changes in the most diverse parts of the body. The disease however is most prevalent in the synovial sheath of the joints, and is characterized by proliferative inflammation. We do not know the actual causes, but only know that we are dealing with a so-called autoimmune or autoaggressive disease, which can lead by an immunological vicious circle to polyarthritic destruction of the afflicted joints.

We are more familiar with the pathogenic mechanism which produces the various typical arthritic deformities. In joints it is mainly a 'pannus' which extends from the synovial sheath over the articular surfaces and destroys the cartilage and the bone beneath it. Softening of the cartilage, or chondromalacia, which is also frequent, is mainly attributed to the action of lysosomal enzymes.

The term 'rheumatoid arthritis' would suggest that the disease is limited to the joints alone. However the longer one devotes oneself to the surgical treatment of this disease, the more one realizes that the 50 per cent incidence ascribed by Ball and Kellgren to a simultaneous affliction of the tendons is not at all exaggerated. In fact, in many cases the tendons play the main part in the development of polyarthritic deformities. The Table 20.1, on which the number of various opera-

TABLE 20.1

Surgical procedures in RA (1962–1977):			3801
1. *Synovectomy in joints and tendon compartments*			1679
Joints upper extremity	1071 ⎫	1321	
lower extremity	250 ⎭		
Tendon compartments hand	318 ⎫		
foot	21 ⎭	339	
Bursae and Baker cyst		19	
2. *Reconstructive surgery*			1976
Arthroplasty, arthrodesis, joint resection, osteotomy, tendon reconstruction			
3. *Other*			146

tions in RA performed at our clinic are recorded, may give an idea on the frequency of tendon involvement.

We can distinguish between tendon involvement which:
1. primarily only affects the synovial sheath;
2. spreads from the synovial sheath to the tendon;
3. primarily affects the tendon itself;
4. spreads from the articular capsule to the tendon.

Tenosynovitis (Fig. 20.1) is the most frequent manifestation of rheumatoid disease of the tendon. Its occurrence, as would

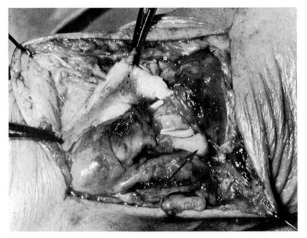

Figure 20.1
Tenosynovitis of the extensor tendons of the fingers. After freeing the posterior annular ligament one can see the thickened synovial membrane which appears to invade the tendons like a snail. Note the rheumatoid nodule in one of the tendons (arrow).

be supposed, is linked with the presence of a synovial sheath. This, in its turn is found in the region of tunnels, under retinacular ligaments, or where the tendon angles around a bony prominence. It is therefore understandable that the hand, with its numerous tendons surrounded by a tendon sheath would be the seat of most tenosynovitic affections. The foot is also more frequently affected by tenosynovitis than is supposed, but certainly less than the hand, although the distribution of tendons is anatomically similar in both. Whether this has to do with the smaller stress the foot tendons are subjected to, or with the incidence of multiple tumefactions being greater in the hand and fingers than in the foot joints, it is something we just do not know. The fact that haemiplegics only show signs of RA on the unparalysed side, or that the joints of the heavily utilized index and third fingers usually show more serious destruction than e.g. the joints of the ring finger, points to a clear connection between the incidence and severity of the disease and the degree of use of the joint. It should be mentioned incidentally that tenosynovitic changes are found in other parts of the body, for instance in the knee in the region of the pes anserinus, or in the shoulder joint in the tendon of the long head of the biceps.

The *diagnosis of rheumatoid tenosynovitis* is based on the identification of *swelling, pain, functional disorders* or *crepitations*. *Swelling* can be observed most frequently where the covering tissue is loose. This could be one of the reasons why tenosynovitis of the extensor compartment should be regarded

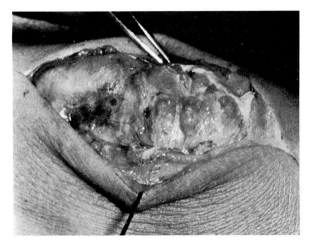

Figure 20.2
Multiple synovial hernias across the posterior annular ligament.

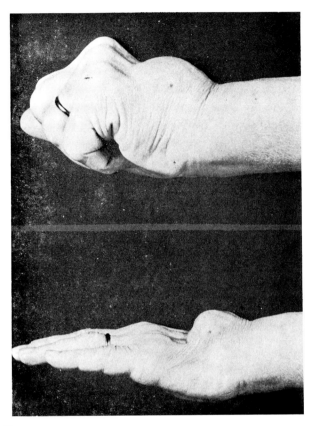

Figure 20.3
Soft and abnormally projecting swelling which does not follow the normal path of the extensor tendons.

as considerably more widespread than that of the flexor compartment. Whether this is really so, is hard to prove, since the very strong volar retinacular ligament and the palmar fascia prevent largely the appearance of inflammatory conditions in depth. One exception is tenosynovitis in the digital canal, which we shall look at in more detail later.

Swellings on the back of the hand are frequently observed; they can arise equally in the wrist which is often the seat of the first symptoms of rheumatoid arthritis, as they can in the extensor tendons. Synovitis of the wrist can be recognized by a diffuse swelling which follows the contours of the wrist joint, predominantly distal to the creaseline of the wrist, i.e. to the radio-carpal line. The fibrous articular capsule prevents a clearly defined swelling from protruding of the soft tissue, such as is characteristic in the case of tenosynovitis of the back of the hand, where we encounter a soft, elastic, more or less fusiform or botuliform thickening, which follows the natural course of the tendons and corresponds to the position and boundaries of the tendon sheaths. The dorsal retinacular ligament subdivides these deformities often into two protruberances, one distal, the other proximal, and lends an hourglass appearance to the whole. In advanced cases, the retinacular ligament is perforated by multiple synovial hernias (Fig. 20.2). In cases where the swelling feels soft, or is abnormally prominent, or its position does not correspond to the normal course of tendons, it is very likely that large fibrinous deposits are present, exactly as it occurs in the case of very active seropositive rheumatoid arthritis (Fig. 20.3 and 20.4). It is pointless trying to puncture such swellings with large needles, nor are cortisone injections of any use: operating is the only remedy. This helps us to understand why patients suffering from polyarthritic tenosynovitis frequently complain of *morning stiffness* of the fingers, which really cannot always be explained by joint involvement. This stiffness, especially the inability to close the fist is characteristic of tenosynovitis of the flexor compartment. As previously mentioned, swelling of the flexor side is not always easy to recognize because of the retinacular ligament and the palmar fascia, but they can occa-

sionally be seen as fusiform protuberances at the lateral borders of the palmar fascia, i.e. in the region of the tendon sheaths of the index and little fingers.

Tenosynovitis of the digital canal is much more frequent than is commonly supposed. We would look for this in cases where the patient is sometimes not able to close his fist actively, whereas it can be closed passively without difficulty. Even a cursory inspection will reveal a general volar protrusion, and

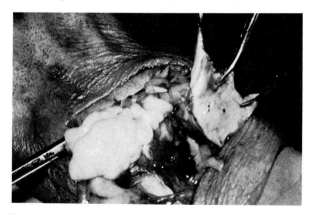

Figure 20.4
Same case as in Figure 20.3: important fibrous deposit protruding from the sheath of the extensor tendons.

palpation will reveal an elastic but firm swelling. In other words, Savill's 'pinch test' or 'fat finger' test is positive and it becomes impossible to lift a fold of the skin, as would be the case under normal conditions. The cause of swellings and functional disorders in these cases is often due to an actual tendinitis accompanying a synovitis. Both the superficial flexor tendon or the deep flexor tendon may be swollen to three to four times its normal size. The tendon is then surrounded by sheath tissue exhibiting all the typical inflammation signs of rheumatoid arthritis. The tendon itself is all the more invaded by this yellowish tissue, which separates the tendinous fibres, impregnates and finally replaces them. This distension of the flexor tendons together with the tenosynovitis which is always present in the digital canal, distal to the metacarpophalangeal joint, is enough to explain the functional disorders already described, i.e. inability to completely close the fist, since this enlarged tendon is incapable of slipping beneath the annular ligament, and is arrested half-way through. These pathological tendinous alterations are by no means uncommon, but seem to be not as frequent as tenosynovitic swellings on the proximal side of the annular ligament, i.e. between the distal fold of the palm and the digital flexor fold. The tumescence is more palpable than visible. Above all however, one can feel (and sometimes even hear) a *crepitation* of the flexor tendons in the inflammed isthmus of the annular ligament, from the hollow of the hand to the digital canal. If the stronger flexors are able to overcome the resistance created by this narrow passage, we have the perfect picture of a *trigger finger*, where extension is no longer actively possible, but only passively. This type of polyarthritic affection occurs in all the fingers, but rarely in the thumb. Diagnosis of less serious cases is more difficult, since actual snapping does not exist, because both flexors and extensors are able to overcome the resistance. In cases such as this, the patient complains of stiff fingers, or pains which can be localized in the hollow of the hand or in the metacarpophalangeal joints. On examination, a grating can be perceived when flexion and extension are repeated. Moreover, a nodular tumescence which is sensitive to pressure can be felt gliding to and fro. This corresponds to a thickening of the tendon situated proximal to the stenosis or even to an actual rheumatic nodule of the tendon, of which we shall speak later.

We should distinguish between this genuine trigger-finger and a blocking of the metacarpo-phalangeal joint, arising for instance from serious destruction of the head of the metacarpals. In such cases we may observe how the finger can be actively flexed, but not extended. This is because movement subluxates the proximal phalanx even further so that it gets caught on the edge of a cavity eroded into the head of the metacarpal and remains stuck in a flexed position. This 'pseudo-triggering' can be cured by simple pressure on the palmar side of the metacarpo-phalangeal joint. The subluxation is then reduced and the possibility of an articular blockade is prevented. In order to avoid disappointment during surgical treatment, it is always advisable to make such an examination before, and also to take an oblique X-ray view (Norgard's ball catching view) to show up any crater-like erosions on the palmar side of the metacarpo-phalangeal joint.

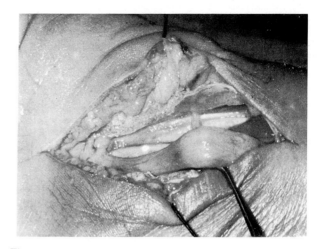

Figure 20.5
Compression of the median nerve in the carpal tunnel. Note the pseudo-neuroma above the compressed area.

Whereas tenosynovitis distal to the lumbrical canal is often associated with the phenomenon of the trigger-finger, more acute tenosynovitis of the digital flexors proximal to the lumbrical canal often shows up as the so-called 'carpal tunnel syndrome', i.e. as a compression of the median nerve (Fig. 20.5). Generally speaking, this is more widespread than is often supposed, and one should always look systematically for it in all rheumatoid arthritis patients. This is especially valid where patients complain of nocturnal paraesthesia or at daytime after manual work, or where thenar atrophy or perception disorders are present.

Even when an electromyogram does not supply absolute proof of median compression, i.e. when a negative EMG does not exclude the existence of a temporary compression of the median nerve, this form of examination should still be made as often as possible. We should also not forget that children often experience serious compression of the nerves without feeling hardly any pain. It is in just such instances that an electromyographic test should be made. Positive Tinel and Phalen tests, and infrequently a visible tumescence proximal to the transverse carpal ligament are further diagnostic indicators. Division of the more proximally situated and thinner lig. carpi volare will cause the median nerve to rise under pressure and we can see it floating on the surface of a gelatinous mass of the considerably swollen tendon sheath. It is only then that it retreats into the actual constriction of the carpal tunnel. Its concomitant vessels appear to be blocked right up at the beginning of the transverse carpal ligament, after which they suddenly look empty. Constrictions of the nerve with variations in calibre of up to 50 per cent are not unusual. This constriction of the nerve is especially visible one to two minutes after servering of the transverse carpal ligament, when the compressed section has a bluish-violet hue and appears infarcted. In cases where there is a 'pseudo-neuroma' proximal to the constriction, the variation in nerve thickness is even more impressive. To the touch, one has the impression that only a portion of the axons can pass through the constricted section of the nerve, or that a massive demyelination had taken place. It is always surprising to note how, even with highly compressed nerves, or with nerves reduced to less than half their normal calibre, the loss of motor activity and sensibility are relatively unimportant, and how especially paresthesia may recover rapidly. In long standing cases motor recovery is not to be expected and full sensory recovery may occur only after several months.

In surveying the above tenosynovitic phenomena, we are impressed with their multiplicity. On the other hand, the *therapeutic principles* in tenosynovitis are much more simple. In principle, surgical treatment should be considered when conservative treatment does not remove swelling and pain within a reasonable period of time, say half to one year.

We are thinking primarily of chrysotherapy as one possibility of basic treatment, but should bear in mind that a subsidence of any swelling under the influence of steroids, whether general or localized, should not be regarded as a cure. It might seem idle to remind one of the dangers of steroids, but one cannot emphasize enough that these are incapable of preventing the progressive destruction of joints and tendons by inflammatory synovitis. Anybody who has had occasion to observe these substances injected directly into the median nerve, where they remain for weeks, or in tendons with subsequent spontaneous rupture, will realize the significance of the axiom '*primum nil nocere*'. Local water soluble steroid injections are effective and justified once or twice with trigger fingers, but surgical treatment should be resorted to after the second or third recurrence of the syndrome. On the other hand, injections can hardly be justified when grotesque swellings would lead one to suspect the existence of large fibrinous masses or rheumatic nodules (Figs. 20.3 and 20.4). Any swelling that has been present for more than a year looks suspiciously like an inflammation, which has spread from the synovial sheath onto the tendon itself (Fig. 20.6).

A positive attitude towards surgical treatment of rheumatoid tenosynovitis can be regarded as justified so much more as:

1. timely treatment leads to a 90 per cent chance of success, the recurrence rate being minimal;

2. it is easier to perform in the earlier than the later stages;

3. in most cases local, i.e. regional or plexus anesthesia can be administered;

4. an ambulatory operation can be performed.

The aim of the operation is:

1. to remove the tissue causing the destruction of the tendon, i.e. synovectomy;

2. decompression of the tendons, with the elimination of pain and the return of normal movement;

3. this contributes in large measure towards preventing a spontaneous rupture of the tendons, which we shall come back to later.

Synovectomy is an important feature in the therapeutic treatment of rheumatoid arthritis, which is apparent from our own statistics (Table 20.1), of 3801 operations performed in RA patients between 1962 and 1977, 1679 were synovectomies, and of these 318 were connected with the tendons of the hand. With tenosynovitis of the *extensor compartment* we start with

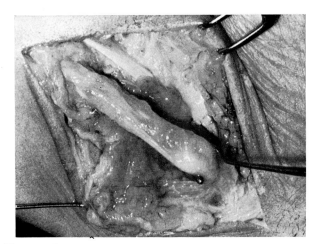

Figure 20.6
Tendon invaded by the inflamed synovial membrane from the sheath.

a straight incision along the third metacarpal and the radius, which gave us better results than the various curved incisions. The dorsal retinacular ligament is exposed, dissection to the ulnar and radial side is carried out without interfering wth the subcutaneous fat pad and sparing the longitudinally running veins. Both the radial and ulnar cutaneous nerve branches are brought into view. The retinacular ligament is severed at the ulnar border in such a way as to form a rectangular flap, opening one by one the different tendinous compartments (Fig. 20.7). Synovectomy of the tendons poses no problems where the tendon is intact, but can become impossible when synovial tissue has completely invaded the tendon (Fig. 20.8). The synovial tissue can often simply be peeled off. At the completion of the operation, the retinacular ligament should be slid underneath the tendons and resutured in its original place. We doubt that Savill was right in simply decompressing the tendon compartments, instead of performing a synovectomy, yet the decompression may be the most important therapeutic agent.

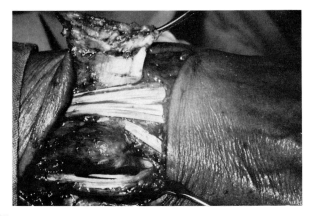

Figure 20.7
Synovectomy of the extensor tendons of the fingers after dissection of the posterior annular ligament. The characteristic tendon extensor proprius of the fifth finger passes in the immediate neighbourhood of the ulnar head which is covered by an inflamed synovial membrane invading a part of the tendon. Spontaneous ruptures occur frequently at this place.

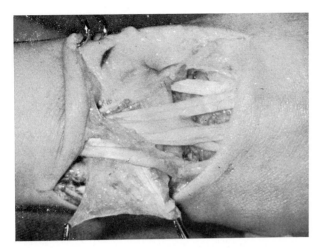

Figure 20.8
After synovectomy of the extensors, the annular ligament is passed below the extensor tendons and above the extensor carpi ulnaris.

We should mention in passing that when a synovitis of the wrist joint is also present, it is possible without much difficulty to proceed with a synovectomy of the radiocarpal and intercarpal joints by a simple rectangular incision of the capsule based distally. We shall return later, in the section dealing with spontaneous ruptures, to the simultaneous resection of an eroded ulnar head.

During postoperative treatment one should remember to get the finger moving the day after the operation. In this way, more or less normal mobility can be achieved within two to three weeks. Active dorsiflexion should be delayed until the wound has healed solidly in order to avoid skin necrosis and bow stringing of the tendons. Isometric finger extension exercises are started in the first postoperative days, the hand being held in neutral or slightly flexed position.

Synovectomy of the flexors follows essentially the same principles and is at the level of the wrist joint identical with an operation for the carpal tunnel syndrome. But contrary to usual operations of this kind, when rheumatoid arthritis is present, the incision should be extended to the forearm. The section of the volar and transverse carpal ligaments is made ulnar to the tendon of the palmaris longus, whose insertion is resected, which helps avoiding a continuous irritation of the scar. In order to perform an extensive synovectomy between the bellies of the digital flexor muscles and the lumbrical canal a wide exposure is necessary. It is not unusual to find the deep flexors stuck together by large adhesions. We do not believe there is any point in separating the deep tendons individually since the tendons themselves would become injured, a condition conducive to even further scar formation. At the termination of a synovectomy, it is always advisable to examine the bottom of the carpal tunnel for other possible causes of compression, such as a cystic protuberance of the radiocarpal joint, or prominent eroded carpal bones, which should be removed and covered with a soft tissue layer.

The operation of a *trigger finger* is identical with synovectomy, distal to the lumbrical canal, i.e. between the fold of the

hand and the annular ligament. We prefer a transverse incision of the distal fold of the palm to a longitudinal, digital one. We resect the tendon sheath amply and try as far as possible to spare the annular ligament, knowing the pathogenetic importance of the direction of pull of the flexor tendons in the creation of ulnar drift of the fingers.

If the pinch test is positive, we combine this operation with a check of the digital canal by making a zig-zag incision (Bruner). The synovectomy (Fig. 20.9a and b) is performed as completely as possible, whilst conserving the pulleys. Unfortunately it is precisely here that serious alterations of the tendon are frequently found, especially in the deep tendon itself, with fibrinoid necrotic tissues penetrating between the bundles of tendinous fibres, and thus partially destroying the tendon. In particularly serious cases a resection of the profundus tendon may be indicated, if this is too severely altered and where no normal gliding of both tendons simultaneously could be expected. The DIP joint has to be fused or stabilized in such a case by tenodesis. Where the sublimis tendon is mainly affected, the whole tendon or—better—just the ulnar slip can be resected.

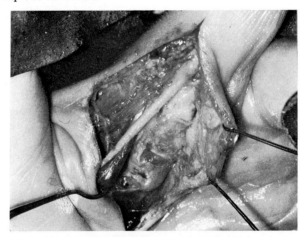

a

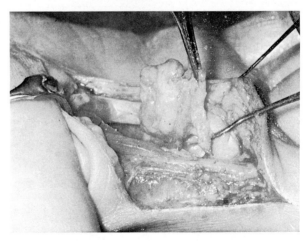

b

Figure 20.9
(a) Severe synovitis extending from the lumbrical canal to the index finger. The digital nerve and the lumbrical muscle are retracted.
(b) Synovectomy of the flexor tendons in the digital canal.

The histology of rheumatoid arthritis does not show any really specific pecularities. At most we could ascribe a certain specificity to rheumatoid granuloma. A central focus of fibrinoid necrosis is surrounded by palisade-like fibroblasts. Such *rheumatoid nodules* can be found in typical places under the skin, particularly on typical pressure joints such as the extensor aspect of the elbow, but they can also be found not infrequently in and on the tendons of the hand. Flatt saw no direct link between the incidence of subcutaneous and tendinous nodules. We found such nodules on the extensor tendons of the finger and on the flexor tendons (Figs. 20.10 and 20.11), where amongst other things they could be the cause of a trigger finger syndrome or of obstructed digital flexion. One patient had very palpable and painful rheumatic nodules on all eight deep tendons at the level of the proximal phalanx. On some of the tendons the nodule lay on the tendon and could easily be peeled off, whereas its neighbours were located right in the middle of the tendon in close connection with other necrotic fibrinoid tissue which penetrated the tendons for a greater part of their length. According to the different findings, surgical removal of tendinous granulomae can be simple or impossible. In advanced cases the only thing possible is a resection until at the healthy part, with an end to end suture, or tenoplasty. It is a rare case indeed, where the necrotic tissue lies in the centre of the long extensor tendon of the thumb, and can easily be scooped out following a longitudinal section of the tendon.

Surgical removal of rheumatic granulomae should be carried out as early as possible, and not when a *spontaneous rupture of tendon* shows up this pathological condition. These spontaneous ruptures occur much more frequently than is commonly supposed in rheumatoid arthritis. Because of the serious accompanying symptoms, and especially because they usually happen painlessly and during routine daily activities, they are often misinterpreted or not noticed. From a functional point of view most spontaneous ruptures of the tendons lead to serious consequences, which is why their early detection and treatment is of paramount importance. According to Page, it

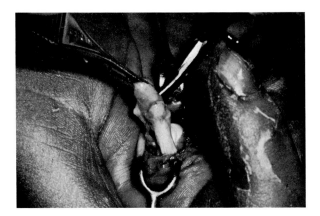

Figure 20.11
A very superficial rheumatoid nodule on the deep flexor tendon of the fifth finger, at the height of the basal phalanx.

is the extensor tendons of the fingers which are affected most frequently, in 90 per cent of all cases. However, it is to be supposed that ruptures of the flexor tendons are not so infrequent, but are more often overlooked as ruptures of the extensor tendons. In any case, and contrary to Page, who does not describe ruptures of the flexor tendons, we have found on five out of 15 operated tendon ruptures, a spontaneous rupture of the flexor pollicis longus.

The following should be considered as the causes of spontaneous ruptures:

1. Weakening of the tendon through:
   (a) infiltrating tenosynovitis; (Fig. 20.6); in advanced cases the tendon loses its white, shiny appearance and looks more like a nerve;
   (b) rheumatic granuloma (centre of fibrinoid necrosis) (Fig. 20.10);
2. Mechanical erosion:
   (a) through a roughened ulnar head (caput ulnae syndrome);
   (b) on the radial tuberosity;
   (c) on several roughened carpal bones (in the carpal tunnel);
   (d) under the retinaculum;
3. A combination of 1 and 2.

The significance of mechanical attrition of the digital extensor tendons has probably been overrated by Vaughan-Jackson, although it certainly does play a role. Moreover Ehrlich has discovered osseous particles in the tendinous tissue of ruptured extensor tendons of the finger. In most cases however there are several factors which lead up to a spontaneous rupture.

Surgical reconstruction of a tendinous rupture depends on its localization and the time it took place. The prognosis will be more favourable the less time has elapsed since the rupture, with little retraction of the proximal stump and the contractility of the muscle fibres being less affected. Moreover, adhesions in the gliding layers beyond the rupture, and defective positions of the joints due to changes in muscular balance may rapidly develop.

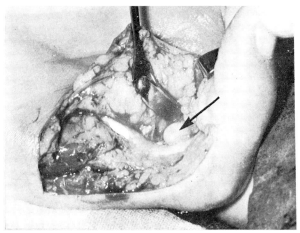

Figure 20.10
Rheumatoid nodule on the deep flexor tendon at the height of the distal palmar crease, giving rise to a permanently flexed finger.

The reconstruction of ruptured tendons is possible:

1. by direct tendon suture, so long as a short time only has elapsed since the rupture;

2. by the use of a tendon graft to bridge a more serious defect;

3. by transposing the distal stump to a tendon with a similar function, or having the same direction as a source of motor power.

Possible sources of energy could be:

1. For the long digital extensor tendon: the neighbouring extensor tendon, the extensor carpi ulnaris, the extensor carpi radialis, longus or brevis. The carpal extensors are by most authors not considered as being good sources of energy as they have a different range of excursion than the finger extensors. Moreover their function is too important as to be sacrificed so easily. The neighbouring extensor tendon should only be used if the angle between both tendons is only small as is the case for the third and fourth finger extensors, whereas the fifth finger extensors, if both are ruptured, should be activated by the extensor indicis proprius. The third or fourth sublimis tendon may be used where two or three finger extensor tendons have to be replaced simultaneously.

2. For the long extensor of the thumb the extensor indicis proprius or as proposed by Verdan, the extensor proprius of the fifth finger, which run a similar course to the ruptured tendon, are the tendons of choice.

3. For the digital flexors: one of the neighbouring flexors should be considered.

Many flexor tendon ruptures are never discovered, if they occur in the carpal tunnel, as the ruptured tendon may become stuck to a neighbouring flexor tendon. If both flexor tendons of a finger are ruptured, then the sublimis tendon of another finger (usually the fourth) may be used as a motor. In exceptional cases where a repair seems to offer little chances an arthrodesis of the PIP and DIP joint may be considered.

4. For the long thumb flexor: if the rupture occurs near the insertion on the terminal phalanx (very exceptionally), a Z-shaped lengthening of the tendon proximal to the carpal tunnel may allow for a re-insertion. Mostly the rupture occurs at eroded prominences of the scaphoid or trapezium. Here the defect can be bridged by a palmaris transplant. Where the thumb flexor is not expected to be working again, a sublimis transplant from the ring finger may be considered. Arthrodesis of the IP and MP joints is indicated when simultaneously severe deformities of these thumb joints exist and where the basal joint of the thumb (CM 1) functions normally.

The literature and also our own experience in this field show that good results can be obtained with all the methods we have described, provided of course the technique and post-operative treatment are good. Operations on tendon ruptures in arthrodesed wrists have shown that satisfactory results are not simply due to a tenodesis effect, but also to an active function of the tendon.

Next to the pathological tendon changes we have described, those where the *tendon* has been *damaged by the inflammed synovial tissue of a neighbouring joint* are also important. There is no place here for further description, but we must mention ulnar deviation of the fingers and the 'boutonnière deformity' as being the most important. At the level of the distal interphalangeal joint, the synovial invasion of the extensor tendons by the affected joint often leads to rupture and to the classic mallet finger.

To conclude this paper on tendon disorders of a polyarthritic nature, I should like to state that 'nothing is really unusual in this disastrous disease, except for those who don't know'.

REFERENCE

GSCHWEND, N. (1968) *Die operative Behandlung der progressiven chronischen Polyarthritis*. Stuttgart: Thieme. (See bibliography).

21. *Spontaneous Tendon Ruptures at the Wrist in Rheumatoid Arthritis*

D. Egloff C. Verdan

Tendon ruptures have been well known for a long time. They were usually attributed to tuberculous synovitis, a low grade form of tuberculosis characterized by granulomas and giant cells of Langhans (Verdan 1952). However there were no areas of caseous necrosis and the tuberculous bacillus was absent. Accordingly, it was thought that this synovitis may be due to a filterable form of the tuberculous bacillus. This idea is very close to the viral conception of rheumatoid arthritis (RA).

It was Vaughan-Jackson who, in 1948, drew attention to tendinous ruptures in RA. This author first described a rupture of the extensor communis of the ring and little fingers in two patients. Thereafter he made a systematic study of the problem.

Before him, in 1940, von Stapelmohr had observed and reported one single case of spontaneous rupture of RA origin in a series of 148 cases which concerned primarily post traumatic ruptures of the extensor pollicis longus.

Until 1955, publications were scarce (Table 21.1). With the five spontaneous ruptures which Laine and Vainio (1955) found while examining 1000 patients suffering from RA, the number of published cases was only 15. The following year. Straub and Wilson (1956) described for the first time some cases of flexor tendon ruptures. In 1959, by a very sophisticated and systematic study, Ehrlich *et al.*, made an original approach to the pathogenesis of these lesions.

Before them, Vaughan-Jackson (1948), Straub (1956) had recognized the importance of the attrition phenomenon in the aetiology of these ruptures. Ehrlich *et al.*, had not only noticed the part of the distal radio-ulnar joint, but the sequence of rupture of the extensor tendons as well.

We owe to Riddell (1963) a study of the results of tendon repair for rupture of the extensor pollicis longus of any cause. He compares two methods of tendon transfer: one of the extensor indicis proprius and one of the extensor carpi radialis brevis. He concludes that, for the repair of the extensor pollicis longus, the transfer of the extensor indicis proprius prevails over the transfer of the extensor carpi radialis brevis.

Moberg (1965) published 13 cases which concerned essentially rupture of flexor tendons, especially of the flexor pollicis longus. The results of surgical treatment show that

TABLE 21.1 Site of Ruptures (literature)

	Finger Ray	Von Stapelmohr 1940	Wadste in 1946	Vaughan-Jackson 1948	Harris 1951	Mathieu-Pierre Weil 1952	Laine et Vainio 1955	Straub et coll. 1956	Ehrlich et coll. 1959	Riddell	Moberg 1965	Mammerfelt et coll. 1969	Total	%	Verdan	%
Abductor longus	I							1					1	0.5		
Extensor brevis	I												0	0		
Extensor longus	I	1	1		5	1	3	1		7	1	20	40	20	4	14
Extensor proprius	II											2	2	1	2	7
Extensor communis	II								2			2	4	2		
Extensor communis	III							1	4		1	8	14	7	3	11
Extensor communis	IV			2			1	2	5		1	19	30	15	7	25
Extensor communis	V			2			1	2	7		1	20	33	17	6	21
Extensor proprius	V							5	6			21	32	15	3	11
Flexor longus	I										7	17	24	12	1	4
Flexor profundus	II							1			2	11	14	7	1	4
Flexor sublimis	III							1				3	4	2		
Flexor profundus	III											1	1	0.5	1	4
Flexor sublimis	III						1						1	0.5		
Flexor profundus	IV											1	1	0.5		
Flexor sublimis	IV												0	0		
Flexor profundus	V											1	1	0.5		
Flexor sublimis	V												0	0		
Total		1	1	4	5	1	6	14	24	7	13	126	202		28	

direct suture as well as graft are possible methods of repair, even in case of severe RA.

Mannerfelt and Norman (1969) published the largest series of tendon ruptures in 1969. Their 66 cases concerned 41 extensor tendons and 25 times flexor tendons. There were 126 tendons in toto. In the same year Nalebuff (1969) established accurate rules for treatment, taking into consideration the type and the number of ruptured tendons.

PATHOGENESIS

According to Vaughan-Jackson (1948), the cause of rupture of his two first cases was the wear and tear of the tendons over the inferior radio-ulnar joint which was itself altered by the rheumatoid disease. He introduced the word 'attrition' to designate this phenomenon. Although it may indeed be true that a single cause can produce a tendon rupture, in most instances several factors contribute to produce the rupture. The following aetiologies can be suggested:

1. attrition;
2. tenosynovitis;
3. tendinitis;
4. adjacent arthritis;
5. vascular impairment of the tendon;
6. local injection of corticoids;
7. physical therapy.

ATTRITION

This term, which has become classic, implies the wear and tear, the rubbing of the tendon when a bony spur is placed along its route. This aetiology is particularly important in some special regions. Backdahl (1963), when he described the caput ulnae syndrome showed the essential role played by the inferior radio-ulnar joint. The sequence of facts can be summarized as follows: the distal extremity of the ulna, site of the rheumatoid inflammatory process, is progressively destroyed, its surface loses its smooth contour and becomes rough. Bony spurs appear and erode the tendon. Furthermore, the joint is destroyed, especially the triangular cartilage. This enables the ulna to luxate dorsalwards. The wear and tear of the tendons is therefore accentuated.

The phenomenon of attrition exists for the flexor tendons as well. Mannerfelt and Norman (1969) have explored the floor of the carpal tunnel radiologically and during surgery. They have been able to determine that attrition was the main cause of rupture in 11 of their 25 cases. They effectively found that the carpal tunnel was perforated by bony spurs, the origin of which were near the articular surfaces between the navicular and trapezium bones. They named this site: 'critical corner'.

The chronological order of rupture is constant. It is the flexor pollicis longus which ruptures first, then the flexor profundus of the index, the sublimis of the index, the profundus of the middle finger, etc. The same type of scheme is found for the extensor tendons. Rupture of the extensor communis of the ring or little finger occurs first. This is followed by rupture of the extensor proprius of the little finger and the other finger extensors, progressing radialward. Therefore it is the tendons of the ulnar aspect which rupture first. It is the opposite for the flexor tendons. Of course the extensor pollicis longus has to be excluded from this rule, because it usually ruptures more distally than the other extensors, near Lister's tubercle.

TENOSYNOVITIS

Lipscomb (1965) has observed that rupture of flexor tendons occurred either in the carpal tunnel or in the digital canal. In these regions the tendons possess a synovial sheath. The same is true for the extensor tendons. The rupture for them occurs exclusively, if we except rupture of their insertions and at the musculo-tendinous junction, where they are surrounded by a synovial sheath. Inflammation of the synovium, tenosynovitis, interferes with tendon gliding, changes the direction of the tendons and favours the extension of the disease to the tendon itself. Backhouse (1971) has drawn special attention to the importance of tenosynovitis. According to this author, lubrication and tendon gliding are impaired. At the distal border of the extensor retinaculum, the tendon is compressed every time it moves. This pump-like mechanism contributes greatly to the alteration of the tendon which results in a rupture.

TENDINITIS

Ehrlich *et al.*, (1959) have studied microscopically the structure of ruptured tendons. They have always found intra-tendinous lesions in the form of a chronic, non-specific inflammation. For Kellgren and Ball (1950), the initial lesion is a fibrinoid necrosis of the collagenous fibres. The likelihood that a tendon can rupture solely because of purely tendinous lesions is, however, very rare. The importance of this factor is hence difficult to assess. The existence of intratendinous nodules had been well demonstrated by these latter authors. They are, however, more often the cause of trigger finger than tendon ruptures. Even so, they cannot be excluded as a possible aetiology of tendon rupture. According to Laine *et al.*, (1955) they are even an important aetiologic factor in the rupture of the extensor pollicis longus.

ADJACENT ARTHRITIS

The importance of the role of the articular synovitis for the finger deformities is well known. Without any specific tendon lesion, it can cause tendinous luxations and ruptures. This occurs when the joint synovium, the collateral ligaments, the lateral fibres of the extensor hood at the MP joint, have been destroyed by the inflammatory pannus. According to the joint involved, the result is an ulnar drift, a buttonhole deformity or a mallet finger.

At the wrist, the arthritis is often underestimated in favour of the attrition, tenosynovitis or intratendinous lesions. However the importance of joint synovitis is revealed by the chronology of the facts of Backdahl's caput ulnae syndrome (1963). Tissue changes caused by the synovitis are numerous. The local inflammation and hypertrophy of the synovium which accompanies it, are in the foreground. A synovitis of the inferior radio-ulnar joint can produce such a thickening of the joint capsule that it herniates at the dorsum of the wrist.

The extensor tendons, particularly the extensor proprius of the little finger and the extensors communis of the little and ring finger, are deflected from their normal course. They are driven radialward just at the distal extremity of the extensor retinaculum. They must go around the head of the ulna which is furthermore often luxated dorsally. They lean against its lateral aspect and it is only after they have passed it that the tendons can resume their course toward their respective insertions. Often there are no bony spurs, the thickening of the joint capsule even forms what could be called a protective pad, the tenosynovitis is virtually absent. The tendinous rupture can be accredited only to the joint synovitis.

VASCULAR IMPAIRMENT OF THE TENDONS

This is an interesting factor which is still not well documented. We know that during the initial phase of RA the inflammatory pannus appears particularly along the vascular tree. It is quite obvious with arthritis of the MP joint where the snail described by Moberg (1966), attacks the bony structures at the margins of the joint, location of the joint capsule insertions and entrance of the vessels. The same phenomenon is observed with the tendons where they are surrounded by a synovial sheath. The pannus grows along the vessels and the vincula. We have then to question whether these pathological tissues will impair not only the arterial blood supply and the venous return but also the lymphatic flow. Verdan and Setti (1972) have clearly shown the serious disorders of the lymphatic vessels in some pathological situations related to rheumatology and old age. However, till now vascular necrosis as a cause of rupture has been established for post-traumatic cases only (Trevor, 1950, Verdan, 1972). Ehrlich *et al.*, (1959) have not found any ischaemic infarct in ruptured tendons during their histological study. Until further investigations it is therefore difficult to consider this factor as an important cause of tendon rupture in RA.

LOCAL INJECTION OF CORTICOIDS

For Moberg (1965) local injection of corticoids can induce tendinous necrosis and be a cause of rupture. According to our operative findings we agree with this interpretation. We believe that one must be cautious with such a treatment.

PHYSIOTHERAPY

If we have included physiotherapy in the list of the possible causes of tendon rupture it is because we think it is wise to give a reminder of its adverse effects. We certainly do not intend to suppress physiotherapy in RA. On the contrary it is often very useful, especially to maintain joint movement and to prevent deformities. However, in cases of advanced disease, one must be very cautious. Otherwise, inappropriate passive movements could provoke ruptures of tendons already partially eroded and cause final deformity, which the patient will not easily forgive.

CLINICAL FACTS

Quite often, the tendinous rupture which appears during a rheumatoid disease is not recognized by the patient as a new feature of his illness. The joint stiffness, the pain and the joint deformations conceal the tendinous lesions from the physician himself. Therefore the injury to the tendinous integrity is often ignored and deformities attributed to purely articular lesions.

However the tendinous symptomatology can be very obvious. This is the case when a patient notices that he cannot extend a finger any more. The exact moment of rupture can sometimes be known if it is accompanied by pain.

On the contrary, we can find a much more insidious symptomatology as with the rupture of a sublimis flexor tendon, which will be manifest only by a weakness of grasp. The rupture of the extensor communis of the index or of the little finger, or of the flexor carpi radialis (Verdan (1976)) are easily missed as their function is taken respectively by the extensor proprius of the index or little finger, the flexor carpi ulnaris and the palmaris longus. With a seriously ill patient, the episode of a tendon rupture is often hidden by the daily symptomatology.

TREATMENT

In the surgery of the rheumatoid hand, the tendon repair is a grade of emergency which comes immediately after the syndrome of nerve compression. Ruptured tendons should be repaired as soon as possible. However, as we have just mentioned, these lesions are clinically not very obvious. They must be looked for by a meticulous and specific examination. Left untreated, the function of the whole hand will stiffen and the result of the tendon repair will be jeopardized. Other tendons will rupture if prophylactic operations are not performed when the repair of the already ruptured tendons is done.

A threat of rupture can be an indication for an operation. The essential operation is, of course, tenosynovectomy. Frequently, however, other operations are done as well. On the back of the wrist the extensor retinaculum is transposed under the tendons. It protects the tendons against an invasion of joint synovitis and assures their ability to glide between the retinaculum and the subcutaneous tissue. The removal of the distal extremity of the ulna belongs to the same group of prophylactic operations as does the removal of Lister's tubercle and the removal of bony spurs in the carpal tunnel. The methods of post-traumatic reconstructive surgery can only rarely be applied to RA. Direct suture is seldom possible as there is always an important gap caused by muscular retraction or more often, by alteration of the tendon at the site of rupture. The natural inclination is, of course, to use a graft. Although Moberg (1965) has shown that the results of this method are as good in RA as in post-traumatic cases, most of the surgeons avoid it. Effectively, a segment of a tendon, without blood supply, is placed in a diseased zone where a tenosynovectomy has just been performed, inevitably leaving behind a certain amount of altered and inflammatory tissue.

In most of the cases one of the following method is used:
1. side to side attachment to a neighbouring intact tendon;
2. tendon transfer;
3. arthrodesis of the impaired joint.

The possibilities for repairing the different tendons are the following:

For the extensor pollicis longus. The transfer of the extensor indicis proprius is actually the most commonly used method. It has many advantages: the operative technique is simple, the gliding amplitude of both tendons is approximately the same, and the angle of approach of the transferred tendon is very similar. However the weakening of the MP extension of the index which this method implies should not be neglected. It can be the cause of an important disability, particularly for a pianist or a surgeon. Furthermore, the extensor indicis proprius might be precious for other reasons. For instance, when the index presents an ulnar drift, its transfer to the radial aspect of the MP joint makes it an abductor which then counteracts the deviation. The decision to use the extensor indicis proprius to repair the extensor pollicis longus must therefore be carefully considered.

If there is any doubt, one can resort to a graft. This method requires the removal of Lister's tubercle and the creation of a pulley to avoid luxation of the graft.

An arthrodesis of the IP joint of the thumb can be useful.

After Michon, Harrisson (1972) has recently described a technique advising the repair of the extensor pollicis longus by the extensor pollicis brevis. This method would have the advantage over the transfer of the extensor indicis proprius, to give a direction of pull which would oppose the tendency of the rheumatoid thumb to become adducted.

Finally Verdan (1972) has shown that the use of the extensor proprius of the little finger is sometimes helpful.

For the extensor communis tendons. The most frequently used method is certainly the side to side attachment to an intact neighbouring tendon. It is, however, not always feasible, especially when the distal stump is too short or when the two tendons do not travel sufficiently in the same direction. This is the case for the extensor communis of the little finger, which can (when the extensor proprius of the little finger is ruptured as well) only with difficulty be anastomosed to its nearest neighbour, the one of the ring finger. It is far more preferable, then, to use the extensor indicis proprius. Severed on the dorsum of the MP joint, it is withdrawn through a little transverse incision at the wrist, rerouted and anastomosed to the distal stump either of the extensor communis or proprius of the little finger. If all the tendons are ruptured, one can resort to transferring a flexor superficialis tendon, most frequently the one of the ring finger which is brought on the dorsum of the hand through the interosseous membrane, according to a method described by Boyes for radial palsy. This method, although technically more difficult, has given us good results. Theoretically it is also possible to use either one of the extensor carpi radialis tendons or the extensor carpi ulnaris. However, it is an unsatisfactory method because it removes one of the prime mechanisms of movement of the wrist and furthermore their amplitude of gliding is too short to adequately replace an extensor communis tendon. Nevertheless, when there is stiffness of the carpus or if an arthrodesis has been performed, this last described method can be very useful.

For the flexor pollicis longus. The transfer of a flexor superficialis tendon is the method of choice. Beforehand, the bony spurs must be removed; an arthrodesis between the navicular

and the trapezium bone might even be necessary, though it is often preferable to perform a simple arthrodesis of the IP joint, especially when this joint is affected by the disease.

For the flexor tendons of the long fingers. If the profundus tendon is intact and the superficialis ruptured, the latter is removed when it impairs the function of the profundus tendon.

If it is only the flexor profundus which is ruptured, it can be repaired by anastomosing its distal stump to the intact superficialis. But if the amplitude of function of the proximal IP joint is satisfactory one can limit the repair to a tenodesis or an arthrodesis of the distal IP joint.

Finally, if both tendons are severed, the profundus can be repaired with the superficialis used as a graft, or a superficialis of a digit where both tendons are intact, can be transferred to the profundus.

CASE REPORTS

Our series includes nine patients. We have done 13 operations for tendinous ruptures at the wrist. The number of ruptured tendons was 28 and the number of repaired tendons 22. The difference is due to the fact that the extensor communis of the little finger, and the extensor proprius of the index or little finger were not repaired when the second tendon of these digits was intact and sufficient to ensure proper function (Figs. 21.1 and 21.2).

Methods of repair. The number of operations is inferior to the number of repaired tendons. Effectively, in two cases, the

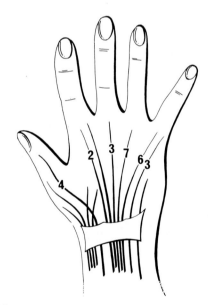

Figure 21.1
Location of extensor tendon ruptures

Extensor communis of the ring finger	: 7
Extensor communis of the little finger	: 6
Extensor pollicis longus	: 4
Extensor proprius of the little finger	: 3
Extensor communis of the middle finger	: 3
Extensor proprius of the index	: 2
Total:	25

TABLE 21.2   Methods of repair

Ruptures	Repairs
1. Extensor pollicis longus	Transfer of the extensor indicis proprius
2. Extensor pollicis longus	Transfer of the extensor indicis proprius
3. Extensor pollicis longus	Transfer of the extensor indicis proprius
4. Extensor pollicis longus	Transfer of the extensor indicis proprius
5. Extensor communis of the ring finger	Transfer of the extensor communis of the little finger
6. Extensor communis of the middle, ring and little fingers	Side by side anastomosis with the extensor communis of the index
7. Extensor communis of the ring finger	Side by side anastomosis with the extensor communis of the middle finger
Extensor communis and proprius of the little finger	Transfer of the extensor indicis proprius
8. Extensor communis of the ring finger	Side by side anastomosis with the extensor communis of the middle finger
Extensor communis and proprius of the little finger	Transfer of the extensor indicis proprius
9. Extensor communis of the ring and little fingers	Transfer of the extensor indicis proprius
Extensor proprius of the little finger	No repair
10. Extensor indicis proprius	No repair
Extensor communis of the middle finger	Side by side anastomosis with the extensor communis of the index
Extensor communis of the ring finger	Side by side anastomosis with the extensor proprius of the little finger
Extensor communis of the little finger	No repair
11. Extensor communis of the middle, ring and little fingers	Transfer of the flexor sublimis of the ring finger
12. Flexor pollicis longus	Transfer of the flexor sublimis of the ring finger
13. Flexor profundus of the index	Side by side anastomosis with the flexor sublimis of the index
Flexor profundus of the middle finger	Side by side anastomosis with the flexor sublimis of the middle finger

tendon used as a substitute, served for the repair of several tendons. The methods of repair are shown in Table 21.2.

We shall report briefly as examples two cases with illustrations. (Case 6 and 11 of Table 21.2).

CASE 6: HÉLÈNE S.

Seropositive RA beginning at age 59. Thermal cure during three weeks at age 68, two months before the first operation: synovectomy of the extensor tendons, transfer of the extensor communis of the little finger to the extensor communis of the ring finger for rupture at the right wrist. Four months later: drop of the middle and ring finger on the opposite side without any traumatic incident. A spontaneous rupture of the extensor communis of the middle and ring finger was diagnosed. At operation the lesions appeared more serious: there was an important synovitis of all the extensor tendons of the long fingers, the extensor communis of the index showed a partial rupture, the extensor indicis proprius was frayed and weak. The extensor communis of the three last fingers was ruptured. The extensor proprius of the little finger was intact although very thin (Fig. 21.3). For the repair, neither the extensor proprius of the index, frayed, nor the extensor proprius of the little finger, too weak, could be used. A graft could not be placed in such a diseased region. Because of lack of time (venous regional anaesthesia) the transfer of a superficialis tendon was impossible. We therefore resorted to a side by side anastomosis of the distal stump of the extensor communis of the three last fingers to the extensor communis of the index. In fact, the distal stump of the little finger was anastomosed with the one of the ring finger, then this unique stump with the one of the middle finger, and finally, the whole was attached laterally to the extensor communis of the index (Fig. 21.4). Approxi-

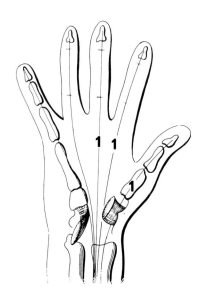

Figure 21.2
Location of flexor tendon ruptures

Flexor pollicis longus	: 1
Flexor profundus of the index	: 1
Flexor profundus of the middle finger	: 1
	Total: 3

mately five years later the SR is 18/44, and the Latex test is positive. We do not observe any tenosynovitis. There is no new tendon rupture. The active extension exists for all fingers, only the ring and little fingers present a small deficiency of extension, of 10 and 20 degrees respectively. On the other side, where the extensor communis of the little finger has been transferred to the extensor communis of the ring finger, active extension

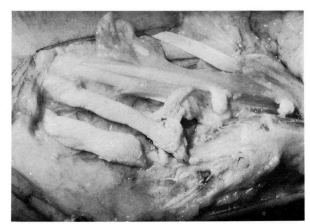

Figure 21.3
Case 6: important synovitis, fraying of the extensor indicis proprius, distal stumps of the ruptured tendons of the extensor communis of the middle and ring fingers.

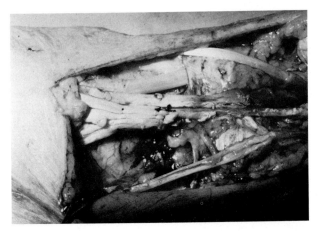

Figure 21.4
Case 6: after synovectomy and tendinous repair. Distal stumps of the extensor communis of the middle, ring and little fingers anastomosed to the extensor communis of the index.

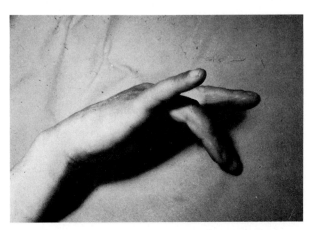

Fugure 21.5
Case 11: preoperative: drop of the middle and ring fingers.

is also possible. There is a deficiency of extension. It is, however, not due to RA but to an associated Dupuytren's disease. The patient is satisfied with the results of the operation mainly because of the improvement of the function.

CASE 11: STEPHAN A

Seronegative RA. Patient operated on at age 34 for a ganglion on the back of the right wrist. Three months later the patient was sent to our clinic because he could not stretch either the middle finger, or the ring finger. (Fig. 21.5). In fact he presents a synovitis of the extensor tendons at both wrists, diagnosis which was confirmed at operation on the right side. It revealed that the extensor communis of the middle and ring fingers were effectively ruptured. However the extensor cummunis of the little finger was also ruptured and the extensor proprius of the index, badly frayed. The extensor proprius of the little finger and the extensor communis of the index were intact. For the repair, the important gap between the proximal and the distal stumps did not allow a side by side anastomosis (Fig. 21.6). We had therefore to resort to a new motor force. The use of one of the extensor carpi radialis was not suitable, because of its inadequate gliding amplitude and because its removal would cause the weakening of the wrist movement, furthermore, it would have had to be prolonged by a graft to reach the distal stumps. A superficialis tendon was therefore used. It was brought on to the dorsum of the hand through interosseous aponeurosis of the forearm and anastomosed to the distal stumps of the extensor tendons of the middle and ring fingers (Fig. 21.7). Three months later a synovectomy of the extensor tendons was performed on the opposite side. There was no tendon rupture. Ten years later the active extension exists for all digits. There is a small deficiency of extension of the middle finger (Fig. 21.8). The disease is not very active (SR 9/22). Latex test negative. However, examination reveals a rupture of the insertion of the profundus tendon of the right index.

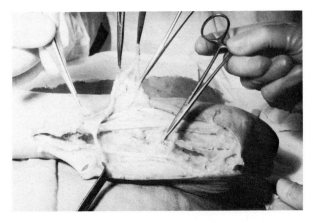

Figure 21.6
Case 11: operation: proximal and distal stumps of the ruptured tendons of the extensor communis of the middle and ring fingers. Notice the important gap.

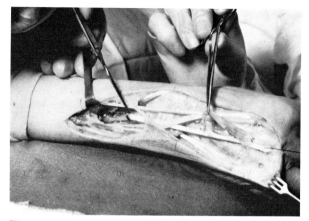

Figure 21.7
Case 11: tendinous repair: the flexor superficialis of the ring finger has been brought on the dorsum of the hand through an opening in the interosseous aponeurosis of the forearm. It will be anastomosed to the distal stumps of the extensor communis of the middle and ring fingers.

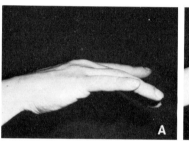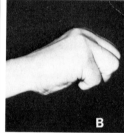

Figure 21.8
Case 11: 10 years after operation. Slight deficiency of extension of the middle finger.

COMMENTS AND ESTIMATION OF OUR RESULTS

Tendon rupture is a frequent lesion. We found it among nine patients of a group of 77 suffering from RA who have been operated on in our clinic during the last 10 years. Our group is, of course, peculiar as it includes only patients who have undergone surgery. However this frequency superior of 10 per cent is in sharp contrast with the statistics Laine and Vainio (1955) published in 1955. It reported only five cases of spontaneous tendon rupture among 1000 patients suffering from RA. Ruptures occur after a long evolution (our average 18 years). It certainly proves the frequent necessity for multiple pathogenesis. We have, however, observed a case of rupture of extensor communis tendons after a very short disease (1 year). This case is number 11 reported in detail. The trauma of the first operation for a ganglion might have accelerated the evolution toward a rupture. Because of lack of accurate information we have not been able to exclude an iatrogenous lesion, which therefore remains another possible explanation. It might have been also a wrong diagnosis of a 'ganglion', instead of a beginning tenosynovitis, which is not rare at all.

As shown in Tables 21.1 and 21.2, ruptures of extensor tendons occur more often than ruptures of flexor tendons. This is true even if we take into consideration the fact that ruptures of superficialis tendons can very well remain undiagnosed. We have encountered incidentally, two ruptures of superficialis tendons during operations for carpal tunnel syndromes. As for the relative frequency among the different extensor tendons our statistics are very close to those of other authors. These are the rupture of the extensor communis of the ring and little finger which is most frequent on the ulnar side and the one of the extensor pollicis longus on the radial side. As for the flexor tendons, our rare cases do not permit of any valuable conclusions in this regard. It might be interesting to notice that we have not observed any rupture either of the extensor carpi ulnaris or radialis, or of the flexor carpi ulnaris or radialis. For the latter, one of us (Verdan 1976) has observed fraying of the tendon on several occasions and a ruptured tendon once. They were, however, not RA cases but had been caused by common arthritis of the joint between the navicular and the trapezium bones.

The estimation of the result by the patients themselves is interesting to know. For the 13 operations, 10 of the patients have considered the results to be positive, two to be indifferent and one to be negative. For this unique failure, the case of a transfer of the extensor indicis proprius for rupture of the extensor pollicis longus, the initial operation had required a secondary correction for tenolysis and shortening of the transferred tendon. Later in the course of the disease a rupture of the flexor longus of the same thumb occurred. It was repaired by transfer of the superficialis tendon of the ring finger. The estimation of the result was therefore more difficult to assess than is usual. However, we ourselves considered this case, as well as one of the cases rated as indifferent by the patient, as a failure. In that case, the transfer of the extensor indicis proprius for a rupture of the extensor pollicis longus had resulted in hyperextension and an important lateral deviation of the distal phalanx. A synovitis of the IP joint was present and was responsible for the failure of the tendinous repair. Taking into consideration the articular mobility, the useful function and the complications, we have rated the other results as good (7) or satisfactory (4). Roughly, the average of the amplitude of active function of the concerned joint was 60 degrees.

Two facts emerge from our observations:

1. The adjustment of the tension of the transferred tendon: this is a phase which is even more delicate in the rheumatoid situation than in the post-traumatic cases. In five cases the tension was found to be insufficient. It is interesting to notice that it always concerned a tendinous transfer, particularly of the extensor indicis proprius and not a side by side anastomosis. The poor conditions of the distal stump, even if macroscopically invisible are possibly the cause of the secondary loosening.

2. It appeared to us that the use of the extensor indicis proprius is not without risks. In four cases out of seven we found a deficiency or weakening of the extension of the index tested against resistance. It can therefore be harmful to remove one of the extensor tendons of the index. We must admit, however, that it has sometimes been difficult to decide whether this deficiency was due to the removal of a tendon, or to the rheumatoid disease itself.

CONCLUSION

Tendon ruptures in rheumatoid disease are not exceptional. The functional impairment it causes is serious as it often occurs when other rheumatoid lesions are already present. They must therefore be looked for systematically so that the diagnosis can be made as early as possible. Appropriate surgical treatment allows not only the repair of the rupture, but the prevention of other ruptures too.

REFERENCES

BACKDAHL, M. (1963) The caput ulnae syndrome in rheumatoid arthritis. A study of the morphology, abnormal anatomy and clinical picture. *Acta rheum. (Amst.)*, **5**, Suppl. 1–75.

BACKHOUSE, K. M., APRIL, G.-L. KAY, COOMES, E.-N., & KATES, A. (1971) Tendon involvement in the rheumatoid hand. *Ann. rheum. Dis.* **30**, 236–242.

DUPLAY, J. (1876) Rupture sous-cutanée du tendon du long extenseur du pouce de la main droite, au niveau de la tabatière anatomique. *Bull. Soc. Chirurgiens, Paris*, **2**, 788.

EHRLICH, G.-E., PETERSON, L.-T., SOKOLOFF, I., & BUNIM, J.-J. (1959) Pathogenesis of rupture of extensor tendons at the wrist in rheumatoid arthritis. *Arthr. and Rheum.*, **2**, 332–346.

HARRIS, R. (1951) Spontaneous rupture of the tendon extensor pollicis longus as a complication of rheumatoid arthritis. *Ann. rheum. Dis.*, **10**, 298–306.

HARRISON, S., SWANNEL, A.-J., & ANSELL, B.-M. (1972) Repair of extensor pollicis longus using extensor pollicis brevis in rheumatoid arthritis. *Ann. rheum. Dis.*, **31**, 490–492.

KELLGREN, J.-H., & BALL, J. (1950) Tendon lesions in rheumatoid arthritis. A clinico-pathological study. *Ann. rheum. Dis.*, **9**, 48–65.

LAINE, V.-A.-I., & VAINIO, K. (1955) Spontaneous ruptures of tendons in rheumatoid arthritis. *Acta orthop. scand.*, **24**, 250–257.

LIPSCOMB, P.-R. (1965) Surgery of the arthritic hand. *Mayo Clin. Proc.*, **40**, 132–164.

MANNERFELT, L., & NORMAN, O. (1969) Attrition ruptures of flexor tendons in rheumatoid arthritis caused by bony spurs in the carpal tunnel. *J. Bone Jt Surg.*, **51-B**, 270–277.

MATHIEU-PIERRE-WEIL & CARRET, L. (1952) Rupture spontanée du tendon long extenseur du pouce d'origine rhumatismale. *Rev. Rhum.*, **7**, 626–628.

MOBERG, E. (1965) Tendon grafting and tendon suture in rheumatoid arthritis. *Amer. J. Surg.*, **109**, 375–376.

MOBERG, E., WASSEN, E., KJELLBERG, S.-R., ZETTERGREN, L., SCHELLER, S. & ASCHAN W. (1966) The early pathologic changes in rheumatoid arthritis. *Act chir. scand.*, **357**, suppl. 142–147.

NALEBUFF, E.-A. (1969) Surgical treatment of tendon rupture in the rheumatoid hand. *Surg. Clin. N. Amer.*, **49**, 811–822.

RIDDELL, D.-M. (1963) Spontaneous rupture of the extensor pollicis longus. *J. Bone Jt Surg.*, **45-B**, 506–510.

VON STAPELMOHR, Sten. (1940) Sur les ruptures tardives du tendon du long extenseur du pouce consécutives aux traumatismes du poignet. *J. int. Chir.*, 5, 163.

VON STAPELMOHR, Sten. (1942) Uber « hohe spät Rupturen » der Sehne des extensor pollicis longus. *Acta chir. scand.*, **86**, 110–128.

STRAUB, L.-R. & WILSON, E.-H. (1956) Spontaneous rupture of extensor tendons in the hand associated with rheumatoid arthritis. *J. Bone Jt Surg.*, **38-A**, 1208–1217.

TREVOR, D. (1950) Rupture of the extensor pollicis longus tendon after Colles's fracture. *J. Bone Jt Surg.*, **32-B**, 370–375.

VAUGHAN-JACKSON, O.-J. (1948) Rupture of extensor tendons by attrition of the inferior radio-ulnar joint: report of 2 cases. *J. Bone Jt Surg.*, **30-B**, 528–530.

VAUGHAN-JACKSON, O.-J. (1959) Attrition ruptures of tendons as a factor in the production of deformities in the rheumatoid hand. *Proc. roy. Soc. Med.*, **52**, 132–134.

VERDAN, Cl. (1952) *Chirurgie réparatrice et fonctionnelle des tendons de la main*. Paris: Expansion Scientifique Française.

VERDAN, Cl. (1972) *Die Eingriffe an Muskeln, Sehnen und Sehnenscheiden. Allgemeine und spezielle Chirurgische Operationslehre*, Wachsmuth W. & Wilhelm A. Berlin: Springer Verlag.

VERDAN, Cl. & SETTI, G.-C. (1972) A study of the lymphatic circulation in flexor tendons. *Proceedings of the 12th Congress of the SICOT. Tel-Aviv, October 9–12–1972*. Amsterdam: Excerpta Medica.

VERDAN, Cl. (1976) Tenosynovitis of the flexor carpi radialis. *Proceedings VIth Congress (1975) of the IPRS, Paris*.

WADSTEIN, T. (1946) Spontaneous rupture of the tendon of the extensor pollicis longus. Transplantation of the extensor indicis proprius. *Acta orthop. scand.*, **12**, 194–202.

22. Trigger Fingers

C. Verdan

Surprisingly enough, not all doctors or even all surgeons are aware of this common affliction; a colleague recently concluded that a sesamoid in the area of the interphalangeal articulation of the thumb was a cause for blocking.

Before the finger blocks, there is often pain on the volar surface of the metacarpophalangeal joint of the thumb, or in the palm just above the level of the proximal pulley of the other four fingers. The functional difficulties increase until finally the distal phalanx of the thumb remains blocked in flexion (Fig. 22.1). Or, for a long finger, active flexion of the middle and distal phalanges seems to stop at a certain angle and the patient, increasing his effort to close his fist, locks the finger in flexion. It remains in the position shown in Fig. 22.2. To extend the finger again, either a great effort of active extension, or, more often, passive extension, provokes a 'click' with a spring effect that can be quite painful.

Note that only active flexion can produce the blocking, whereas active or passive extension can relieve it.

The thumb is the most often affected, followed by the long and ring fingers (Fig. 22.2). It commonly occurs in the morning upon waking and decreases or even disappears during the day. It is the result of stenosis of the fibrous ring of the basal pulley that thereby constricts the flexors.

In the *thumb* this occurs in the inextensible zone of the sesamoid sling, producing a tendinous nodule distally. This nodule follows the movements of the tendon and is the source of the blockage. Usually this small tendinous nodule is felt to disappear after surgical liberation.

In the *fingers*, this retraction of the fibrous ring (i.e. the first pulley) constricts the two tendons where profundus perforates superficialis. Often a local exudate is produced in the small synovial sac which can be compared with a preputial organ (Fig. 22.3).

In alternating flexion-extension movements the examiner can feel in the patient's palm the gliding of a fusiform nodule passing through the fibrous ring and remaining blocked in the palm; straightening of the finger is then impossible. Several fingers may be affected simultaneously or successively, especially in diabetics.

We must underline the fact that these trigger fingers are not of the same origin as those caused by granulomatous nodules in the synovial sheath, frequent in rheumatoid arthritis (cf. Gschwend; also Egloff and Verdan).

In the *thumb*, this syndrome also occurs in infants and young children, but the distal phalanx is totally blocked in flexion (rarely also in extension); these cases must not be confused with congenital camptodactyly, because if they are not operated upon the skeletal growth will be abnormal and the late correction of the thumb necessarily incomplete. This is a congenital stenosis of the fibrous ring of the proximal pulley.

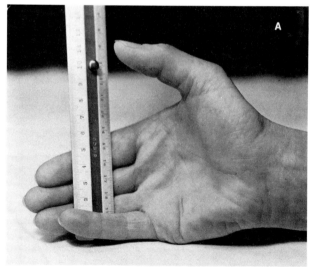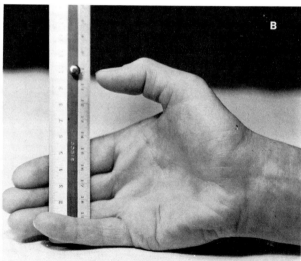

Figure 22.1
'Trigger thumb'; woman aged 43, working in a precious stones factory. Trauma (?) six months prior. Persistent pain, then locking. (A) Active flexion of the distal phalanx is stopped.

(B) Suddenly the distal phalanx flexes completely (with pain) and remains locked in this position.

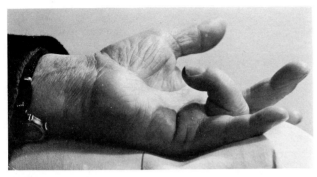

Figure 22.2
'Trigger finger', left ring finger; housewife aged 67. Slowly developing pain on palmar surface of the MP joint. Suddenly episodes of locking in flexion.

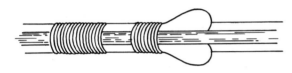

Figure 22.3
Sketch of the synovial tunnel, a kind of preputial organ on the upper extremity of the digital sheath of the middle three fingers. The short fibrous ring (the first pulley), which is inserted on the metacarpophalangeal volar plate, must be excised during the operation for a trigger finger.

REFERENCES

For references see Chapter 23.

TREATMENT

In the early stages, endosynovial injections of corticoids can alleviate or cure this syndrome; once it is well established, however, it is best to operate. Operations on the tendons themselves are to be avoided. Excision of the basal fibrous ring succeeds in freeing the tendinous nodule such that it no longer catches during movements. It has been suggested that the centre of the tendon be excised (or even a centrally located calcification observed sometimes in the flexor pollicis longus) but this trauma to the endotendon can only weaken it or cause reactionary oedema that complicates the situation.

Surgical incisions will be placed:

1. for the *thumb*: in the metacarpophalangeal flexion crease, care being taken not to damage the collateral nerves and arteries. As for de Quervain's stenosing tenosynovitis, it is best to inject local anaesthesia in the subcutaneous tissue such that the skin is lifted and the pedicles protected;

2. for the *four fingers*: the incisions are slightly different for each finger. They must permit direct access to the small basal pulley, taking into account the creases of the skin.

   (a) For the *middle finger* one can use the last few centimetres, of the distal palmar crease, directed obliquely towards the second web space.

   (b) For the *ring* and *little fingers* the incision is parallel to the distal palmar crease, placed a few millimetres distally.

   (c) For the *index* an oblique incision along existing creases is best; the operation is only rarely needed for this finger.

23. De Quervain's Stenosing Tenosynovitis

C. Verdan

In 1895 de Quervain described a painful affliction of the radial styloid process 'tenosynovitis stenosans fibrosa'. More common in women, it limits the thumb's movement and provokes pain radiating to the thumb and the forearm with the slightest effort (especially torsion).

According to de Quervain (1895 and 1921): 'The lesion consists of a shrinkage of the osteofibrous groove containing the common sheath of abductor pollicis longus and extensor pollicis brevis. Objective symptoms are pain when pressure is applied locally and a thickening of the fibrous pulley. Exposure under local anaesthesia shows the tendons caught in their

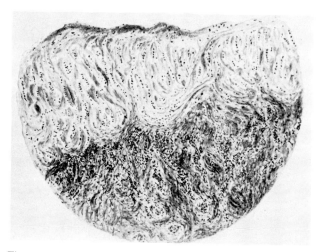

Figure 23.1
Fibro-cartilage nodules filling the upper half of the section under the mesothelium.

synovial sheath by the pressure of the shrunken ring. Slitting the latter liberates the tendons and relieves the pain. Histological examination shows fibrous thickening of the wall in long-standing cases and a slight globocellular infiltration in early ones.'

Without considering aetiology, stenosing tenosynovitis can afflict patients with rheumatoid arthritis as well as those never having shown signs of any such illness. Frequently it is associated with other degenerative connective tissue alterations (Lipscomb 1965) such as 'trigger-finger', rhizomyelic arthrosis of the thumb, carpal tunnel syndrome, Heberden or Bouchard nodules, scapulo-humeral periarthritis, etc. However, it also does afflict young adults with no other 'rheumatismal' illnesses.

The histological alterations of the fibrous ring have been described by von Albertini. In the sheath's wall, underneath the mesothelium are transverse fibrocartilage nodules. They form a constrictive zone that is characteristic of the late stage of this affliction (Fig. 23.1).

Clinically this thickening is often visible as a longitudinal spindle and can be felt as a very hard cuff on the radial styloid process which is painful on pressure and percussion.

'Inflammation of the styloid process' of acrostealgic origin similar to lateral epicondylitis of the elbow (tennis elbow) has been diagnosed; I personally have never seen a case that was not, in reality, de Quervain's stenosing tenosynovitis.

Active extension-abduction and forced passive flexion of the thumb ray with the wrist in ulnar abduction are particularly painful. Note however that there is no question of 'trigger-finger' as it has sometimes been described.

TREATMENT

Early or mild cases can be relieved or cured by local injections of corticoids, but long-standing ones should always be operated. Seen during the operation, the newly formed fibrous tissue is very hard and upon section is white and cartilaginous. The underlying tendons are compressed by this ring and to compensate are wider above and below the groove. Obviously, this wider part is caught in the stenosis during the slightest movement.

SURGICAL TECHNIQUE

The primary risk is damage to the cutaneous sensitive branches of the radial nerve which are numerous at this level. The small, very painful neuromas that may result can be more troublesome than the tenosynovitis.

A longitudinal or oblique incision crossing the creases of the skin is contraindicated; it will widen and often becomes keloid. A transversal incision in the creases almost completely disappears, especially when placed on the radiopalmar side of the wrist. The aesthetic result is excellent. To be sure that the incision is safe, the subcutaneous tissues should be well infiltrated with local anaesthetic so as to raise the skin up and away from the nerves. When using narcosis, regional venous anaesthesia, or axillary blocks, an infiltration of physiological solution should be used to lift up the skin.

The incision should be placed slightly distal to the radial styloid process such that lifting the upper edge of the wound exposes the thickened ring. The ring is then sectioned longitudinally along one of its insertions; the sheath is thus opened over 1½ to 2 cm and its roof lifted and excised along the other insertion. I believe this is preferable to a simple incision which leaves two mobile flaps that can be the source of further fibrosis.

Now, using a tendon hook, one must verify which tendons are in the sheath. Normally there should be two tendons, the abductor pollicis longus and extensor pollicis brevis, but this is only rarely the case.

Often there are one, or many, aberrant tendons that are in fact multiple bundles of abductor pollicis longus or extra tendons whose insertions vary; sometimes even the abductor pollicis brevis has become digastric.

Extensor pollicis brevis (tested by its function of extending the proximal phalanx on the metacarpal) can be in a separate sheath located dorsal to the first. It also must be liberated by excision of the roof since pain can also arise at this level. The fibrous ridge separating the grooves can also be removed.

Putting the tendons back again is followed by single plane suture of the skin using mattress sutures. The hand and thumb are immobilized, in a slightly compressive bandage and an aluminium splint, for five to six days. This can be replaced the second week by a lighter bandage before removal of the sutures.

Complete cure is nearly always the result, with light work possible two weeks, and heavy work one month after the operation.

REFERENCES

ALBERTINI, A. Von. Spezielle Pathologie der Sehnen, Sehnenscheiden und Schleimbeutel. In *Handbuch der Speziellen Patholigischen Anatomie und Histologie.* vol. 9, p. 508, Henke-Lubarsch.

DE QUERVAIN, F. (1895) Uber eine Form von chronischer Tendovaginitis. *Korresp.—Bl. schweiz. Arz.,* **25,** 389.

DE QUERVAIN, F. (1921) Tendovaginitis Stenosans fibrosa. *Münch. med. Wschr.,* **5.**

LIPSCOMB, P.-R. (1965) Surgery of the arthritic hand, St. Bunnell memorial lecture. *Mayo Clin. Proc.,* **40,** 137–164.

VERDAN, Cl. (1952) *Chirurgie réparatrice et fonctionnelle des tendons de la main.* Paris: Expansion Scientifique.

WINTERSTEIN, O. (1930) Uber Sehnenscheiden Stenosen. *Ergebn. Chir. Orthop.,* **23,** 151.

REHABILITATION

24. Rehabilitation after Tendon Injuries to the Hand

C. B. Wynn Parry

In this chapter the management of the hand after surgery for tendon lesions is described in detail. The conventional division of flexor tendon lesions into those at the wrist and those in 'No-man's land' or as Verdan has wittily described it, 'chasse gardée', has been adopted, and lesions of the extensor tendons divided into those at the wrist and over the dorsum of the hand, and those in the finger. The author's experience extends over some 20 years at the Services' rehabilitation centres. These centres offer a full day's programme of rehabilitation on a residential basis. The majority of patients are recovering from fractures, dislocations or orthopaedic operations or with neurological and rheumatological disorders. Injuries to the hand are common and of the 350 patients at the two centres, there are rarely less than 25 with hand disabilities. The centres have generous space for gymnasia where class exercises and games are carried out under the supervision of highly specialized remedial gymnasts, a large open physiotherapy department, a hydrotherapy pool, occupational therapy with a full range of light, heavy and engineering workshops, for restoration of function, work assessment and retraining when necessary. Patients can be transferred from hospital at an early stage after surgery and are under the close supervision of a team of surgeons, specialists in physical medicine and remedial therapists.

Under full time, rehabilitation patients regain a higher standard of recovery more quickly than if only treated for a short period daily, or denied any form of planned rehabilitation (Wynn Parry, 1966).

LESIONS AT THE WRIST

Simple lesions of the tendons at the wrist present no problems and normally do not require formal rehabilitation.

If all flexor tendons have been cut, most surgeons excise the sublimis and suture only the profundus to avoid adherence of tendons to each other or to the skin, causing a flexion deformity at the proximal interphalangeal joints.

After multiple tendon suture mobilization is usually allowed three weeks after surgery and some 10 days of active exercises under the supervision of a physiotherapist is all that is required. Severe lacerating wounds at the wrist, involving all tendons and nerves, often result in adherence of the tendons to each other and to the skin. In these circumstances, intensive rehabilitation is essential if any sort of reasonable function is to be obtained. Oil massage is given gently at first, progressing to stronger and deeper massage with circular, transverse and longitudinal movements to break down the adhesions.

Following 10 minutes of such massage, slow, gentle, passive stretch is put on the tendons whilst supporting the MP joints and trying gradually to extend the PIP joints. This is done at first with the MP joints in full flexion; as the deformity resolves, increasing extension of the MP joints can be allowed during this manœuvre. After the slow gentle stretch a plaster splint is applied to the palmar surface of the forearm, palm and fingers, and bandaged on, being maintained in this position between each treatment session.

A plaster splint is worn at night, which gives some $\frac{3}{4}$ full correction. A fully correcting splint would be too painful to be worn in the night. In the early stages of recovery, plasters may need to be changed once or even twice a day, later, every other day, and then twice a week.

The plasters are used to maintain the movement gained by physiotherapy—they are not *corrective* in the sense of causing continuous stretch. We strongly oppose the type of splint that produces active stretch with pulleys, elastics or springs as these tend to produce more deformity than that which they attempt to correct.

This treatment should not be painful: the secret is slow, gentle correction, to obtain only a degree or two of mobilization at a time. This, however, is cumulative and over a period of several weeks, even very severe deformities can be corrected.

The surgical team for whom we work feel that such conservative measures are superior to tenolysis and dissection of fibrous tissue, which is always a much more formidable prospect than would appear from clinical examination through the intact skin.

Following these physiotherapy sessions, active exercises, games and occupational therapy are prescribed, all to encourage general flexion and function of the hand.

CASE HISTORY

Figure 24.1, illustrates a patient who cut all flexor tendons and both median and ulnar nerves at the wrist. Secondary suture of the nerves was undertaken and he started rehabilitation five weeks later. There was gross adherence at the wrist causing the limitation of flexor tendon excursion. Intensive oil massage, slow stretches and serial plasters were required, as well as occupational therapy, games and exercises. The following illustrations show the progress. The patient made an excellent tendon and neurological recovery and was back at work, eight months after injury, as an electrical fitter.

LESIONS IN THE PALM AND FINGERS

In the mid-palm, suture of the flexor tendons gives good results, particularly if sublimis is excised and the lumbrical

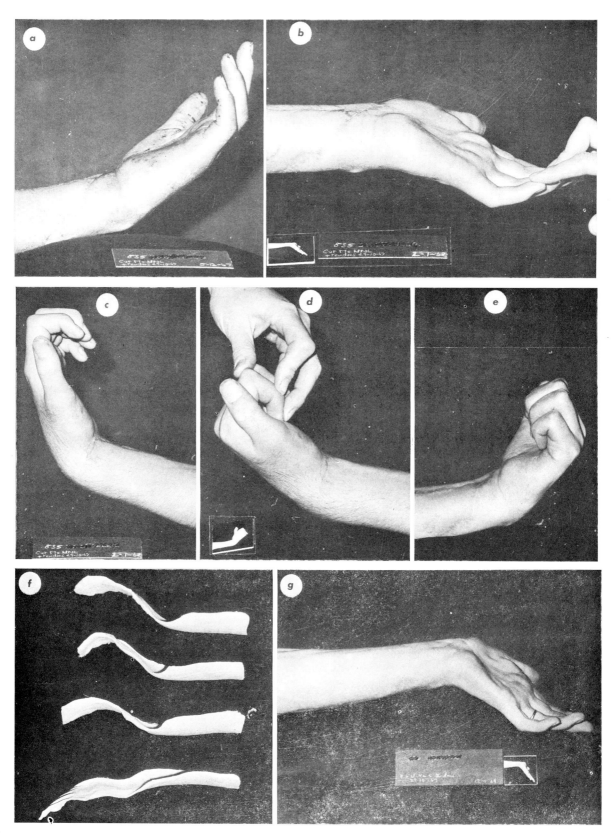

Figure 24.1
(a) Appearance of hand five weeks after secondary suture of both nerves and all tendons at the wrist. There was virtually no movement at any of the interphalangeal joints and gross adherence at the wrist. (b) Passive extension one month after starting rehabilitation. (c) and (d) Active flexion and passive flexion one month after starting rehabilitation. (e) Active flexion 13 weeks after start of treatment. (f) Serial plasters used in correction of deformity. (g) Active extension one year after injury.

wrapped round the sutured profundus so that adherence does not occur. No more formal rehabilitation is usually necessary than for simple lesions at the wrist. (When tendons are involved in severe crush or blast injuries the management is entirely different and is discussed on p. 177). The management of lesions in the distal part of the palm and in the fibrous flexor sheath, however, present complex problems, the solution to which is still a matter for much debate and controversy. It is usually claimed that suture of both tendons in the fibrous flexor sheath is not feasible, for there is so little room within the sheath that the slightest additional tissue in the form of scarring leads to adherence and a stiff finger. For this reason, it has been common practice to excise both tendons and put in a free graft. In the opinion of most authorities, this is the treatment of choice, unless the surgeon is especially skilled and all the conditions ideal for primary suture in the flexor tendon sheath.

However, results of flexor tendon grafts even in the best hands still give rise to concern, for the proportion of excellent results remains unsatisfactory and one cannot expect full finger flexion with the tip of the finger flexing to the distal palmar crease in more than 75 per cent of patients. For this reason a number of experienced surgeons have been undertaking suture of the tendon in the fibrous flexor sheath provided that the wound is clean, seen early within the first six hours and the surgeon is skilled. Bolton (1969) has reported a number of patients in which such ideal criteria existed and virtually full function with the finger touching the distal crease resulted.

FLEXOR TENDON GRAFTS

The length of time for which a finger is immobilized after flexor tendon grafting varies from surgeon to surgeon, but an average time is 17 to 21 days during which time the finger is kept completely at rest. Some surgeons take the finger out of plaster at the tenth day and allow active exercises, but most keep the finger completely immobile for up to three weeks. It has been shown that there is no advantage in early movement and indeed a tendon does not gain its vascular supply before the third week, and there is therefore a definite danger in starting movements before the third week. Often there will be some local oedema in the finger and it is important to remove this as early as possible to prevent fibrosis. This means that the hand may need to be kept in elevation at night and indeed during the day, in between sessions of exercise and physiotherapy. For this purpose a special sling has been devised at our Unit which allows the hand to be put in any position of elevation. Figure 24.2 shows the sling and shows how it can be adjusted by putting the buckles in different positions.

The skin may be scaly and it is often helpful for the physiotherapist to give some light oil massage to the skin.

For the first two weeks active exercises only are allowed in which the physiotherapist supports the finger at the MP, the PIP and the DIP joints and encourages the patient to flex at each joint in turn. Resistance can be given after five weeks to the other fingers and such facilitation encourages the graft to

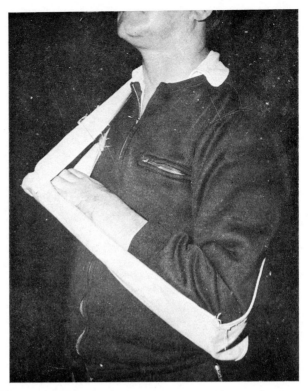

Figure 24.2
Special sling allowing the hand to be kept in elevation at various levels by the strap and buckles. The forearm rests on a firm base provided by half an aluminium back splint.

work more strongly. It is unwise to give resistance to the affected finger before the sixth week. Thereafter resistance can gradually be increased, first with the physiotherapist preventing the movement and then giving active resistance.

There is usually some degree of adherence of the graft, either in the finger or in the palm, and more often than not it is necessary to give some light massage to loosen these adhesions. This can be given twice a day and may become gradually more vigorous after the sixth week. Friction is best given when the graft is put under tension and is more effective than trying to relieve adherence in the relaxed position. In the early stages oil massage is advisable: later, lanolin can be given as this can produce a deeper effect. At the start of formal rehabilitation some two or three weeks after grafting, there is usually a flicker of movement at the terminal interphalangeal joint and up to 10 degrees at the proximal interphalangeal joint. The finger is usually held in about 30 degrees flexion at the PIP joint, and 10 to 20 degrees flexion at the DIP joint. There is no doubt that if the finger is put in marked flexion during the stage of immobilization after grafting, it is extremely difficult to gain reasonable function. Flexion of more than 30 degrees at the PIP joint is likely to lead to a permanent flexion deformity. Some surgeons are in the habit of bandaging the finger right down in full flexion in the palm and in our experience such cases do extremely badly. We have never seen, in our unit, a patient whose hand was so splinted, regain anything like reasonable function.

As well as active exercises between the third and sixth week, specific hand games can be played in the physiotherapy department. Games involving string, such as cat's cradles and knotting, making houses with cards, games with matches and simple ball games are all useful as is any activity involving picking up objects. Occupational therapy is most important, for here the patient is using his hand for functional and absorbing activities.

The following techniques are used in the various stages after grafting in the occupational therapy department at our centres:

OCCUPATIONAL THERAPY

At the Services' centre, activities have to be selected which young Servicemen will accept: traditional occupational therapy crafts such as weaving, basketry, etc, are rejected, though there may be a place for their use in routine hospital practice for women. Men prefer using tools and lathes. When possible we try to provide activity which will help in the upkeep of the unit. Thus the Gestetner duplicating machine is most useful for providing copies of forms for the administrative work of the centre and the handle of the machine can be padded to provide light repetitive grip in the early stages of activity after tendon surgery. Printing presses have been devised with adaptations which can be quickly and easily adjusted for most hand movements, various grip attachments provide large handle grip, span grip, disc attachments, narrow tubular grips and bilateral grips. Handles can be covered with material enabling the patient to feel more easily with sensory impairment, for example, rough surfaces such as a roller can be covered with cotton string and provide a better sense of grip than a smooth shiny metal handle. Work can be varied in resistance from light to very heavy work. Type setting using composing stick and various sized tweezers provides light resistance. For general office work, preparation of card and paper can be carried out on various guillotines with similar adaptations to those on the printing presses.

Brushmaking: Wire-twisting on a special machine provides hand movement with resistance, and brushes can be made for the hospital or centre.

Cardboard Box Manufacture: Gripping of small hand tools is involved in making boxes—small craft knives, stapling machines and rulers and these can often be produced in bulk for local manufacturers and the profit put back into the department.

Polythene bag sealing provides light work for co-ordination to feed polythene into the machine. Movement is mainly at the MP joints and opposition of the thumb for pinch grip. This activity can provide covers for books and documents as well as a variety of sizes of bag.

Ornamental Brick making: This provides work in the later stages of treatment where resistance is necessary, but it can be graded from light to very hard depending on the moulds used, and the weight of cement in the box 'shaper'. Bricks can be sold for garden reconstruction.

Painting and Decorating: A 'do-it-yourself' room is much appreciated where patients can paint walls; various grips are provided for each stage, i.e. for cleaning down the walls, filling and preparing surfaces and scraping.

Cement mixing: This gives really heavy work required in the later stages of tendon rehabilitation. Once more, depending on the nature of the disability, the grips can be specifically constructed to achieve accurate tendon movement. Shovel handles can be altered, different working methods used and the weight of shovels varied. Flag stones, garden seats can be made for the hospital.

Gardening: Provided the patient enjoys gardening, a wide variety of hand movements are provided in the garden. Watering, use of trowel, planting out in the greenhouse in the early stages as well as digging, fencing, mowing in the later stages.

Wrought Iron: This is a useful activity in the later stages of treatment, metal strips are cut to a specific length, shaped round a jig and assembled prior to welding. Applications can be decorative or functional and this activity is very popular (Figure 24.3).

Carpentry offers a wide range of hand movement and uses many different hand movements: gripping with a saw, rotation with screwdrivers, cylinder grip with a hammer. Controlled finger movements with a chisel.

Games: Whenever possible rehabilitation should be made as enjoyable as possible and so a wide variety of games are provided all using specific hand movements. These include blow football using rubber bulb syringes for grip, flip football, using a leather bag on the hand, which encourages extensor movements of the fingers, draughts of varied weights, car race game, beat the clock (Fig. 24.4), rod football in which the handles of the rod carry small wooden figures and can be of varying shape to suit the stage of disability and magnetic jigsaw puzzles providing light pinch grip (the board can be put upon the wall so that patients with oedema can work in elevation). In general, a dynamic occupational therapy department will consider any application for work that might be useful for the hospital or centre and relate it to the specific problem of the patient's hand provided the activity is interesting and easily set up. Local contracts can provide a valuable source of revenue to the depart-

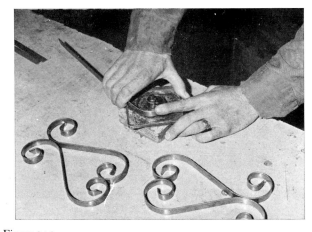

Figure 24.3
Wrought Iron Work.

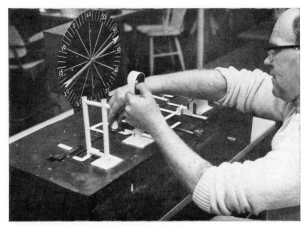

Figure 24.4
The lever in the patient's right hand has to be moved through a series of gates, each operated by a different hand movement against the clock.

ment. Therapists should be encouraged to use their ingenuity to develop new activities and games, and to relate these wherever possible to the patient's interests, work or hobbies, using many different hand movements: gripping with a saw, rotation with screwdrivers, cylinder grip with a hammer, controlled finger movements with a chisel.

SPECIALIZED PHYSIOTHERAPY

One of the most valuable techniques for encouraging movement in a flexor tendon after grafting are the so called proprioceptive neuro-muscular facilitation techniques. These techniques represent comparatively recent developments in physiotherapy and are a logical and functional way of exercising a muscle. The principles of these techniques in the re-education of weak muscles and restoration of joint range are well established and widely accepted as an essential part of routine physiotherapy teaching. Consequently, all physiotherapists now have a mastery of these methods but as many doctors are still unfamiliar with these an explanation of their rationale will be presented here. Briefly, the principles are as follows: Maximum activity in a muscle depends on maximum discharge of the anterior horn cells that supply that muscle. In order to obtain maximum discharge of the anterior horn cells, all available influences must be brought to bear that work on those anterior horn cells. When a muscle has been immobilized for any length of time, such as after a tendon graft, or after a fracture whilst in plaster, the central inhibitory state is heightened in the anterior horn cells that supply that muscle and it is more difficult to excite, a common example is after knee injuries when the quadriceps may be quite markedly inhibited. It is therefore important to try and make available all possible influences on the anterior horn cell to lower its heightened inhibitory state. Increasing sensory inflow and irradiation of activity from neighbouring anterior horn cells are the two most valuable methods.

Increased sensory inflow can be produced by:

1. Stretch: increasing stretch activates the muscle spindle system resulting in an inflow of afferent impulses into the cord

and sets the bias of the spindle system to a more sensitive level, reducing the central inhibitory state.

2. Pressure on the proprioceptive end organs in tendon and joint as well as traction on the joint will also increase sensory inflow.

3. Visual effects. The patient is asked to watch the movements and 'feel' the pattern that is being encouraged—this is reinforced by the physiotherapist's commands, given in a forceful positive manner.

4. Ice cubes rubbed on the muscle also increase the inflow and can be useful, provided sensation is normal.

Irradiation: If the anterior horn cells lying adjacent to those supplying the muscle to be treated are stimulated to discharge, there will be an overflow of electrical activity that will lower the central inhibitory state of those cells. This is known as irradiation. A well known example of this is in the re-education of a weak quadriceps muscle, when the patient is asked to dorsiflex the ankle as he tries to contract the quadriceps. The cell columns supplying the anterior tibialis lie close to those supplying the quadriceps and their electrical activity irradiates to those cells supplying the quadriceps and increases their discharge.

When the triceps is weak, a stronger contraction can be elicited by irradiation from cells supplying the extensors of shoulder, wrist and fingers than by a simple prime mover action. Thus the therapist asks the patient for a strong extensor thrust of the whole upper limb against her resistance, at the same time putting the elbow joint slightly on the stretch and stimulating the stretch receptors in the triceps tendon manually (Fig. 24.5).

Successive induction: Where there has been maximum voluntary contraction of an antagonist, there is facilitation of the agonist. Thus, after a strong maximum contraction of the wrist and finger flexors, it is easier for the extensors to contract as there has been an alternation of central inhibitory and excitatory states in the spinal cord.

Pattern re-education: Kabat (1961) has shown that normally

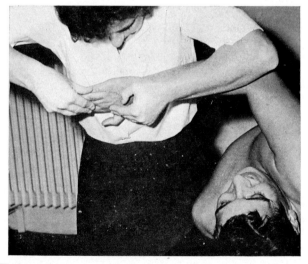

Figure 24.5
PNF Techniques in re-education of extensor tendons.

muscles work in spiral and diagonal patterns. Thus bringing the hand to the mouth involves a diagonal movement from the side across the body and almost all functional activities such as dressing, using tools, swinging rackets or clubs involve rotational movements and diagonal patterns. The 'Swedish drill' types of exercise that were popular in the earlier part of this century were unphysiological as well as boring. The new proprioceptive techniques are physiological and capture the patient's interest as he can see clearly how they relate to daily life. Moreover it is possible to exhaust a patient in as little as two minutes and thus these manœuvres are highly efficient in physiotherapist's time and impressive to the patient.

TECHNIQUES

Irradiation is always from strong muscles to weak and so in re-educating weak hand muscles the shoulder and elbow are worked first and then the wrist, fingers and thumb.

Furthermore, the moving part is felt by the patient most and thus the shoulder is pivoted and fixed. Maximum movement is encouraged distally, as the manœuvre increases in force so only the weak part is allowed to move. Thus in re-educating weak finger flexors, as after suture or graft, the diagonal flexion adduction internal rotation pattern is used, and at the start, the whole upper limb is brought across the body and then out away from the body in extension abduction external rotation. The shoulder is then fixed and the power is concentrated on the elbow, then the wrist and then the fingers.

Repeated contractions are used to reinforce the activity of the weak muscles. Hold/relax techniques allow relaxation between each isometric maximum contraction reinforcing each contraction.

Each patient has his own best line of activity or 'groove' and the diagonal patterns vary slightly from patient to patient so the physiotherapist has to find the groove for each patient which varies with his body structure.

For opposition of the thumb the best position to work is in extension, adduction, internal rotation; for adduction, flexion adduction, external rotation; for palmar abduction, extension, abduction and internal rotation.

For re-education of the fingers, indicis and medialis are worked as a unit as are annularis and minimus, which rotate towards the palm in flexion and derotate in extension and must therefore be worked in this diagonal pattern.

Ice. Ice towels applied to the part for 10 minutes before treatment are valuable for reducing spasm and oedema. The ice must cover the whole muscle and be changed frequently, according to how long it takes to achieve the required effect. If oedema is a problem, ice towels in elevation before re-education are very useful.

These techniques are of particular value when tendons become stuck or markedly adherent and are valuable when the patient finds difficulty in moving the finger due to pain or poor motivation.

Use of splints. One of the problems of the rehabilitation of flexor tendon grafts, can be the splinting effect at the metacarpophalangeal joint when the patient attempts to flex the IP

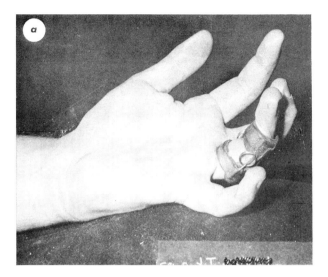

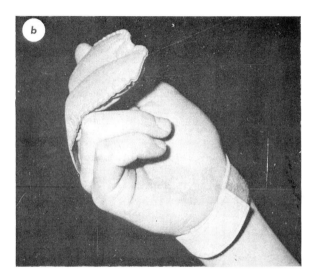

Figure 24.6
(a) 'Capener' Splint to encourage flexion. (b) Double finger stall to encourage movement by using assistance of adjacent normal finger for multiple grafts.

joints. This is due to the overaction of the intrinsic muscles acting at the MP joint. This is often seen when there has been too long a delay between the original injury and the flexor tendon grafting, when the patient gets in the habit of flexing the finger by the intrinsic muscles working at the MP joint only. To try and overcome this the MP joint is held in extension and the patient concentrates on moving the IP joints only. Once resistance is given, the splinting effect often returns and it has been found useful at this stage to provide a form of lively splint, such as the spring wire 'Capener' splint (Fig. 24.6a). A double finger stall can often be helpful to overcome this splinting effect and indeed double or triple finger stalls are valuable whenever patients find difficulty in flexing the IP joints and can be introduced at the sixth or seventh week if recovery is slow (Fig. 24.6b).

COURSE

In an uncomplicated flexor tendon graft there should, by the sixth week, be 30 degrees movement at the PIP joint and 10 to 15 degrees at the DIP joint. By the eighth week there should be at least 45 degrees at the PIP joint and some 20 to 30 degrees at the DIP joint. It may be some months before full flexion is obtained and, of course, in many cases full flexion in which the IP joints can be brought down to the distal palmar crease, never returns; however a reasonable result demands an extension deformity at the PIP joint of no more than 30 degrees and the ability of the patient to touch the palm (Stewart Harrison, 1969).

Individual work is of extreme importance in the re-education of flexor tendon grafts. Occupational therapy and gym activities are vital but there is never any substitute for the physiotherapist giving individual attention at each IP joint and progressing treatment particularly by PNF techniques.

The simple uncomplicated flexor tendon graft should be fit to return to work eight weeks after surgery. This implies five to six weeks of active rehabilitation. There is no doubt that in adults the best results are obtained if intensive treatment is given daily for at least half a day and if possible for a full day, for by this means the quickest result will be obtained and the maximum amount of movement will be regained. The results of flexor tendon grafts cannot be assessed for at least a year after surgery, for movement continues to increase and power to improve as time goes on, particularly if the patient uses the hand. Manual workers usually obtain better results than clerical or sedentary workers. For this reason patients who are in sedentary trades and who do not make demands on their hand, require a more intensive and a longer period of rehabilitation than those who use their hand at work, for their rehabilitation can be work itself from the eighth week onwards. It is wiser not to let people return to really heavy manual work for 8 to 10 weeks after surgery, in case they put too much strain on the graft.

In our experience, lesions of the little finger take longer to recover, perhaps because there is no tendon on the ulnar side to help mass flexion movements.

COMPLICATIONS

There are a number of circumstances in which results of flexor tendon grafts may not be satisfactory, and may lead to restricted function. These are:

1. Abnormalities of the circulation, particularly where digital arteries have been severed.

2. Involvement of the digital nerves.

3. Marked fibrosis—some patients have a capacity for forming fibrous tissues very easily and this may hinder movement in the graft.

4. Injuries in which there has been a tearing or wrenching strain or rupture of the tendon rather than clean division.

5. Crush injuries when the hand is caught in machinery.

6. Infection is liable to lead to fibrosis and therefore limitation of movement.

7. Cases where suture or grafting has been undertaken at a later stage and there has been more than two months between injury and surgery.

8. Patients in whom immobilization has been prolonged for more than four weeks and particularly where the finger has been held in marked flexion.

9. Patients in which there have been multiple injuries: although multiple tendon grafting can give good results, rehabilitation is more difficult and takes longer.

10. Motivation is of extreme importance; if the patient wants to get better and is prepared to work hard he will obviously get a much better result than those patients who expect the physiotherapist to do all the work for them.

11. The quality of surgery is obviously of extreme importance, the more experienced the surgeon and the more skilled he is, the better the result. This is a field in which surgery is best left to the expert and is not the province of the orthopaedic surgeon who makes an occasional foray into hand surgery.

Should tenolysis be necessary it is important to establish active rehabilitation straight after surgery; that means the next day if possible, and certainly well before the stitches come out. Although there are many causes of stiffness and lack of movement after flexor tendon grafts, the management and the problem these present are basically the same—that is restoration of gliding motion of the tendon by reducing the adherence, encouraging movements at the stiff joints and trying to regain movement in joints which have become permanently stiff. And the principles remain the same whether the cause of stiffness is excessive fibrosis, severe infection, stretching of the tendon sheaths in a tearing injury, or involvement of the digital nerves giving lack of proprioceptive feed-back.

Adherence of the Graft. If the graft has become adherent it is important to try and relieve this by intensive lanolin massage, four times a day, followed by intensive active work against resistance. Clearly this cannot be done until at least six weeks after the graft. Intensive treatment of this sort can often mobilize an adherent tendon and even quite surprisingly stiff fingers can become mobile in a matter of three to four weeks after intensive treatment of this sort. If adherence has caused oedema, it is important to eradicate this oedema at the earliest possible moment for if this is allowed to persist it will lead to more fibrous tissue being laid down and an even stiffer finger. The best way to relieve oedema is by elevating the hand and by applying ice. Heat, particularly in the form of wax baths is contraindicated where there is oedema for this causes more swelling. Ice treatment is of great value: crushed ice is applied in towelling to the part affected, which must be elevated for increasing periods, starting with five minutes and increasing to 10 or 15 minutes after a few days' treatment. This is followed by massage and active exercises. The limb is elevated between treatment sessions and kept in elevation above the head at night.

Stiff IP joints. If there is a permanently stiff IP joint in flexion serial plasters may be required to try and obtain extension, though if the patient has no more than a 30 degree extension lag this is acceptable for function.

If the flexion deformity is 45 degrees or more, the finger will usually get in the way; the extent to which this interferes with function can be found out by trial at the patient's work, or a mock-up of his work in the occupational therapy department, and if so, it will become necessary to try and obtain more extension. Often this can be obtained by intensive oil massage, slow gentle stretches given by the physiotherapist with the finger fully supported, and then the application of a plaster of Paris splint to the palmar surface of the finger. Some workers have found that putting the finger actually into a plaster cylinder for a few days may be a more effective way (though one is loath to immobilize a finger for more than a few hours at a time) as one is concerned to obtain power in the graft as well as active movement.

These techniques can often successfully overcome very severe flexion deformities, but it is important that they be used in the relatively early stages. If a finger has been stiff for this reason for more than three months, it is extremely unlikely that conservative treatment will overcome a flexion deformity, and it may then be necessary to carry out some form of surgery on the IP joints, such as the Curtis procedure and if this is unsuccessful it may be necessary to amputate the finger.

Digital nerve involvement. It has been our experience that patients who have sustained severance of the digital nerves take longer to regain reasonable function than those in whom the digital nerve has been intact. Long term assessment of a group of patients with digital nerve involvement did not show that they had any decrease in final range of function (Morley, 1956), but the experience of physiotherapists treating such patients is that they are more difficult to rehabilitate for they lack the sensory feed-back that will tell them how strongly their muscle is contracting and what position the joint is under various circumstances. It is therefore important to know if somebody has sustained a digital nerve lesion for they will need more intensive and individual work and may require a long period under full time rehabilitation.

Ultrasonics. Claims have been made for ultrasonic therapy as a means of relieving fibrosis and adherence in circumstances where there is excessive fibrosis; thus patients with crush injuries of the hand, stiff fingers after flexor tendon grafting and after burns, have been treated with ultrasonics and good results have been claimed. As far as we know there has been no controlled study published in which a group of patients were treated solely with ultrasonics and compared with a group treated with the traditional measures of oil massage, slow stretches, serial plasters and active exercises. Our impression is that ultrasonics can occasionally accelerate the relief of fibrosis, but that it is in no way a substitute for the traditional measures, and until such a control study is available we see no call to replace them with ultrasound.

Rupture of the graft. Occasionally, during rehabilitation, a snap may be heard and movement may immediately be lost, and it is often thought that this indicates tearing or snapping of the graft. In fact, such a circumstance is extremely rare, and the majority of cases in which such a situation arises are due to snapping of an adhesion. Under these circumstances the finger should immediately be rested for two or three weeks and then graduated active exercises started without resistance for a further two weeks. In almost all cases good function will

return, but if it is clear that there is no movement at all at such a stage, then exploration and regrafting may be necessary. Usually, in such cases, after a week of immobilization, it is permissible to ask the patient to try and get active movement and if the graft has not been snapped, there will be a flicker of movement at one or both joints. This indicates that further immobilization will be successful.

Sometimes one sees a remarkable range of movement quite soon after flexor tendon grafting, for example we have seen a number of patients in whom there has been 30 degrees movement at the PIP joint and 20 degrees at the DIP joint at four weeks after grafting. Such patients are likely to stretch the graft at a later stage, and indeed we are suspicious of a patient with much movement at an early stage, and prefer to see a small range of movement gradually increasing as the weeks go by. A rapid recovery of movement in the early stages usually means the graft has not got a secure bed and is thus more vulnerable.

SUTURE

Controversy rages and will rage for many years to come on the question as to whether primary grafting, delayed primary grafting, secondary grafting, or primary or secondary suture of the flexor tendons in the tendon sheath is the treatment of choice. So much depends on the availability of a skilled surgeon and on good aftercare, and it is very difficult to compare results from one surgeon to another. Our experience over the last 10 years in which a number of patients have been referred to us in which suture has been carried out rather than grafting suggests that the results are as good.

The rehabilitation after tendon suture is similar to that after grafting. In the last 15 years we have had personal experience of rehabilitating 320 patients with flexor tendon grafts and sutures. The majority have been grafts but in recent years there have been more sutures performed and we have figures for 30 primary sutures of profundus in the sheath. The average time between operation and surgery has been three weeks in both and the average stay at the Rehabilitation Centre three weeks and the range of movement was 53 degrees at PIP and 25 degrees at DIP joints on discharge in both the patients treated by grafting and by suture. However, one is comparing patients in which the ideal situation exists in the case of sutures. If there are complicating factors, the case is most likely to be treated by secondary grafting, so it should not be concluded from these figures that suture is the treatment of choice.

In cases where there were complications such as infections, fibrosis, digital nerve involvement, multiple tendon grafts, the average stay at the centre was eight weeks before function was judged to be adequate for the patient's job. The average range in this series, was found to be 22 degrees at DIP, and 50 degrees at PIP joints. In some patients only a flicker was obtained at the DIP joint but a good range at the PIP joint (45 degrees or more). The finger almost always touched the palm, grip was strong and function good.

The following case histories illustrate some of these points.

LACK OF POSTOPERATIVE REHABILITATION

A.K. is an 18-year-old civilian apprentice engineer who cut the FPD to right indicis and minimus in an accident at work. Four months later a PL graft was carried out to right indicis and six months later to right minimus. No formal rehabilitation was given. Eighteen months later a tenolysis on both tendons was carried out for lack of movement. He was referred to MRU two weeks later. Movements were:

Indicis DIP 30–31. PIP 55–75. MP 0–65 finger to palm 5 cm.
Minimus DIP 0–5. PIP 0–45 MP 0–65, finger to palm 4.5 cm.

Intensive treatment was given and 5 weeks later movements were:

Indicis DIP 20–35 PIP 20–85. MP full.
Minimus DIP 10–35. PIP 0–75. MP full. Grip was 70 per cent normal.

He was assessed in the workshops and found fully fit for his job. This case illustrates two points: the danger of not providing rehabilitation after tendon grafting, and the good results that can be obtained with intensive treatment despite a long delay after grafting, given a co-operative and motivated patient.

DELAY IN SURGERY

D.I., a 24-year-old fireman, cut his right medialis on a broken beer glass, dividing FSD and FPD but not the digital nerves. Skin suture was performed. Four months later he sought advice as the finger was getting in his way and palmaris longus grafting was performed: 26 days later he was admitted to MRU. There was 10 degrees movement at DIP, (0–10), 30 degrees at PIP (0–30) with, as expected, a poor grip. Routine rehabilitation was given and eight weeks later, movements were 0–80 at MP, 0–80 at PIP and the finger could touch the palm ¾ inch from the mid-palmar crease. He was assessed and found fully fit for duty.

On review six months after discharge he had almost normal flexion (Fig. 24.7). This case illustrates the excellent results that can be obtained despite a long delay between injury and grafting.

In one of our patients the delay between injury and grafting was eight years—10 degrees at DIP and 30 degrees at PIP only resulted but grip was full and function excellent.

BLAST INJURIES

G.McN., a 25-year-old surface worker, sustained deep wounds of the palmar surface of his hand when a varnish bottle he was holding exploded. Skin suture was effected the same day. It was not clear, owing to gross oedema and pain, what structures had suffered and he was transferred to MRU 20 days after injury with deep scarring in the palm, some residual oedema and lack of activity in FPD index. EMG studies showed absent sensory potentials on the index finger. Intensive oil massage, slow stretches, active work in physiotherapy and gymnastics and workshop activities were given.

Two months after injury, he returned to hospital where very dense scarring was dissected out. The medial digital nerves to the thumb and both digital nerves to the indicis, were sutured, FSD to index excised and FPD sutured with silk.

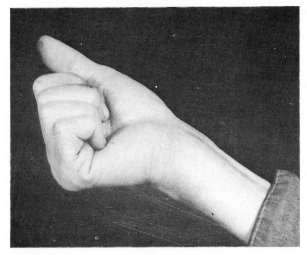

Figure 24.7
End result in Patient DI 11 months after grafting medialis.

Twenty-one days later he returned to MRU with 20 degrees movement (30–50) of DIP joint, 15 degrees movements (30–65) at PIP.

Two months later the scar in the palm was supple and non-adherent. DIP had active range of 45 degrees (15–60). PIP of 50 degrees (40–90). Grip was 7 lb on affected side and 12 lb on normal side. Sensation was returning. He was tested on his job and found fit for all but heavy lifting and returned to duty. This case illustrates the value of intensive treatment in conditions where gross scarring follows blast injuries.

MULTIPLE GRAFTS

J.R.O., an air wireless fitter sustained lacerations to his hands from a panga in a fight with terrorists.

He had sustained the following injuries:

1. To the right hand: A large cut the whole way through the first inter-osseous space opening the carpo-metacarpal joint of the thumb and dividing the extensor pollicis brevis. Right indicis: Cut through the volar aspect at proximal phalangeal level dividing both flexor tendons and both digital nerves. Right medialis: Cut at the level of the proximal phalanx dividing both flexor tendons and the digital nerve on the ulnar side of the finger. Annularis: Cut at proximal phalangeal level severing both flexor tendons. Minimus: Cut at level of distal interphalangeal joint severing long flexor and both digital nerves and opening joint. These injuries were treated as follows:

The injury to the right interosseous space was treated by suture of the muscle with fine catgut and suture of the extensor pollicis brevis with 3.0 Mersilene. The injuries to the fingers were treated by simple skin suture only, as the surgeon was not able to identify the digital nerves and did not wish to carry out a formal exploration at this stage.

2. To the left hand: There was a cut severing the extensor tendon of the long finger and 2 other cuts of small importance on the hand.

This injury was treated with tendon suture with 3.0 Mersilene and the metacarpophalangeal joint splinted with plaster of Paris.

He was transferred to England and sent straight to the MRU for preoperative mobilization as the IP joints were stiff. There was no active movement at any PIP joint on the right hand. Full mobility and reasonable power in the intrinsics was restored in three weeks. The right indicis and medialis were then grafted, using plantaris, sublimis being sacrificed, and he was readmitted to MRU three weeks later. At this stage indicis showed 10 degrees active movement (25–35)— medialis 10 degrees (35–45) and there was a flicker at the DIP joints.

Intensive rehabilitation included a triple finger stall, enclosing the two grafted fingers and progressive work in gymnasium, physiotherapy and occupational therapy.

Seven weeks later there was full extension of indicis PIP and 75 degrees active flexion, 10 degrees lack of full extension medialis and 65 degrees active flexion. There was 15 degrees active movement from full extension at the DIP joints. Power was 50 per cent of normal. He was returned to hospital at this stage for grafting of annularis using palmaris longus.

Three weeks later he returned to MRU for routine rehabilitation which included the use of a triple finger stall.

Six weeks later movements recorded were:

           Index   PIP   0–90
                      DIP   0–30
           Medialis   PIP   20–90
                      DIP   0–45
           Annularis PIP   20–40
                      MP   0–30
Power 60 per cent of normal.

He was set a trade test inviting use of hammer, files, hacksaws, soldering iron, drills, screwdriver, punches, shears and pliers and completed it satisfactorily and was therefore returned to full duty seven months after injury.

RUPTURES

In ruptures of the tendon, for example at rugby, range of movement was limited after grafting. This is due to the damage done by tearing and the profuse fibrosis that follows along the whole length of the tendon sheath. In the best result, movements were 45 degrees at DIP and 55 degrees at PIP but several had virtually no movement at DIP and 30 degrees only at PIP, while in one, the DIP had to be arthrodesed. However, all had acceptable function, only one of 12 having to change his trade due to stiffness of the finger.

INFECTION

H.P.M., a 42-year-old supplier, put his right hand through a window, severing extensor tendons to right middle and ring fingers, which were repaired by primary suture, and severing flexors to annularis and minimus at the level of the PIP joints and the digital nerves and arteries to these fingers. Three weeks later he was readmitted to hospital with gross infection of the affected fingers.

He was admitted to MRU for mobilization prior to tendon grafting. This required two months' intensive oil massage,

stretching, active exercise and games for there was gross scarring in the palm, oedema of the fingers and only 20 degrees passive range in the IP joints from 30–50. Subsequently, the right annularis was grafted using palmaris longus but the minimus was left, owing to the gross scarring and stiffness of the IP joints. Twenty days later he was readmitted to MRU with 27–35 active range at PIP and 27–31 at DIP root. The minimus was stuck at 40 degrees at DIP and 45 degrees at PIP joint. Seven weeks later, after intensive treatment, which included the use of a double finger stall, movements of annularis were 20–60 at DIP and 10–80 at PIP. The finger was able to be flexed to within 3.5 cm of the palm, grip was 60 per cent of normal.

He was found fully fit for duty and minimus was not in the way.

MULTIPLE DISORDERS

There are various circumstances under which tendons may be damaged incidentally—to a severe hand lesion. These include crush injuries, blast injuries, Dupuytren's Contracture, multiple fractures or fracture dislocations. Tendons may either be divided or, more commonly, bound down by massive fibrosis or adhere to callus. Each severe hand injury of this sort presents its own particular problem but the general principles are the same—attempts to mobilize the tendons and skin by frequent sessions of active massage, the use of stretch plasters, Plastazote wedges to increase the excursion of the thumb web and interdigital spaces, intensive active exercises and functional activities in the occupational therapy workshop.

The more severe the lesion the more important it is to institute full time intensive treatment. Massive scarring causing a 'frozen hand' is not amenable to surgery other than skin cover when appropriate. Even very severe stiffness can be remarkably improved by conservative measures.

SUTURE

F.C.H., a 20-year-old sheet metal worker, cut his right medialis on a bottle just distal to the MP joint. Nine weeks later the finger was explored and both tendons found to be cut and bound down by fibrous tissue. The distal ends of FSD and FPD were sutured to the distal end of profundus with wire. Five weeks later he came to the MRU with active range at DIP of 10–15, Passive 10–45, Active at PIP 10–80, Passive 10–80.

Seven weeks later, movements after routine rehabilitation were DIP 30–60. PIP 5–90, the finger just touched the palm, grip was 11 lb on affected side 15 lb on normal side.

He was assessed and found fully fit for duty (Fig. 24.8).

FLEXOR TENDON INJURIES TO THE THUMB

These can be treated either by suture or graft. Complications such as infection, excess scarring, adherence, occur as in lesion of the fingers and in such circumstances, the usual management is required including oil massage and stretches. However results of flexor tendon injury to the thumb are usually good whether there are complicating factors or not. The main cri-

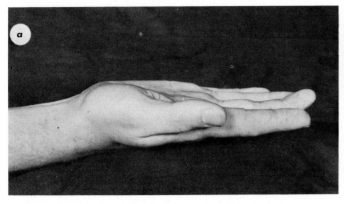
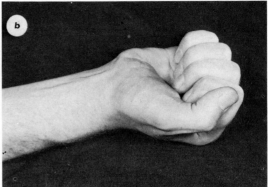

Figure 24.8
(a) Extension. (b) Flexion in patient FCH three months after suture of medialis.

terion for good thumb function is a strong pinch in opposition to the finger tips and this does not require more than 30 degrees active flexion at the IP joint. Power is relatively easy to restore by physiotherapy and occupational therapy as already described.

The average range of movement obtained at the IP joint after three weeks rehabilitation in uncomplicated cases was 60 degrees and 35 degrees in cases where infection or scarring complicated the case.

CASE HISTORY

Patient J.T.D. cut his flexor pollicis longus and digital nerves on 24 July 1968. Palmaris graft was carried out on 21 November 1968 and the nerves sutured.

He started rehabilitation on 1 January 1969 when it was noted that the tendon graft was adherent to the scar in the thumb. Active range was 8 degrees at the IP joint. After intensive treatment he was discharged three weeks later with 48 degrees at the IP joint and a grip of 10 lb compared with 14 lb on the normal side. He returned to his job as an Air Frame Fitter two months after grafting (Fig. 24.9).

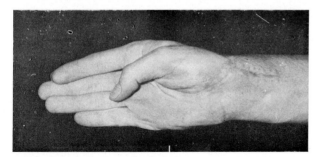

Figure 24.9
Result two months after grafting of Flexor Pollicis Longus.

EXTENSOR TENDONS INJURIES

Injuries to the extensor tendons at the wrist or over the dorsum of the hand usually do not present a problem of rehabilitation unless there is adherence of the extensor mechanism in fractures, crush injuries, infection or burns. In such a situation the principles are the same as in complex flexor tendon injuries: oil massage, to overcome the adherence and intensive active exercises with graded resistance, occupational therapy and games. Extensor tendon injuries in the finger can offer considerable problems in rehabilitation, particularly if adherence occurs over the dorsal surface of the finger.

Here it may be impossible to obtain active movement at the IP joints and the aim of treatment is to develop strong grip. It is less easy to provide specific physiotherapy for extensor tendons than it is for flexor tendons. Flexion and grip are easier and stronger movements to retrain.

PNF techniques are of particular value in re-educating extensor function using flexion, abduction, external rotation patterns and extension, abduction and internal rotation patterns to obtain a maximum extensor movement of shoulder, elbow, wrist, finger and thumb, by irradiation.

Games such as jacks, cat's cradle with string, tiddly winks, matches, pennies, are all valuable in the physiotherapy department to encourage the extensor tendons to contract (Fig. 24.10).

Electrical stimulation can be most valuable for extensor tendons, to give the patient the idea of the movement but only as an assistance, never to replace the patient's active efforts.

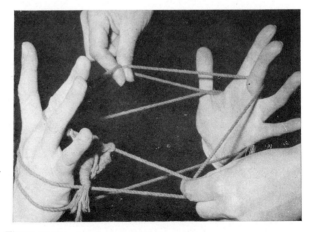

Figure 24.10
Games with string are useful for re-educating extensor tendons.

The patient should be encouraged to contract his muscles with the current, and then, intermittently, the current is turned off and the patient tries to activate the tendon by himself. The stimulus is then reapplied. As the session progresses the patient may often find he is much more successful in initiating movement than at the beginning.

In our experience, electrical stimulation is of no value for re-education of flexor tendon grafts or sutures but has a definite place in the management of extensor tendon injuries.

The management of mallet finger, boutonnière deformities and swan neck lesions is primarily surgical.

Rehabilitation can offer methods of regaining power and range of movement both before and after surgery, but we are not impressed by attempts to correct these deformities by conservative means such as lively splints or the possibility of overcoming marked degrees of lag by exercise alone.

ILLUSTRATIVE CASE HISTORIES

C.D., a woman driver, was involved in a road traffic accident, sustaining fracture of the parietal bone, and ruptured the extensor tendon of the left indicis over the proximal phalanx. Three weeks later a $\frac{1}{4}$ inch gap was repaired in the tendon and some glass splinters removed. She was put in plaster of Paris and started rehabilitation 15 days later. There was 22 degrees

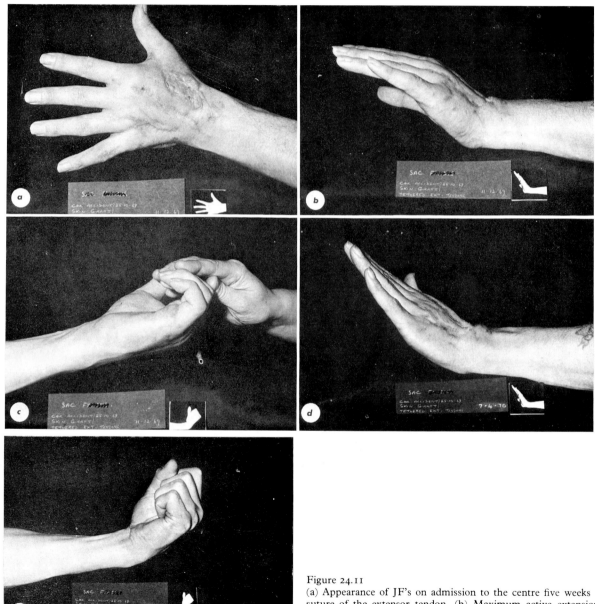

Figure 24.11
(a) Appearance of JF's on admission to the centre five weeks after suture of the extensor tendon. (b) Maximum active extension on admission. (c) Maximum passive flexion on admission. (d) Full extension five months after injury. (e) Full flexion five months after injury.

active flexion of the PIP joint which lacked 10 degrees extension.

Nine days' intensive exercises gave her full passive range of movement and good power but she still had an extension lag at the PIP joint. She was supplied with a Capener splint and allowed to return to duty as a driver wearing the splint all day.

On review 8 weeks later she had overcome the lag fully.

CONCLUSION

It will have become clear from what has been said in this chapter that the results of treatment in tendon lesions depends on a variety of factors: whether the lesion is in so called 'No-man's land', if it involves infection, digital nerve involvement, associated fractures or crushing, a long period between injury and treatment or poor motivation. But our experience leads us to believe that the two overriding factors are skilled surgery and proper rehabilitation. Only a surgeon versed in the techniques of hand surgery with a wide experience and critical outlook can obtain the best results and it is the writer's opinion that the occasional surgeon who does not make a special study of the hand cannot hope to be as successful as the dedicated hand specialist. Rehabilitation can help a first-class surgeon to achieve a first-class end result. Often, rehabilitation can offer much better function after indifferent surgery than no rehabilitation at all. Certainly the more complications that exist the more important is intensive full time skilled rehabilitation, using all the resources of modern physiotherapy and occupational therapy, in order to regain function.

Physiotherapy and occupational therapy can offer the surgeon a means of obtaining the maximum range of passive movement and muscle power preoperatively in order to facilitate postoperative recovery and can provide the means to regain function after surgery quicker and to a higher standard than if the patient is left to his own devices. But such treatment must be realistic, active, dynamic, related to the patient's interests and work and supervised in detail from day to day.

The operation is only one event, albeit the most important one, in a chain of circumstances, starting with the preparation of the hand for surgery in the best state and continuing until the patient has adequate function for all the varied activities to which he wishes to put his hand.

REFERENCES:

BOLTON, H. (1970) *The Hand* **2,** 56.
HARRISON STEWART, S. (1969) *The Hand* **1,** 106.
KABAT (1961) *Therapeutic Exercise.* ed. S. Licht. New York: S. Licht.

MORLEY, G. H. (1956) *Brit. J. Plast. Surg.,* **8,** 300.
WYNN PARRY, C. B. (1966) *Rehabilitation of the Hand.* London: Butterworths.

INDEX